S0-BZF-303

Your *Clinics* subscription just got better!

You can now access the FULL TEXT of this publication online at no additional cost! Activate your online subscription today and receive...

- Full text of all issues from 2002 to the present
- Photographs, tables, illustrations, and references
- Comprehensive search capabilities
- Links to MEDLINE and Elsevier journals

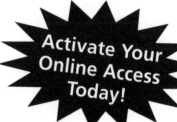

Activate Your Online Access Today!

Plus, you can also sign up for E-alerts of upcoming issues or articles that interest you, and take advantage of exclusive access to bonus features!

To activate your individual online subscription:

1. Visit our website at **www.TheClinics.com**.

2. Click on "Register" at the top of the page, and follow the instructions.

3. To activate your account, you will need your subscriber account number, which you can find on your mailing label (note: the number of digits in your subscriber account number varies from six to ten digits). See the sample below where the subscriber account number has been circled.

This is your subscriber account number

```
************************************3-DIGIT 001
FEB00   J0167   C7   123456-89   10/00   Q: 1

J.H. DOE, MD
531 MAIN ST
CENTER CITY, NY  10001-001
```

4. That's it! Your online access to the most trusted source for clinical reviews is now available.

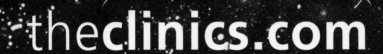
theclinics.com

ELSEVIER

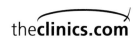

THORACIC SURGERY CLINICS

Advances in Anesthesia and
Pain Management

GUEST EDITOR
Jerome M. Klafta, MD

CONSULTING EDITOR
Mark K. Ferguson, MD

February 2005 • Volume 15 • Number 1

SAUNDERS

An Imprint of Elsevier, Inc.
PHILADELPHIA   LONDON   TORONTO   MONTREAL   SYDNEY   TOKYO

W.B. SAUNDERS COMPANY
A Division of Elsevier Inc.

The Curtis Center • Independence Square West • Philadelphia, Pennsylvania 19106

http://www.theclinics.com

THORACIC SURGERY CLINICS   Volume 15, Number 1
February 2005   ISSN 1547-4127
Editor: Catherine Bewick   ISBN 1-4160-2796-3

The ideas and opinions expressed in *Thoracic Surgery Clinics* do not necessarily reflect those of the Publisher. The Publisher does not assume any responsibility for any injury and/or damage to persons or property arising out of or related to any use of the material contained in this periodical. The reader is advised to check the appropriate medical literature and the product information currently provided by the manufacturer of each drug to be administered to verify the dosage, the method and duration of administration, or contraindications. It is the responsibility of the treating physician or other health care professional, relying on independent experience and knowledge of the patient, to determine drug dosages and the best treatment for the patient. Mention of any product in this issue should not be construed as endorsement by the contributors, editors, or the Publisher of the product or manufacturers' claims.

Thoracic Surgery Clinics (ISSN 1547-4127) is published quarterly by the W.B. Saunders Company. Corporate and editorial offices: The Curtis Center, Independence Square West, Philadelphia, PA 19106-3399. Accounting and Circulation Offices: 6277 Sea Harbor Drive, Orlando, FL 32887-4800. Periodicals postage paid at Orlando, FL 32862, and additional mailing offices. Subscription prices are $175.00 per year (US individuals), $255.00 per year (US institutions), $88 per year (US students/individuals), $225.00 per year (Canadian individuals), $315.00 per year (Canadian institutions), $113 per year (Canadian and foreign students/individuals), $225.00 per year (foreign individuals), and $315.00 per year (foreign institutions). Foreign air speed delivery is included in all *Clinics'* subscription prices. All prices are subject to change without notice. POSTMASTER: Send address changes to *Thoracic Surgery Clinics*, W.B. Saunders Company, Periodicals Fulfillment, Orlando, FL 32887-4800. **Customer Service: 1-800-654-2452 (US). From outside of the US, call 1-407-345-4000.** E mail: hhspcs@harcourt.com.

Reprints. For copies of 100 or more, of articles in this publication, please contact Commercial Rights Department, Elsevier Inc., 360 Park Avenue South, New York, NY 10010-1710. Tel: (212) 633-3813, Fax: (212) 633-3820, e-mail: reprints@elsevier.com

Thoracic Surgery Clinics is covered in *Index Medicus* and *EMBASE/Excerpta Medica*.

Printed in the United States of America.

CONSULTING EDITOR

MARK K. FERGUSON, MD, Professor of Surgery, Section of Cardiac and Thoracic Surgery, The University of Chicago, Chicago, Illinois

GUEST EDITOR

JEROME M. KLAFTA, MD, Associate Professor and Associate Chair for Education, Department of Anesthesia and Critical Care, University of Chicago, Chicago, Illinois

CONTRIBUTORS

JAY B. BRODSKY, MD, Professor, Department of Anesthesia, Stanford University School of Medicine, Stanford, California

JAVIER H. CAMPOS, MD, Professor of Anesthesia; Clinical Director, Department of Anesthesia; and Director of Cardiothoracic Anesthesia, University of Iowa Health Care, Iowa City, Iowa

T. LINDA CHI, MD, Associate Professor, Department of Diagnostic Imaging, The University of Texas M. D. Anderson Cancer Center, Houston, Texas

JEFFREY A. CLARK, MD, Assistant Professor, Department of Anesthesiology, Dartmouth Hitchcock Medical Center, Lebanon, New Hampshire

CHARL J. DE WET, MBChB, Assistant Professor, Department of Anesthesiology and Division of Cardiothoracic Surgery, Washington University School of Medicine, St. Louis, Missouri

MICHAEL A. ERDEK, MD, Assistant Professor; Director, Adult Inpatient Pain Service; and Director, Divisional Quality Improvement, Division of Pain Medicine, The Johns Hopkins University School of Medicine, Baltimore, Maryland

DAVID FERSON, MD, Professor, Department of Anesthesiology and Pain Medicine, The University of Texas M. D. Anderson Cancer Center, Houston, Texas

ALLAN GOTTSCHALK, MD, PhD, Associate Professor, Department of Anesthesiology and Critical Care Medicine, The Johns Hopkins Hospital, Baltimore, Maryland

KATHERINE P. GRICHNIK, MD, Associate Clinical Professor, Department of Anesthesiology, Duke University Medical Center, Duke University Health Care Systems, Durham, North Carolina

PHILIP M. HARTIGAN, MD, Assistant Professor of Anesthesia, Harvard Medical School; and Director, Thoracic Anesthesia, Department of Anesthesiology, Perioperative and Pain Medicine, Brigham and Women's Hospital, Boston, Massachusetts

ERIC JACOBSOHN, MBChB, MHPE, FRCPC, Associate Professor, Department of Anesthesiology and Division of Cardiothoracic Surgery; and Medical Director, Cardiothoracic Intensive Care Unit, Washington University School of Medicine, St. Louis, Missouri

MICHAEL R. JOHNSTON, MD, FRCSC, Associate Professor, Division of Thoracic Surgery, Department of Surgery, University of Toronto; and The University Health Network, Toronto General Hospital, Toronto, Ontario, Canada

JOHN P. LAWRENCE, MD, Associate Professor of Anesthesia, Director of Anesthesiology Residency, Director of Cardiothoracic Anesthesia Fellowship, and Director of Cardiothoracic Anesthesia, Department of Anesthesia, University of Cincinnati, Cincinnati, Ohio

KEVIN McCONNELL, MD, Resident Physician, Department of Surgery, Washington University School of Medicine, St. Louis, Missouri

E. ANDREW OCHROCH, MD, Assistant Professor, Department of Anesthesia, University of Pennsylvania Health System, Philadelphia, Pennsylvania

ALESSIA PEDOTO, MD, Instructor in Anesthesia, Harvard Medical School; and Staff Anesthesiologist, Department of Anesthesiology, Perioperative and Pain Medicine, Brigham and Women's Hospital, Boston, Massachusetts

PETER D. SLINGER, MD, FRCPC, Professor, Department of Anesthesia, University of Toronto; and The University Health Network, Toronto General Hospital, Toronto, Ontario, Canada

PETER S. STAATS, MD, Associate Professor, The Johns Hopkins University School of Medicine, Baltimore, Maryland; and Private Practice, Shrewsbury, New Jersey

ERIN A. SULLIVAN, MD, Associate Professor of Anesthesiology, Director, Cardiothoracic Anesthesiology, and Associate Chief of Anesthesiology, University of Pittsburgh Medical Center Presbyterian Hospital, Pittsburgh, Pennsylvania

AVERY TUNG, MD, Associate Professor, Department of Anesthesia and Critical Care, and Director of Critical Care Services, Burn Unit, University of Chicago, Chicago, Illinois

CONTRIBUTORS

CONTENTS

FORTHCOMING ISSUES

RECENT ISSUES

THORACIC
SURGERY
CLINICS

Thorac Surg Clin 15 (2005) ix

Preface

Advances in Anesthesia and Pain Management

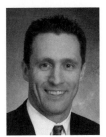

Jerome M. Klafta, MD
Guest Editor

This year approximately 40 million anesthetics will be administered in the United States. In just the past decade, estimates for the number of deaths attributed to anesthesia have dropped 25-fold from 1 in 10,000 anesthetics to fewer than 1 in 250,000. Remarkably, this decline is reported during a time when the definition of an operable candidate has expanded considerably.

A century and a half after the first administration of ether at the Massachusetts General Hospital, and just 55 years since the introduction of the double-lumen endotracheal tube, anesthesiology in general—and thoracic anesthesiology in particular—have changed dramatically and continue to evolve. Many of the advances in anesthesiology discussed in this issue of the *Thoracic Surgery Clinics* are relevant for all types of surgeries. Among these advances are new devices for awareness monitoring, supraglottic airway devices, breath-by-breath analysis of respiratory gases, multimodal pain therapy, and techniques for prevention of acute lung injury. Other developments are specific to anesthesia for thoracic surgery, such as improved lung separation techniques, a refined understanding of the pathophysiology of one-lung ventilation, and evidence-based perioperative management of patients with end stage lung disease. Several articles depict state-of-the-art anesthetic management for lung volume reduction, lung transplantation, and other thoracic operations. Because the comorbidities of patients who need thoracic surgery have a tremendous impact on the approach to anesthesia, current strategies in preoperative evaluation and postoperative intensive care are also considered.

As a clinician, teacher, and residency program director, I have always been energized and enlightened by interdisciplinary collaboration. I was therefore especially enthusiastic to share the advances that have been made in my field of anesthesiology and pain management with my surgical colleagues. The authors and I recognize that this issue is not only an opportunity to inform but also a chance to enrich the symbiotic relationship between surgeons and anesthesiologists, a relationship that ultimately serves our patients. We sincerely hope that our efforts foster a better understanding of the nuances, capabilities, and challenges of anesthesiology and pain management in 2005.

I thank all of the authors for their outstanding contributions and Dr. Mark Ferguson for his gracious invitation to serve as Guest Editor of this issue.

Jerome M. Klafta, MD
Department of Anesthesia and Critical Care
University of Chicago
5841 S. Maryland Ave., MC 4028
Chicago, IL 60637, USA
E-mail address: jklafta@airway.uchicago.edu

ELSEVIER
SAUNDERS

Thorac Surg Clin 15 (2005) 1 – 10

The Evolution of Thoracic Anesthesia

Jay B. Brodsky, MD

Department of Anesthesia, H3580, Stanford University School of Medicine, Stanford, CA 94305, USA

The modern era of safe, routine intrathoracic surgery is relatively recent; it began in the 1930s. Although basic techniques for thoracic surgery had been developed earlier, successful operations within the chest could not be performed until some major problems in anesthetic management, which often are taken for granted today, had been solved. The foremost obstacle in the development of thoracic surgery as a specialty was the "pneumothorax problem." Opening the pleural cavity to ambient pressure resulted in collapse of the lung and paradoxical respirations, a situation that could not be tolerated by a spontaneously breathing patient.

Major advances in thoracic surgery coincided with changes in anesthetic practice. Developments and improvements in airway intubation techniques and devices, controlled ventilation, newer and safer anesthetic agents, accurate intraoperative monitoring, and control of postoperative pain all have enabled innovative and more complex surgical procedures to be performed safely.

Starting with the introduction of inhalation anesthesia in the 1840s, by the beginning of the twentieth century, successful surgery within the abdominal cavity had become commonplace. The evolution of general surgery followed the routine practice of asepsis, the ability to administer blood and intravenous fluids, the availability of radiography and endoscopy techniques for diagnosis, and, most importantly, the administration of inhalational and regional anesthesia.

Although the morbidity and mortality of abdominal operations were much greater than would be acceptable today, a patient undergoing a laparotomy

for a bowel resection in 1930 had a reasonable chance of surviving the operative experience. This was not the situation for procedures within the chest. Before the 1930s, there was reluctance by thoracic surgeons to perform any but the simplest operation. Although thoracotomy was technically possible, the prognosis for any patient undergoing a major intrathoracic resection was extremely poor.

The inability to operate successfully within the chest was the result of limitations in anesthetic practice. Anesthetic techniques for thoracic surgery had not changed significantly from what they had been 50 years earlier. In 1937, an authoritative surgical textbook described a technique of thoracic anesthesia that was essentially unchanged from a description published in another text in 1908 [1].

"Pneumothorax Problem"

In an anesthetized, spontaneously breathing patient with an intact chest wall, both lungs remain expanded during inspiration. Opening the chest causes a sudden collapse of the operative lung. The patient soon becomes tachypneic and cyanotic. The mediastinum shifts toward the nonoperative lung. As the patient attempts to breathe, the collapsed lung expands and contracts, but respirations are "paradoxical" (ie, the lung becomes smaller on inspiration and larger on expiration). The term *penduluft* described the transfer of air from the exposed collapsed lung to the healthy lung while the patient attempted to breathe.

Although general surgeons had adequate time and relatively satisfactory conditions in which to operate, thoracic surgeons did not. The lung moved up and down so violently with the patient struggling for each

E-mail address: Jbrodsky@stanford.edu

1547-4127/05/$ – see front matter © 2005 Elsevier Inc. All rights reserved.
doi:10.1016/j.thorsurg.2004.08.005

breath that attempts at anything other than the simplest resection were technically difficult. Within a few minutes, the patient became hypotensive from loss of venous return, and unless the procedure was discontinued immediately and the chest closed quickly, the patient would die. Because surgery had to be accomplished so rapidly, operations that could be performed successfully under these conditions were few and limited.

Before the 1930s, the major indications for thoracic surgery were empyema and tuberculosis. Lung infection was treated by thoracoplasty with rib resection, decortication, and drainage. The surgical treatment of tuberculosis consisted of creation of a pneumothorax. Because procedures within the chest had to be done quickly, pulmonary resection in the early 1930s was performed with a snare or tourniquet technique. Reoperation was necessary several days later to remove necrotic tissue. The dangers of infection, hemorrhage, and air leak were great and

resulted in significant morbidity and mortality. In cases in which the lung was adherent to the chest wall, there seemed to be fewer problems. The beneficial effect of an adherent lung even prompted some surgeons to inject irritants into the pleural cavity several days before an open thoracotomy.

Several ingenious, but ultimately impractical, solutions were advanced to deal with the "pneumothorax problem." One approach was a negative-pressure chamber, the idea of the surgeon von Mikulicz and his assistant Sauerbruch [2]. In 1904, they proposed keeping an animal's entire body inside a negative-pressure chamber at -15 cm H_2O, while the head remained outside the chamber (Fig. 1). Lung expansion could be maintained with the chest open. Sauerbruch later performed thoracotomies in a large airtight chamber with the pressure reduced below atmospheric pressure. The patient's head and the anesthesiologist were on the outside, while the patient inside the chamber continued to breathe unassisted.

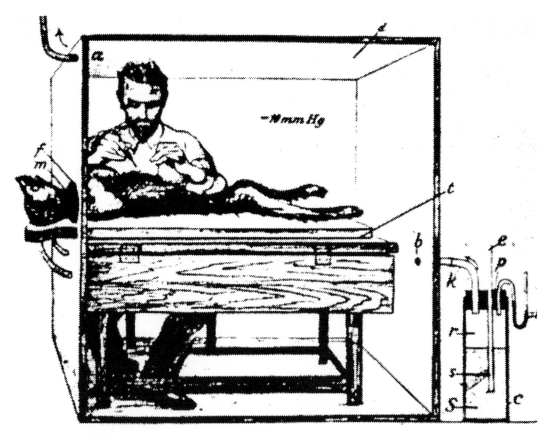

Fig. 1. Sauerbruch first performed thoracotomies on animals and later on patients in a large airtight, negative-pressure chamber. Lung expansion was maintained with an open chest while the patient continued to breathe spontaneously without assistance. (*From* Mushin WW, Rendell-Baker L, editors. The principles of thoracic anesthesia. Springfield [IL]: Charles C Thomas; 1953; with permission.)

Brauer took a different and less successful approach. He described a technique in which the lung was kept expanded by placing only the patient's head in a positive-pressure chamber. Spontaneous, unassisted respiration could continue, but oxygenation, carbon dioxide elimination, and cardiac filling were inadequate with this method [3].

Positive-pressure ventilation

With the benefit of hindsight, it now is recognized that the aforementioned techniques were dead-end approaches to the "pneumothorax problem." Modern thoracic surgery awaited the development of tracheal intubation and positive-pressure ventilation [4]. Tracheal ventilation had been described in the nineteenth century, but it was almost completely ignored by the influential surgeons of that period, particularly due to Sauerbruch's advocacy of his negative-pressure chamber method.

In the 1880s, in the United States, O'Dwyer [5] developed a practical method of "blind" oral tracheal intubation for the treatment of diphtheria (Fig. 2). At about the same time, another physician, Fell, attached a bellows system to an intubating cannula to provide positive-pressure ventilation for drug overdose patients.

The prominent American surgeon Matas first applied the combined Fell-O'Dwyer apparatus to treat traumatic pneumothorax, then later performed surgery using positive-pressure ventilation and general anesthesia. At the turn of the twentieth century, he wrote with brilliant foresight that "the procedure that promises the most benefit in preventing pulmonary collapse in operations on the chest is the artificial inflation of the lung and the rhythmical maintenance of artificial respiration by a tube in the glottis directly connected with a bellows" [6]. Matas expressed dismay that his colleagues had failed to apply these techniques, which he noted had been used in the physiology laboratories for decades in the artificial respiration of animals.

In 1916, Giertz, a former colleague of Sauerbruch, showed with open-chest animal experiments that rhythmic inflation of the lungs was more effective than either negative-pressure chamber or continuous positive-pressure chamber ventilation. Sauerbruch, even long past the 1930s, continued to oppose any change from negative-pressure to intermittent positive-pressure ventilation. He greatly influenced and in doing so delayed the modern practice of thoracic surgery, even though all the necessary components

(laryngoscopy, endotracheal tubes, a positive-pressure ventilating system) had been available for years. A few surgeons did adopt the Fell-O'Dywer apparatus for thoracic surgery, but most did not, perhaps because this technique required expertise

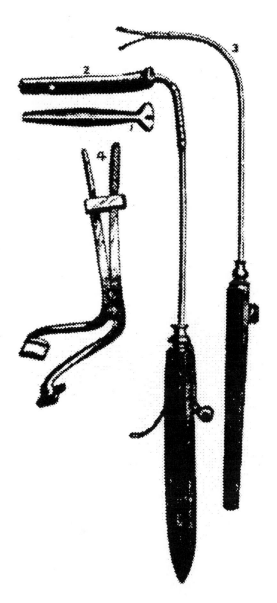

Fig. 2. O'Dwyer's instruments for laryngeal intubation of patients with diphtheria. The tracheal tube (1) was designed to lie in the larynx with the expanded upper end resting on the vocal cords. The tube (2) is shown in place on the introducer (3). A mouth gag also is shown (4). (*From* Mushin WW, Rendell-Baker L, editors. The principles of thoracic anesthesia. Springfield [IL]: Charles C Thomas; 1953; with permission.)

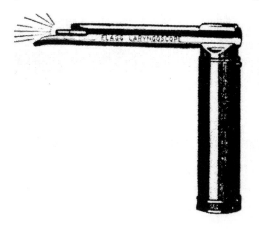

Fig. 3. The Flagg laryngoscope (1932) was the prototype of modern instruments. It featured a battery in the handle and a bulb at the tip of the blade. (*From* Mushin WW, Rendell-Baker L, editors. The principles of thoracic anesthesia. Springfield [IL]: Charles C Thomas; 1953; with permission.)

in "blind" tracheal intubation and a "deeper" state of anesthesia.

Tracheal intubation

Kirstein [7] had introduced direct laryngoscopy in 1895. Jackson modified and improved Kirstein's instrument and techniques. The Jackson laryngoscope could be used to deliver an air-ether combination by intratracheal insufflation that could render the patient apneic [8,9]. Elsberg [10], who is credited with performing the first thoracotomy in 1910, used intratracheal positive-pressure ventilation via a Jackson laryngoscope.

World War I was a major impetus for the development of anesthetic and surgical techniques for all types of trauma, including thoracic injuries. The pioneering anesthetists Magill and Rowbotham proposed the routine use of endotracheal anesthesia for maxillofacial surgery [11]. Uncuffed, wide-bore rubber tubes were placed "blindly," that is, without laryngoscopy either orally or nasally. Despite the success of endotracheal anesthesia, however, open-drop and mask anesthesia continued to be the techniques used for most procedures, including thoracic surgery.

The modern laryngoscope was described by Flagg [12] in 1932 (Fig. 3). The laryngoscope allowed easier endotracheal tube placement and was the prototype for the many modern laryngoscopes that have followed. The Macintosh laryngoscope blade, introduced in 1943, remains in use to day [13].

Anesthetic technique

As previously noted, the usual indication for thoracic surgery was infection. Cross-contamination from the diseased to the healthy lung was a major problem. The anesthetic practice was to keep the level of anesthesia "light" because it was considered essential that the patient maintain the cough reflex. To retain an active cough reflex, the use of spinal and regional anesthesia alone was advocated for thoracotomy [14].

The most popular general anesthetic technique in the first third of the twentieth century was open drop ether or chloroform. The patient breathed spontaneously, and the depth of respirations controlled the level of anesthesia. With deeper planes of anesthesia, minute ventilation was reduced, and less ether or chloroform was delivered. This method was satisfactory for most operations, but it was inadequate for thoracic surgery because of the "pneumothorax problem." With open drop anesthesia, the thoracic surgeon had only a short time to complete the procedure and close the chest if the patient was to survive. General anesthesia also could be provided by delivery of gases (oxygen with nitrous oxide) via an airtight mask with spontaneous respiration or intratracheal insufflation of anesthetic gases using a Jackson laryngoscope.

In 1928, Guedel and Waters [15] described an endotracheal tube with an inflatable cuff (Fig. 4). They noted that a cuffed endotracheal tube could protect the lungs from gastric aspiration. Because

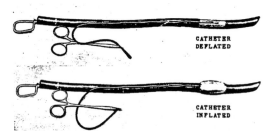

Fig. 4. The Guedel and Waters intratracheal catheter (endotracheal tube) was introduced in 1928. It was constructed of rubber, was 14 inches long, and had 1/16-inch-thick walls with an inside lumen diameter of 3/8 inch. The cuff either was cemented in place or could be removed. The cuff was inflated with a measured quantity of air from a syringe. Forceps were used to clamp the tube to the inflated cuff. A metal stylet was placed inside the lumen to stiffen the tube while it was being advanced. (*From* Mushin WW, Rendell-Baker L, editors. The principles of thoracic anesthesia. Springfield [IL]: Charles C Thomas; 1953; with permission.)

ventilation could be controlled and airway secretions could be removed with suctioning, the depth of general anesthesia could be deepened. The patient's lungs were hyperventilated to eliminate spontaneous respirations, and even deeper levels of anesthesia could be used to induce diaphragmatic immobility and complete apnea.

The cuffed endotracheal tube combined with positive-pressure ventilation was the long-awaited clinical breakthrough that provided a practical solution to the "pneumothorax problem." With rhythmic controlled ventilation to both lungs, *penduluft* breathing could be avoided during open chest operations.

One-lung ventilation

In 1931, only 3 years after the introduction of the cuffed endotracheal tube, Gale and Waters [16] described a technique for selective one-lung ventilation. Their publication ushered in the modern era of anesthesia for thoracic surgery. They intubated the trachea with a cuffed rubber endotracheal tube using direct laryngoscopy. The tube was advanced "blindly" into the bronchus of the healthy lung. After being positioned properly, the large-volume cuff at the tube's distal end was inflated to the point where it not only sealed the intubated bronchus, but also extended over into the carina and obstructed ventilation to the bronchus of the diseased lung. Only the healthy lung was ventilated, while the operated lung gradually collapsed from absorption atelectasis (Fig. 5).

The advantages of this method were immense. For the first time, the thoracic surgeon was provided with an immobile surgical field, usually adequate ventilation of the healthy lung, the absence of cardiovascular collapse from sudden pneumothorax, and the prevention of secretions from entering into the trachea and dependent healthy lung. These remain the basic objectives in the current practice of one-lung ventilation for thoracic surgery. From this point, progress proceeded rapidly, although in many instances the acceptance of new ideas, new equipment, or a new technique into everyday clinical practice was not immediate.

In 1935, Archibald [17] described a bronchial blocker for the control of secretions during one-lung ventilation. A rubber catheter with an inflatable distal balloon was inserted into the bronchus of the diseased lung. Radiographs were used to confirm and readjust the blocker's position. Lung tissue beyond the inflated balloon collapsed. The following year, Magill

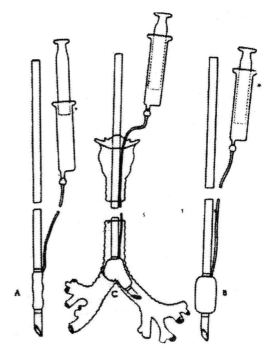

Fig. 5. Gale and Waters technique for one-lung ventilation. A cuffed endotracheal tube (*A*) was advanced into the healthy lung's bronchus. When inflated (*B*), the cuff sealed off the healthy bronchus allowing positive-pressure ventilation, but also extended over and obstructed ventilation to the operated lung (*C*). (*From* Mushin WW, Rendell-Baker L, editors. The principles of thoracic anesthesia. Springfield [IL]: Charles C Thomas; 1953; with permission.)

[18] designed a blocker that could be positioned accurately in the bronchus under direct vision by means of an endoscope passed down the blocker tube's lumen.

With the introduction by Gale and Waters of one-lung ventilation using a cuffed endotracheal tube in 1932 and Magill's improved bronchial blocker in 1936, advances in surgical techniques for intrathoracic operations began in earnest. The anesthesiologist could ventilate an apneic, nonmoving patient's lung, while providing the surgeon with a quiet operative field. The surgeon had sufficient time to perform the operation. By today's standards, relatively rapid surgery was still necessary because of continued perfusion ("shunt") of blood through the nonventilated lung, which still could result in life-threatening hypoxemia.

The 1930s saw the development of ligation techniques for airway and vascular structures, surgical techniques that reduced the incidence of air leak, tension pneumothorax, and hemorrhage. Pleural drainage and postoperative use of a closed chest thoracostomy tube also were described during this period. Nissen reported the first successful pneumonectomy, for bronchiectasis, in 1931 [19]. The first successful pneumonectomy for a malignancy was by Graham in 1933 [20].

Single-lumen endobronchial tubes and bronchial blockers

In 1936, Rovenstine [21] used a double-cuffed, single-lumen endobronchial tube that he advanced "blindly" into the bronchus of the ventilated lung. Inflating only the proximal balloon of Rovenstine's tube provided two-lung ventilation, whereas inflating both cuffs allowed only one-lung ventilation of the healthy lung (Fig. 6). He recommended endobronchial intubation for one-lung ventilation to control secretions during lung resection and to provide the surgeon with a quiet surgical field.

Many other endobronchial tubes [22–24] and endobronchial tubes with a combined bronchial blocker [25–28] were introduced into anesthetic practice.

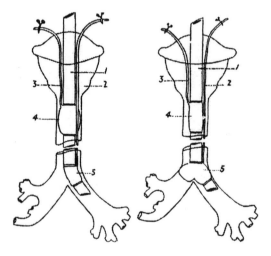

Fig. 6. In 1936, Rovenstine described a double-cuffed, single-lumen endobronchial tube that was advanced "blindly" into the bronchus of the ventilated lung. The upper cuff (4) was inflated first for two-lung ventilation. When the lower cuff (5) was inflated, it allowed only single-lung ventilation of the healthy lung, while blocking ventilation to the diseased lung. (*From* Mushin WW, Rendell-Baker L, editors. The principles of thoracic anesthesia. Springfield [IL]: Charles C Thomas; 1953; with permission.)

Crafoord [29] even used a ribbon gauze tampon to block the bronchus and control secretions. Each of these devices was advanced into the bronchus either "blindly" or with a rigid bronchoscope.

These rubber tubes have since been replaced, but today's techniques for bronchial blockade remain essentially unchanged from techniques first used in the 1930s. For many years, the Fogarty embolectomy catheter was popular as a bronchial blocker [30]. Other balloon-tipped catheters, including pulmonary artery and wedge catheters and even the Foley urinary catheter, have been used as blockers. All bronchial blockers work on the principle that when ventilation to a lung or lobe is obstructed, the unventilated portion of that lung eventually collapses secondary to absorption atelectasis.

The limitations and positioning difficulties of these bronchial blockers have been an impetus for refinements in their design. A combined endotracheal tube and bronchial blocker, the Univent tube, was introduced in the 1980s [31,32]. It is a large endotracheal tube with a small anterior channel containing a thin balloon-tipped tube. The latter can be advanced into the bronchus as a blocker. If postoperative ventilation is planned, reintubation is unnecessary because at the completion of surgery the blocker can be deflated and withdrawn into the tube's main body, which can be used as an endotracheal tube.

More recently, several balloon-tipped plastic tubes have been designed specifically for bronchial blockade. The most innovative is a wire-guided endobronchial blocker [33]. With this device, one-lung ventilation can be achieved in almost any patient, even someone requiring awake, nasal fiberoptic intubation. A wire loop at the tip of the blocker is coupled to a pediatric bronchoscope, and the bronchoscope is advanced into the bronchus under direct vision through an endotracheal tube. The blocker's balloon has low-pressure properties, in contrast to other balloon-tipped catheters, such as the Fogarty catheter, which are not designed for bronchial blockade and have high-pressure balloons, which can damage the airway.

Bronchial blockers do not permit suctioning or reexpansion and then recollapse of the operated lung during surgery. Blood, pus, or tumor material can collect, and cross-contamination is possible when the blocker balloon is deflated. Bronchial blockade generally is indicated for situations when placement of a double-lumen tube is impractical or impossible, as may occur in an adult patient with a "difficult" airway or a child whose trachea is too small for a double-lumen tube.

Double-lumen tubes

In 1949, Carlens [34] described a double-cuffed, double-lumen tube that was intended to be used for differential bronchospirometry. The following year, Bjork and Carlens [35] used the double-lumen tube for selective one-lung anesthesia. Modifications of the Carlens tube soon followed [36–38].

Surgeons and anesthesiologists soon recognized the advantages of these tubes [39,40]. A double-lumen tube allows safe, effective one-lung ventilation; provides a quiet surgical field; and protects the dependent healthy lung from aspiration while the patient is in the lateral position. The operated lung can be collapsed, reinflated, and recollapsed safely at will during the procedure. The bronchus of the collapsed lung can be suctioned through the non-ventilating lumen to remove blood and secretions before the lung is reexpanded.

Despite the many advantages of rubber double-lumen tubes, difficulty with intubation and placement and high airway resistance during one-lung ventilation initially restricted their use. The Robertshaw tube, which was introduced in 1962, solved some of these problems [41]. The Robertshaw double-lumen tube lacks the carinal hook of the Carlens and White tubes. The carinal hook was helpful for accurate "blind" placement of these double-lumen tubes, but often was implicated as a cause of serious airway trauma. The Robertshaw tube has wider lumens and a more molded curvature to reduce kinking and to improve gas flow.

Disposable, plastic double-lumen tubes in use since the early 1980s generally have replaced the older rubber tubes [42]. Their plastic construction allows greater ease and safety in intubation and placement. The plastic material is thinner than rubber so that their lumens are larger than rubber tubes of equivalent circumference. Larger lumens offer less resistance to airflow during one-lung ventilation. It is easier to pass a suction catheter or fiberoptic bronchoscope down a plastic double-lumen tube. The presence of water vapor, blood, and secretions is visible through the clear plastic. In contrast to the low-volume, high-pressure cuffs of the rubber tubes, plastic double-lumen tubes have high-volume, low-pressure cuffs that reduce the risks of airway trauma [43].

Fiberoptic bronchoscopy

Double-lumen tubes were advanced into the bronchus and positioned "blindly." The introduction of flexible fiberoptic bronchoscopy into clinical practice occurred in the 1970s and first was used for double-lumen tube placement in the 1980s [44]. A fiberoptic bronchoscope allows tubes to be positioned under direct vision, reducing the risks of trauma and hypoxemia from tube malposition and increasing the safety of one-lung ventilation.

Controlled intraoperative ventilation

The successful introduction of controlled ventilation for intrathoracic operations required clinical acceptance of laryngoscopy, tracheal intubation, and positive-pressure ventilation. The first experimental ventilator, the Spiropulsator was described by a Swedish otolaryngologist, Freckner, in 1934 and used by Crafoord [45] in surgery soon afterward. Intermittent positive-pressure ventilation became practical, however, only after the introduction of curare for muscle relaxation in 1942 [46]. Use of curare in thoracic surgery was reported in 1947 [47].

Skeletal muscle paralysis from neuromuscular blocking drugs produces apnea and allows intraoperative control of ventilation with much lighter planes of general anesthesia. A technique combining oxygen and nitrous oxide with morphine was developed that allowed unrestricted use of electrocautery during surgery. This technique significantly reduced bleeding, a major cause of complications in operations for pulmonary infections.

General acceptance of intraoperative controlled positive-pressure ventilation did not occur until after the polio epidemic in Denmark in 1952. The Engstrom volume-controlled ventilator, which had been used successfully in the management of polio victims, was applied for postoperative care of thoracic surgical patients [48]. The success of mechanical ventilation outside the operating room convinced anesthesiologists that these machines could be useful during surgery. Widespread acceptance of mechanical ventilation for delivering anesthetics did not occur until the 1960s.

Initially, controlled ventilation was with either ether or cyclopropane anesthesia. These agents were safe and potent, although highly explosive. In 1956, the first modern inhalational anesthetic, halothane, was developed specifically to meet the needs of the surgeon and patient [49]. In contrast to ether and cyclopropane, it was nonflammable so that electrocautery could be used safely. Halothane also is sufficiently potent, eliminating the need for nitrous oxide and allowing high concentrations of oxygen to be used during one-lung anesthesia. Over the ensuing years, halothane was replaced by newer and improved halogenated anesthetics. These have included methoxyflurane and enflurane in the 1960s and 1970s and isoflurane, sevoflurane, and desflurane in the 1980s and 1990s.

Intraoperative monitoring

Routine intraoperative monitoring before 1960 was basic, consisting of an ECG, cuff blood pressure measurements, and an esophageal stethoscope. The 1960s witnessed the introduction into clinical practice of invasive monitoring. Arterial blood gases could be measured during thoracotomy to guide the management of one-lung ventilation. For the first time, anesthesiologists could measure accurately and manipulate physiologic variables, such as central venous and pulmonary artery pressure [50]. The current era is characterized by effective, safe, noninvasive monitoring. The widespread application of capnography and oximetry have reduced greatly the incidence of adverse intraoperative events, and their application during one-lung ventilation has eliminated the need for invasive monitors in many patients [51]. Anesthesiologists can assess accurately ventilation and cardiovascular status continuously and can intervene when necessary.

Maximizing oxygenation during one-lung ventilation

Even with a double-lumen tube, controlled ventilation, and inspired oxygen of 100%, the persistent "shunt" to the unventilated lung can produce dangerously low oxygen tensions during one-lung ventilation. Positive end-expiratory pressure and continuous positive airway pressure, techniques initially developed for management of patients in respiratory failure, were applied during one-lung ventilation in the 1980s [52]. Positive end-expiratory pressure to the ventilated lung or continuous positive airway pressure to the collapsed lung or the combination of the two can optimize oxygenation during thoracotomy, allowing the surgeon time to complete even the most difficult surgical procedure [53].

Postoperative analgesia

Morbidity and mortality after thoracic operations have declined dramatically since the 1980s [54].

Among the most important factors for reducing complications have been advances in the management of postthoracotomy pain.

The lateral thoracotomy incision is intensely painful. If inadequately treated, postthoracotomy pain can lead to postoperative pulmonary dysfunction and the vicious cycle of hypoventilation, atelectasis, hypoxemia, and often pneumonia. Systemic opioids traditionally have been the mainstay for treating this pain. The therapeutic window for systemic opioids is narrow, however, because overmedication would produce hypoventilation, whereas undermedication would prevent deep breathing and coughing.

In their comprehensive review of postthoracotomy analgesia, Kavanagh et al [55] discussed the many analgesic regimens (systemic opioids, spinal and epidural opioids, ketamine, nonsteroidal anti-inflammatory drugs, intercostal nerve blocks, cryoanalgesia, transcutaneous electric nerve stimulation, intrapleural local anesthetics, epidural and paravertebral local anesthetics) currently in use. Because each of these methods has its advocates, an optimal analgesic technique acceptable to everyone is still elusive. Most anesthesiologists and surgeons would agree, however, that the use of epidural opioids combined with local anesthetics has been another major contribution to the evolution of anesthesia for thoracic surgery.

Behar et al [56] first reported the benefit of epidural morphine for pain management in 1979. This report was followed by rapid acceptance of spinal (intrathecal and epidural) opioid analgesia for pain control after all types of operations [57]. Spinal local anesthetics previously had been used for postthoracotomy pain, but the high incidence of associated hypotension made this method less than ideal.

In 1984, Shulman et al [58] performed a prospective study comparing thoracotomy patients receiving epidural and intravenous morphine. The epidural group had superior pain relief and better postoperative pulmonary function than the control group receiving systemic morphine. Stenseth et al [59] reported that 91% of his patients undergoing thoracotomy were "satisfied" with their analgesia and 83% were "pain-free" after epidural morphine.

During the 1980s and 1990s, the use of lumbar and thoracic epidural analgesia, either with opioids alone or with opioids combined with local anesthetics, revolutionized the postoperative management of thoracic surgical patients. No other treatment modality has been proved superior. Some have even argued that every thoracotomy patient "deserves" epidural analgesia [60]. After thoracotomy, a comfortable, spontaneously breathing patient has fewer complications and recovers more quickly. Predictable postthoracotomy analgesia has allowed more complex procedures to be performed on more fragile patients.

Summary

The specialty of thoracic surgery has evolved along with the modern practice of anesthesia. This close relationship began in the 1930s and continues today. Thoracic surgery has grown from a field limited almost exclusively to simple chest wall procedures to the present situation in which complex procedures, such as lung volume reduction or lung transplantation, now can be performed on the most severely compromised patient.

The great advances in thoracic surgery have followed discoveries and technical innovations in many medical fields [61]. One of the most important reasons for the rapid escalation in the number and complexity of thoracic surgical procedures now being performed has been the evolution of anesthesia for thoracic surgery. There has been so much progress in this area that numerous books and journals are devoted entirely to this subject [62–65].

The author has been privileged to work with several surgeons who specialized in noncardiac thoracic surgery. As a colleague of 25 years, the noted pulmonary surgeon James B.D. Mark wrote, "Any operation is a team effort... (but) nowhere is this team effort more important than in thoracic surgery, where near-choreography of moves by all participants is essential. Exchange of information, status and plans are mandatory" [66]. This team approach between the thoracic surgeon and the anesthesiologist reflects the history of the two specialties. With new advances in technology, such as continuous blood gas monitoring and the pharmacologic management of pulmonary circulation to maximize oxygenation during one-lung ventilation, in the future even more complex procedures may be able to be performed safely on even higher risk patients.

References

[1] Mushin WM, Rendell BL, editors. The principles of thoracic anaesthesia: past and present. Springfield (IL): Charles C Thomas; 1953.

[2] Naef AP. The mid-century revolution in thoracic and cardiovascular surgery: Part 1. Interactive Cardiovasc Thorac Surg 2003;2:219–36.

[3] Meyer JA. Unterduck and Uberdruck, 1904. Ann Thorac Surg 1989;47:933–8.

[4] Fell SC. A history of pneumonectomy. Chest Surg Clin N Am 1999;9:267–90.

[5] O'Dwyer J. Intubation of the larynx. N Y Med J 1885;42:145–7.

[6] Matas R. The history and methods of intralaryngeal insufflation for the relief of acute surgical pneumothorax, with a description of the latest devices for the purpose. Trans South Surg Gynecol Assoc 1900;12:52–84.

[7] Kirstein A. Autosckopie des larynx und der trachea. Berl Klin Wchnschr 1895;32:476–8.

[8] Meyer W. Some observations regarding thoracic surgery on human beings. Ann Surg 1910;52:34–57.

[9] Jackson C. The technique of insertion of intratracheal insufflation tubes. Surg Gynecol Obstet 1913;17:507–9.

[10] Elsberg CA. Clinical experiences with intratracheal insufflation (Meltzer), with remarks upon the value of the method for thoracic surgery. Ann Surg 1910;52:23–33.

[11] Magill IW. Endotracheal anaesthesia. Proc R Soc Med 1929;22:83–7.

[12] Flagg PJ. Intratracheal inhalation anesthesia in practice. Arch Otolaryngol 1932;15:844–59.

[13] Macintosh RR. A new laryngoscope. Lancet 1943;1:205.

[14] Shields HJ. Spinal anesthesia for thoracic surgery. Anesth Analg 1935;14:193–8.

[15] Guedel AE, Waters RM. A new intratracheal catheter. Anesth Analg 1928;7:238–9.

[16] Gale JW, Waters RM. Closed endobronchial anesthesia in thoracic surgery. J Thorac Surg 1931;1:432–7.

[17] Archibald E. A consideration of the dangers of lobectomy. J Thorac Surg 1935;4:335–51.

[18] Magill IW. Anaesthetics in thoracic surgery with special reference to lobectomy. Proc R Soc Med 1936;29:643–53.

[19] Brewer III LA. The first pneumonectomy: historical notes. J Thorac Cardiovasc Surg 1984;88:810–26.

[20] Graham AE, Singer JJ. Successful removal of the entire lung for carcinoma of the bronchus. JAMA 1933;101:1371–4.

[21] Rovenstine EA. Anaesthesia for intrathoracic surgery: the endotracheal and endobronchial techniques. Surg Gynecol Obstet 1936;63:325–30.

[22] Mushin WW, editor. Thoracic Anaesthesia. Philadelphia: FA Davis; 1963.

[23] Gordon W, Green R. Right lung anaesthesia: anaesthesia for left lung surgery using a new right endobronchial tube. Anaesthesia 1957;12:86–93.

[24] Pallister WK. A new endobronchial tube for left lung anaesthesia with specific reference to reconstructive pulmonary surgery. Thorax 1959;14:55–7.

[25] Oech SR. A cuffed endotracheal tube with an incorporated endobronchial blocker. Anesthesiology 1955;16:468–9.

[26] Vellacott WN. A new endobronchial tube for bronchopleural fistula repair. Br J Anaesth 1954;26:442–4.

[27] Macintosh R, Leatherdale RA. Bronchus tube and bronchus blocker. Br J Anaesth 1955;27:556–7.

[28] Green R. Endobronchial tube and blocker for right upper lobe. Anaesthesia 1958;13:349–52.

[29] Crafoord C. On the technique of pneumonectomy in man. Acta Chir Scand 1938;81:1–142.

[30] Ginsberg RJ. New technique for one-lung anesthesia using an endobronchial blocker. J Thorac Cardiovasc Surg 1981;82:542–6.

[31] Inoue H, Shohtsu A, Ogawa J, et al. Endotracheal tube with movable blocker to prevent aspiration of intratracheal bleeding. Ann Thorac Surg 1984;37:497–9.

[32] Kamaya H, Krishna PR. New endotracheal tube (Univent tube) for selective blockade of one lung. Anesthesiology 1985;63:342–3.

[33] Arndt GA, Buchika S, Kranner PW, DeLessio ST. Wire-guided endobronchial blockade in a patient with a limited mouth opening. Can J Anaesth 1999;46:87–9.

[34] Carlens E. A new flexible double-lumen catheter for bronchospirometry. J Thorac Surg 1949;18:742–6.

[35] Bjork VO, Carlens E. The prevention of spread during pulmonary resection by the use of a double-lumen catheter. J Thorac Surg 1950;20:151–7.

[36] Bryce-Smith R. A double-lumen endobronchial tube. Br J Anaesth 1959;31:274–5.

[37] Bryce-Smith R, Salt R. A right-sided double lumen tube. Br J Anaesth 1960;32:230–1.

[38] White GM. A new double lumen tube. Br J Anaesth 1960;32:232–4.

[39] Jenkins AV, Clarke G. Endobronchial anaesthesia with the Carlens catheter. Br J Anaesth 1958;30:13–8.

[40] Newman RW, Finer GE, Downs JE. Routine use of the Carlens double-lumen endobronchial catheter: an experimental and clinical study. J Thorac Cardiovasc Surg 1961;42:327–39.

[41] Robertshaw FL. Low resistance double-lumen endobronchial tubes. Br J Anaesth 1962;34:576–9.

[42] Burton NA, Watson DC, Brodsky JB, Mark JB. Advantages of a new polyvinyl chloride double-lumen tube in thoracic surgery. Ann Thorac Surg 1983;36: 78–84.

[43] Fitzmaurice BG, Brodsky JB. Airway rupture from double-lumen tubes. J Cardiothorac Vasc Anesth 1999; 13:322–9.

[44] Benumof JL. Fiberoptic bronchoscopy and double-lumen tube position. Anesthesiology 1986;65:117–8.

[45] Crafoord C. Pulmonary ventilation and anesthesia in major chest surgery. J Thorac Surg 1940;9:237–53.

[46] Griffith HR, Johnson GE. The use of curare in general anesthesia. Anesthesiology 1942;3:418–20.

[47] Stephens HB, Harroun P, Beckert FE. The use of curare in anesthesia for thoracic surgery. J Thorac Surg 1947;16:50–62.

[48] Bjork VO, Engstrom C-G. The treatment of ventilatory insufficiency after pulmonary resection with tracheot-omy and prolonged artificial ventilation. J Thorac Surg 1955;30:356–67.

[49] Raventos J. The action of fluothane: a new volatile anaesthetic. Br J Pharmacol 1956;11:394–410.

[50] Brodsky JB. What intraoperative monitoring makes sense? Chest 1999;115(5 Suppl):101S–5S.

[51] Brodsky JB, Shulman MS, Swan M, Mark JB. Pulse oximetry during one-lung ventilation. Anesthesiology 1985;63:212–4.

[52] Capan LM, Turndorf H, Patel C, Ramanathan S, Acinapura A, Chalon J. Optimization of arterial oxygenation during one-lung ventilation. Anesth Analg 1980;59:847–51.

[53] Cohen E, Eisenkraft JB, Thys DM, Kirschner PA, Kaplan JA. Oxygenation and hemodynamic changes during one-lung ventilation: effects of CPAP10, PEEP10, and CPAP10/PEEP10. J Cardiothorac Anesth 1988;2:34–40.

[54] Cerfolio RJ, Allen MS, Trastek VF, et al. Lung resection in patients with compromised pulmonary function. Ann Thorac Surg 1996;62:348–51.

[55] Kavanagh BP, Katz J, Sandler AN. Pain control after thoracic surgery: a review of current techniques. Anesthesiology 1994;81:737–59.

[56] Behar M, Magora F, Olshwang D, Davidson JT. Epidural morphine and the treatment of pain. Lancet 1979;1:527–9.

[57] Rawal N, Sjostrand U, Dahlstrom B. Postoperative pain relief by epidural morphine. Anesth Analg 1981; 60:726–31.

[58] Shulman M, Sandler AN, Bradley JW, et al. Postthoracotomy pain and pulmonary function following epidural and systemic morphine. Anesthesiology 1984; 61:569–75.

[59] Stenseth R, Sellevold O, Breivik H. Epidural morphine for postoperative pain: experience with 1085 patients. Acta Anaesthesiol Scand 1985;29:148–56.

[60] Slinger PD. Pro: every postthoracotomy patient deserves thoracic epidural analgesia. J Cardiothorac Vasc Anesth 1999;13:350–4.

[61] Sabiston Jr DC. Foreword. In: Wolfe WG, editor. Complication in thoracic surgery: recognition and management. St. Louis: Mosby-Year Book; 1992.

[62] Marshall BE, Longnecker DE, Fairley HB, editors. Anesthesia for thoracic procedures. Boston: Blackwell Scientific Publications; 1988.

[63] Benumof JL. Anesthesia for thoracic surgery. 2nd edition. Philadelphia: WB Saunders; 1995.

[64] Cohen E, editor. The practice of thoracic anesthesia. Philadelphia: JB Lippincott; 1995.

[65] Kaplan JA, Slinger PD, editors. Thoracic Anesthesia. 3rd edition. Philadelphia: Churchill Livingstone; 2003.

[66] Brodsky JB, editor. Problems in anesthesia: thoracic anesthesia. Philadelphia: JB Lippincott; 1990.

**ELSEVIER
SAUNDERS**

Thorac Surg Clin 15 (2005) 11 – 25

**THORACIC
SURGERY
CLINICS**

Preoperative Assessment: An Anesthesiologist's Perspective

Peter D. Slinger, MD, FRCPC[a],*, Michael R. Johnston, MD, FRCSC[b]

[a]*Department of Anesthesia, University of Toronto, and The University Health Network, Toronto General Hospital,
3EN 200 Elizabeth Street, Toronto, ON, Canada, M5G 2C4*
[b]*Division of Thoracic Surgery, Department of Surgery, University of Toronto, and The University Health Network,
Toronto General Hospital, 10EN 200 Elizabeth Street, Toronto, ON, Canada, M5G 2C4*

Preoperative anesthetic assessment before chest surgery is a continually evolving science and art. Advances in anesthetic management, surgical techniques, and perioperative care have expanded the population of patients now considered to be "operable" (Fig. 1) [1]. This article focuses on preanesthetic assessment for pulmonary resection surgery in cancer patients. The principles described apply to all other types of nonmalignant pulmonary resections and to other chest surgery. The major difference is that in patients with malignancy, the risk-to-benefit ratio of canceling or delaying surgery pending other investigation or therapy is always complicated by the risk of further spread of cancer during any extended interval before resection. This is never completely "elective" surgery.

Although 87% of patients with lung cancer die of their disease, the 13% cure rate represents approximately 26,000 survivors per year in North America. Surgical resection is responsible for essentially all of these cures. A patient with a "resectable" lung cancer has a disease that is still local or locoregional in scope and can be encompassed in a plausible surgical procedure. An "operable" patient is someone who can tolerate the proposed resection with acceptable risk [2]. Several general points should be appreciated in the assessment of pulmonary resection patients, as follows:

1. *Anesthesiologists are not gatekeepers.* It is rarely the anesthesiologist's function to assess these patients to decide who is or is not an operative candidate. In most situations, the anesthesiologist sees the patient at the end of a referral chain from chest or family physician to surgeon. At each stage, there should have been a discussion of the risks and benefits of surgery. It is the anesthesiologist's responsibility to use the preoperative assessment to identify patients at elevated risk and to use that risk assessment to stratify perioperative management and focus resources on the high-risk patients to improve their outcome. This is the primary function of the preanesthetic assessment.

2. *Short-term versus long-term survival.* Although there has been a large amount of research done on long-term survival (6 months – 5 years) after pulmonary resection surgery there has been a comparatively small volume of research on the short-term (<6 weeks) outcome of these patients. This research area is currently active, however, and several studies can be used to guide anesthetic management in the immediate perioperative period, when it has an influence on outcome.

3. *Disjoint assessment.* Until more recently, preanesthetic management was part of a continuum in which a patient was admitted preoperatively for testing and the management plan evolved as test results returned. Currently the reality of practice patterns in anesthesia has changed such that a patient commonly is assessed initially in an outpatient clinic and often not by the member of the anesthesia staff who actually will administer the anesthesia. The actual contact with the responsible anesthesiologist may be

---

* Corresponding author.
E-mail address: peter.slinger@uhn.on.ca (P.D. Slinger).

only 10 to 15 minutes before induction. It is necessary to organize and standardize the approach to preoperative evaluation for these patients into two temporally disjoint phases: the initial (clinic) assessment and the final (day-of-admission) assessment. Elements vital to each assessment are described in this article.

4. *"Lung-sparing" surgery.* Thoracic surgeons now are trained to perform lung-sparing resections, such as sleeve-lobectomies or segmentectomies. The postoperative preservation of respiratory function has been shown to be proportional to the amount of functioning lung parenchyma preserved [3]. To assess patients with limited pulmonary function, the anesthesiologist must understand these newer surgical options in addition to the conventional lobectomy or pneumonectomy.

Prethoracotomy assessment naturally involves all of the factors of a complete anesthetic assessment, including past history, allergies, medications, and upper airway. This article focuses on the additional information beyond a standard anesthetic assessment that the anesthesiologist needs to manage a pulmonary resection patient.

Assessment for perioperative complications

To assess patients for thoracic anesthesia, it is necessary to have an understanding of the risks specific to this type of surgery. The major causes of perioperative morbidity and mortality in the thoracic surgical population are respiratory complications. Major respiratory complications are atelectasis, pneumonia, and respiratory failure, which occur in 15% to 20% of patients and account for most of the expected 3% to 4% mortality [4]. The thoracic surgical population differs from other adult surgical populations in this respect. For other types of surgery, cardiac and vascular complications are the leading cause of early perioperative morbidity and mortality. Cardiac complications, including arrhythmia and ischemia, occur in 10% to 15% of thoracic surgery patients [5].

Respiratory function

The best assessment of respiratory function comes from a detailed history of the patient's quality of life. A completely asymptomatic patient with no limitation of activity and full exercise capacity probably

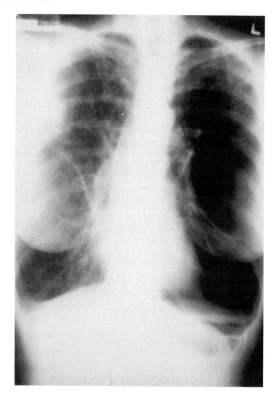

Fig. 1. Preoperative chest x-ray of a 55-year-old woman with severe bullous emphysema and a carcinoma of the right upper lobe. Preoperative forced expiratory volume in 1 second = 25% predicted. Although this woman's pulmonary function does not meet traditional minimal criteria for a lung operation, she now is considered a potential candidate for bilateral combined cancer resection and emphysema surgery. (*From* Slinger PD, Johnston MR. Preoperative evaluation of the thoracic surgery patient. In: Kaplan JA, Slinger PD, editors. Thoracic anesthesia. 3rd edition. Philadelphia: Churchill Livingstone; 2003. p. 1–23; with permission.)

does not need screening cardiorespiratory testing before pulmonary resection. Owing to the biology of lung cancer, these patients are a small minority of the patient population.

Because the anesthesiologist who will manage the case often has to assimilate a great deal of information about the patient in a short time, it is useful to have objective standardized measures of pulmonary function that can be used to guide anesthetic management and to have this information in a format that can be transmitted easily between members of the health care team. Much effort has been expended to try to find a single test of respiratory function that has sufficient sensitivity and specificity to predict outcome for all pulmonary resection patients. It is now clear that no single test ever will accomplish this.

Many factors determine overall respiratory performance [6,7]. It is useful to think of the respiratory function in three related but independent areas: respiratory mechanics, gas exchange, and cardiorespiratory interaction.

Respiratory mechanics

Many tests of respiratory mechanics and volumes show correlation with postthoracotomy outcome, including forced expiratory volume in 1 second (FEV_1), forced vital capacity (FVC), maximal voluntary ventilation (MVV), and residual volume-to-total lung capacity ratio (RV/TLC). It is useful to express these as a percent of predicted volumes corrected for age, sex, and height (eg, $FEV_{1\%}$). Of these, the most valid single test for postthoracotomy respiratory complications is the predicted postoperative FEV_1 (ppo-$FEV_{1\%}$), which is calculated as follows:

$$ppoFEV_{1\%} = \text{preoperative } FEV_1\%$$
$$\times \, (1 - \% \text{ functional lung tissue}$$
$$\text{removed}/100)$$

One method of estimating the percent of functional lung tissue is based on a calculation of the number of functioning subsegments of the lung removed (Fig. 2). Nakahara et al [4] found that patients with a $ppoFEV_1$ greater than 40% had no or minor postresection respiratory complications. Major respiratory complications were seen only in the subgroup with $ppoFEV_1$ less than 40% (although

Lung Subsegments

Total Subsegments = 42

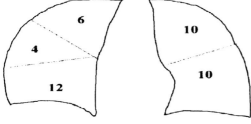

Example: Right lower lobectomy
Postoperative FEV1 decrease = 12/42 (29%)

Fig. 2. The number of subsegments of each lobe is used to calculate the predicted postoperative pulmonary function. (*From* Slinger PD, Johnston MR. Preoperative evaluation of the thoracic surgery patient. In: Kaplan JA, Slinger PD, editors. Thoracic anesthesia. 3rd edition. Philadelphia: Churchill Livingstone; 2003. p. 1–23; with permission.)

not all patients in this subgroup developed respiratory complications), and 10 of 10 patients with $ppoFEV_1$ less than 30% required postoperative mechanical ventilatory support. These key threshold $ppoFEV_1$ values, 30% and 40%, are useful to remember when managing these patients. The schema of Fig. 2 may be overly complicated, and it can be useful simply to consider the right upper and middle lobes combined as being approximately equivalent to each of the other three lobes with the right lung 10% larger than the left. These data of Nakahara et al are from work done in the 1980s, and more recent advances, particularly the use of epidural analgesia, have decreased the incidence of complications in the high-risk group [8]. $ppoFEV_1$ values of 40% and 30% remain useful, however, as reference points for the anesthesiologist. $ppoFEV_1$ is the most significant independent predictor of complications among a variety of historical, physical, and laboratory tests for these patients [5].

Lung parenchymal function

As important to the process of respiration as the mechanical delivery of air to the distal airways is the subsequent ability of the lung to exchange oxygen and carbon dioxide between the pulmonary vascular bed and the alveoli. Traditionally, arterial blood gas data (eg, $PaO_2 < 60$ mm Hg or $PaCO_2 > 45$ mm Hg) have been used as cutoff values for pulmonary resection. Cancer resections now have been done successfully [5] or combined with volume reduction in patients who do not meet these criteria [9], although they remain useful as warning indicators of increased risk. The most useful test of the gas exchange capacity of the lung is the diffusing capacity for carbon monoxide (DLCO). Although the DLCO initially was thought just to reflect diffusion, it actually correlates with the total functioning surface area of alveolar-capillary interface. This simple noninvasive test, which is included with spirometry and plethysmography by most pulmonary function laboratories, is a useful predictor of postthoracotomy complications. The corrected DLCO can be used to calculate a postresection (ppo) value using the same calculation as for the FEV_1. A ppoDLCO less than 40% predicted correlates with increased respiratory and cardiac complications and is to a large degree independent of the FEV_1 [10].

Cardiopulmonary interaction

The final and perhaps most important assessment of respiratory function is an assessment of the cardiopulmonary interaction. All patients should have some assessment of their cardiopulmonary reserves. The traditional, and still extremely useful, test in ambulatory patients is stair climbing [11]. Stair climbing is done at the patient's own pace but without stopping and usually is documented as a certain number of flights. There is no exact definition for a "flight," but 20 steps at 6 inches/step is a frequent value. The ability to climb 3 flights or more is closely associated with decreased mortality and somewhat associated with morbidity. Less than 2 flights is very high risk.

Formal laboratory exercise testing has become more standardized and more valid and is currently the gold standard for assessment of cardiopulmonary function. Among the many cardiac and respiratory factors that are tested, the maximal oxygen consumption (VO_2max) is the most useful predictor of postthoracotomy outcome. Walsh et al [12] showed that in a high-risk group of patients (mean preoperative $FEV_1 = 41\%$ predicted), there was no perioperative mortality if the preoperative VO_2max was greater than 15 mL/kg/min. This is a useful reference number for the anesthesiologist. Only 1 in 10 patients with a VO_2max greater than 20 mL/kg/min had a respiratory complication. Exercise testing can be modified in patients who are not capable of stair climbing by using bicycle or arm exercises. Complete laboratory exercise testing is labor intensive and expensive. Several alternatives to exercise testing have been shown to have potential as replacement tests for prethoracotomy assessment.

The 6-minute walk test shows an excellent correlation with VO_2max and requires little or no laboratory equipment [13]. A 6-minute walk test distance of less than 2000 ft correlates to a VO_2max less than 15 mL/kg/min and correlates with a decrease in oximetry (SpO_2) during exercise. Patients with a decrease of SpO_2 greater than 4% during exercise (stair climbing 2 or 3 flights or equivalent) [14,15] are at increased risk of morbidity and mortality. The 6-minute walk test and exercise oximetry may replace VO_2max for assessment of cardiorespiratory function in the future. Both of these tests are still evolving, and for the present exercise testing remains the gold standard. Postresection exercise tolerance can be estimated based on the amount of functioning lung tissue removed. An estimated ppoVO_2max less than 10 mL/kg/min may be one of the few remaining absolute contraindications to pulmonary resection. In a small series reported by Bollinger et al [16], mortality was 100% (3/3 patients) with a ppoVO_2max less than 10 mL/kg/min.

After pulmonary resection, there is a degree of right ventricular dysfunction that seems to be in proportion to the amount of functioning pulmonary vascular bed removed [17]. The exact etiology and duration of this dysfunction are unknown. Clinical evidence of this hemodynamic problem is minimal when the patient is at rest, but is dramatic when the patient exercises, leading to elevation of pulmonary vascular pressures, limitation of cardiac output, and absence of the normal decrease in pulmonary vascular resistance usually seen with exertion [18].

Ventilation/perfusion scintigraphy

Prediction of postresection pulmonary function can be refined further by assessment of the preoperative contribution of the lung or lobe to be resected using ventilation/perfusion (V/Q) lung scanning [19]. If the lung region to be resected is nonfunctioning or minimally functioning, the prediction of postoperative function can be modified accordingly. This assessment is particularly useful in pneumonectomy patients and should be considered for any patient who has a ppoFEV$_1$ less than 40%.

Split-lung function studies

A variety of methods have been described to try to simulate the postoperative respiratory situation by unilateral exclusion of a lung or lobe with an endobronchial tube/blocker or by pulmonary artery balloon occlusion of a lung or lobe artery [20]. These and other varieties of split-lung function testing also have been combined with exercise to try to assess the tolerance of the cardiorespiratory system to a proposed resection. Although these tests currently are carried out and used to guide therapy in certain individual centers, they have not shown sufficient predictive validity for widespread universal adoption in potential lung resection patients. One possible explanation for some predictive failures in these patients may be that lack of a pulmonary hypertensive response to unilateral occlusion may represent a sign of a failing right ventricle misinterpreted as a good sign of pulmonary vascular reserve. Lewis et al [21] showed that in a group of patients with chronic obstructive pulmonary disease (COPD) (ppo-FEV_1<40%) undergoing pneumonectomy, there were no significant changes in the pulmonary vascular pressures intraoperatively when the pulmonary artery was clamped, but the right ventricular ejection fraction and cardiac output decreased. Echocardiography may offer more useful information than vascular pressure monitoring in these patients [22].

It is conceivable that the future combination of unilateral occlusion studies with echocardiography may be a useful addition to this type of preresection investigation.

Flow-volume loops

Flow-volume loops can help identify the presence of a variable intrathoracic airway obstruction by evidence of a positional change in an abnormal plateau of the expiratory limb of the loop [23]. This change can occur as a result of compression of a main conducting airway by a tumor mass. Such a problem may warrant that general anesthesia be induced after an awake intubation or with maintenance of spontaneous ventilation [24]. In an adult patient capable of giving a complete history who does not describe supine exacerbation of cough or dyspnea, flow-volume loops are not required as a routine preoperative test.

Combination of tests

No single test of respiratory function has shown adequate validity as a sole preoperative assessment [5]. Before surgery, an estimate of respiratory function in three areas—mechanics, parenchymal function, and cardiopulmonary interaction—should be made for each patient. These three aspects of pulmonary function form the "three-legged stool" that is the foundation of prethoracotomy respiratory assessment (Fig. 3). These data can be used to plan intraoperative and postoperative management (Fig. 4) and to alter these plans when intraoperative surgical factors necessitate that a resection become more extensive than foreseen.

If a patient has a ppoFEV$_1$ greater than 40%, it should be possible for the patient to be extubated in the operating room at the conclusion of surgery, assuming the patient is alert, warm, and comfortable (*AWaC*). Patients with a ppoFEV$_1$ less than 40% usually constitute about one fourth of an average thoracic surgical population. If the ppoFEV$_1$ is greater than 30% and exercise tolerance and lung parenchymal function exceed the increased risk thresholds, extubation in the operating room should be possible depending on the status of associated diseases (see later). Patients in this subgroup who do not meet the minimal criteria for cardiopulmonary and parenchymal function should be considered for staged weaning from mechanical ventilation postoperatively so that the effect of the increased oxygen consumption of spontaneous ventilation can be assessed. Patients with a ppoFEV$_1$ of 20% to 30% and favorable predicted cardiorespiratory and parenchymal function can be considered for early extubation if thoracic epidural analgesia is used (see later).Otherwise, these patients should have postoperative staged weaning from mechanical ventilation. The validity of this approach has been confirmed by the National Emphysema Treatment Trial, which found an unacceptably high mortality for lung volume reduction surgery in patients with preoperative FEV$_1$ and DLCO values less than 20% predicted [25]. In the borderline group (ppoFEV$_1$ of 30–40%), the presence of several associated factors

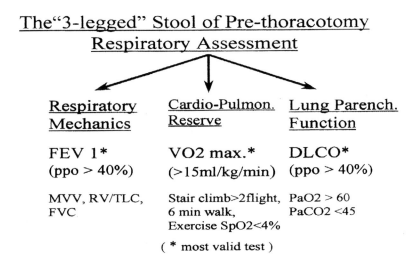

Fig. 3. The "3-legged" stool of prethoracotomy respiratory assessment. *Most valid test (see text).

Post-thoracotomy Anesthetic Management:

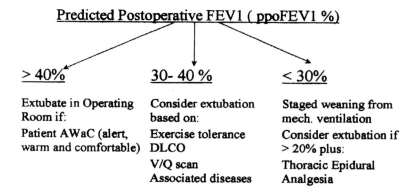

Fig. 4. Anesthetic management guided by preoperative assessment and the amount of functioning lung tissue removed during surgery.

and diseases that should be documented during the preoperative assessment enter into the considerations for postoperative management.

Intercurrent medical conditions

Age

There does not seem to be any maximal age that is a cutoff to pulmonary resection. If a patient is 80 years old and has a stage I lung cancer, their chances of survival to age 85 are better with the tumor resected than without. The operative mortality in a group of patients 80 to 92 years old was 3%, a respectable figure, in a series reported by Osaki et al [26]. The rate of respiratory complications (40%) was double that expected in a younger population, however, and the rate of cardiac complications (40%), particularly arrhythmias, was nearly triple that which should be seen in younger patients. Although the mortality from lobectomy in the elderly is acceptable, the mortality from pneumonectomy (22% in patients >70 years old) [27], particularly right pneumonectomy, is excessive. Presumably the reason is the increased strain on the right heart caused by resection of the proportionally larger vascular bed of the right lung.

Cardiac disease

Cardiac complications are the second most common cause of perioperative morbidity and mortality in thoracic surgical patients.

Ischemia

Because most pulmonary resection patients have a smoking history, they already have one risk factor for coronary artery disease [28]. In 2002, the second iteration of the American College of Cardiology/ American Heart Association guideline update for perioperative cardiovascular examination for non-cardiac surgery was published. The multidisciplinary authors of this document deem elective pulmonary resection surgery as an "intermediate risk" procedure in terms of perioperative cardiac ischemia [29]. "High-risk" procedures include major emergency surgery, aortic surgery, and peripheral vascular surgery [29]. The overall documented incidence of postthoracotomy ischemia is 5% and peaks on day 2 to 3 postoperatively [30]. This is approximately the risk that would be expected from a similar patient population having major abdominal, orthopedic, or other procedures. Beyond the standard history, physical examination, and ECG, routine screening for cardiac disease does not seem to be cost-effective for all prethoracotomy patients [31]. Noninvasive testing is indicated in patients with major (unstable ischemia, recent infarction, severe valvular disease, significant arrhythmia) or intermediate (stable angina, remote infarction, previous congestive failure, or diabetes) clinical predictors of myocardial risk and in elderly patients [28,32]. Therapeutic options to be considered in patients with significant coronary artery disease are optimization of medical therapy, coronary angioplasty, or coronary artery bypass, either before or at the time of lung resection [33]. Timing of lung resection surgery after a myocardial infarction is always a difficult decision. Based on the data of Rao et al [34] and generally confirmed by clinical practice, limiting the delay to 4 to 6 weeks in a medically stable and fully investigated and optimized patient seems acceptable after myocardial infarction.

When cardiology consultation is sought, a specific question, such as "is this patient's medical regimen optimized," should be asked. "Clearance" for surgery is not particularly helpful, unless it provides a description of the patient's pathology (including the results of diagnostic tests) and makes a statement about the intended cardiologic plan (eg, "the patient has severe three-vessel coronary artery disease not amenable to revascularization, and she is currently optimized medically").

Arrhythmia

Dysrhythmias, particularly atrial fibrillation, are a well-recognized complication of all pulmonary resection surgery [35]. Factors known to correlate with an increased incidence of arrhythmia are the amount of lung tissue resected, age, intraoperative blood loss, and intrapericardial dissection [36,37]. Prophylactic therapy with digoxin has not been shown to prevent these arrhythmias. Diltiazem has shown some promise, however [38].

Renal dysfunction

Renal dysfunction after pulmonary resection surgery is associated with a high incidence of mortality. Golledge and Goldstraw [39] reported a perioperative mortality of 19% (6/31) in patients who developed any significant elevation of serum creatinine in the postthoracotomy period compared with 0% (0/99) in patients who did not show any renal dysfunction. The factors, which were highly associated ($P < .001$) with an elevated risk of renal impairment, are as follows:

1. Previous history of renal impairment
2. Diuretic therapy
3. Pneumonectomy
4. Postoperative infection
5. Blood loss requiring transfusion

Other factors that were statistically significant but less strongly associated with renal impairment included preoperative hypertension, chemotherapy, ischemic heart disease, and postoperative oliguria (<33 mL/h). Nonsteroidal anti-inflammatory drugs (NSAIDs) were not associated with renal impairment in this series, but are a concern in any thoracotomy patient with an increased risk of renal dysfunction. The high mortality in pneumonectomy patients from either renal failure or postoperative pulmonary edema emphasizes the importance of fluid management in these patients [40] and the need for close and intensive perioperative monitoring, particularly in patients on diuretics or with a history of renal dysfunction.

Chronic obstructive pulmonary disease

The most common concurrent illness in thoracic surgical patients is COPD, which incorporates three disorders—emphysema, peripheral airways disease, and chronic bronchitis. Any individual patient may have one or all of these conditions, but the dominant clinical feature is impairment of expiratory airflow [41]. Assessment of the severity of COPD traditionally has been on the basis of the FEV_1 percent of predicted values. The American Thoracic Society currently categorizes stage I as greater than 50% predicted (this category previously included *mild* and *moderate* COPD), stage II as 35% to 50%, and stage III as less than 35%. Stage I patients should not have significant dyspnea, hypoxemia, or hypercarbia, and other causes should be considered if these are present. Advances in the understanding of COPD that are relevant to anesthetic management are discussed next.

Respiratory drive

Major changes have occurred in understanding of the control of breathing in COPD patients. Many stage II or III COPD patients have an elevated $PaCO_2$ at rest. It is not possible to differentiate these "CO_2 retainers" from nonretainers on the basis of history, physical examination, or spirometric pulmonary function testing. This carbon dioxide retention seems to be related more to an inability to maintain the increased work of respiration (W_{resp}) required to keep the $PaCO_2$ normal in patients with mechanically inefficient pulmonary function and not primarily due to an alteration of respiratory control mechanisms. It previously was thought that chronically hypoxemic/hypercapnic patients relied on a hypoxic stimulus for ventilatory drive and became insensitive to $PaCO_2$; this explained the clinical observation that COPD patients in incipient respiratory failure could be put into a hypercapnic coma by the administration of a high concentration of oxygen (FIO_2). Actually, only a minor fraction of the increase in $PaCO_2$ in such patients is due to a diminished respiratory drive because minute ventilation is basically unchanged [42]. The $PaCO_2$ increases because a high FIO_2 causes a relative decrease in alveolar ventilation and an increase in alveolar dead space by the redistribution of perfusion away from lung areas of relatively normal V/Q matching to areas of low V/Q ratio because regional hypoxic pulmonary vasoconstriction is decreased and due to the Haldane effect [43]. Supplemental oxygen must be administered to these patients postoperatively, however, to prevent the hypoxemia associated with the unavoidable decrease in functional residual capacity (FRC). The attendant increase in $PaCO_2$ should be anticipated and monitored. To identify these patients preoperatively, all stage II or III COPD patients need an arterial blood gas assessment.

Nocturnal hypoxemia

COPD patients desaturate more frequently and severely than normal patients during sleep [44]. This desaturation is due to the rapid and shallow breathing pattern that occurs in all patients during REM sleep. In COPD patients breathing air, this desaturation causes a significant increase in the respiratory dead space-to-tidal volume (VD/VT) ratio and a decrease in alveolar oxygen tension (PAO_2) and PaO_2. This condition is not the sleep apnea–hypoventilation syndrome. There is no increased incidence of sleep apnea–hypoventilation syndrome in COPD. In 8 of 10 COPD patients studied, the oxygen saturation decreased to less than 50% at some time during normal sleep, and this was associated with an increase in pulmonary artery pressure [45]. This tendency to desaturate, combined with the postoperative decrease in FRC and opioid analgesia, places these patients at high risk for severe hypoxemia postoperatively during sleep.

Right ventricular dysfunction

Right ventricular dysfunction occurs in 50% of COPD patients [46]. The dysfunctional right ventricle, even when hypertrophied, is poorly tolerant of sudden increases in afterload [47], such as the change from spontaneous to controlled ventilation [48]. Right ventricular function becomes crucial in maintaining cardiac output as the pulmonary artery pressure increases. The right ventricular ejection fraction does not increase with exercise in COPD patients as it does in normal patients. Chronic recurrent hypoxemia is the cause of the right ventricular dysfunction and the subsequent progression to cor pulmonale. Patients who have episodic hypoxemia despite normal lungs (eg, central alveolar hypoventilation, sleep apnea–hypoventilation syndrome) [49] develop the same secondary cardiac problems as COPD patients. Cor pulmonale occurs in 40% of adult COPD patients with an FEV_1 less than 1 L and in 70% with FEV_1 less than 0.6 [45]. It is now clear

that mortality in COPD patients is related primarily to chronic hypoxemia [50]. The only therapy that has been shown to improve long-term survival and decrease right heart strain in COPD is oxygen. COPD patients who have resting PaO_2 less than 55 mm Hg and patients who desaturate to less than 44 mm Hg with usual exercise should receive supplemental home oxygen [40]. The goal of supplemental oxygen is to maintain a PaO_2 of 60 to 65 mm Hg. Compared with patients with chronic bronchitis, emphysematous COPD patients tend to have a decreased cardiac output and mixed venous oxygen tension, while maintaining lower pulmonary artery pressures [46]. Pneumonectomy candidates with a $ppoFEV_1$ less than 40% should have transthoracic echocardiography to assess right heart function. Elevation of right heart pressures places these patients in a very high risk group [22].

Combined cancer and emphysema surgery

The combination of volume reduction surgery or bullectomy and lung cancer surgery has been reported in emphysematous patients who previously would not have met minimal criteria for pulmonary resection owing to the concurrent lung disease (see Fig. 1) [51,52]. Although the numbers of patients reported are small, the expected improvements in postoperative pulmonary function have been seen, and the outcomes are encouraging. This situation offers an extension of the standard indications for surgery in a small, well-selected group of patients.

Special preoperative considerations

Preoperative therapy of chronic obstructive pulmonary disease

There are four treatable complications of COPD that must be actively sought and therapy begun at the time of the initial prethoracotomy assessment: atelectasis, bronchospasm, chest infection, and pulmonary edema. Atelectasis impairs local lung lymphocyte and macrophage function, predisposing to infection [53]. Pulmonary edema can be difficult to diagnose by auscultation in the presence of COPD and may present abnormal radiologic distributions (eg, unilateral, upper lobes) [54]. Bronchial hyperreactivity may be a symptom of congestive failure [55]. All COPD patients should receive maximal bronchodilator therapy as guided by their symptoms. Only 20% to 25% of COPD patients respond to corticosteroids. In a patient who is poorly controlled on sympathomimetic and anticholinergic bronchodilators, a trial of corticosteroids may be beneficial [56]. It is not clear if corticosteroids are as beneficial in COPD as they are in asthma.

Physiotherapy

Patients with COPD have fewer postoperative pulmonary complications when a perioperative program of intensive chest physiotherapy is initiated preoperatively [57]. Physiotherapy is one of the few evidence-based techniques that decrease respiratory complications in high-risk patients. It is uncertain if this benefit applies to other pulmonary resection patients. Among the different modalities available (eg, cough and deep breathing, incentive spirometry, positive end-expiratory pressure [PEEP], continuous positive airway pressure [CPAP]), there is no clearly proven superior method [58]. The important variable is the quantity of time spent with the patient and devoted to chest physiotherapy. Family members or nonphysiotherapy hospital staff can be trained easily to perform effective preoperative chest physiotherapy, and this should be arranged at the time of the initial preoperative assessment. Even in the most severe COPD patient, it is possible to improve exercise tolerance with a physiotherapy program [59]. Little improvement is seen before 1 month. Among COPD patients, those with excessive sputum benefit the most from chest physiotherapy [60].

A comprehensive program of pulmonary rehabilitation involving physiotherapy, exercise, nutrition, and education has been shown consistently to improve functional capacity for patients with severe COPD [61]. These programs usually are of several months' duration and generally are not an option in resections for malignancy. For nonmalignant resections in patients with severe COPD, however, rehabilitation should be considered. The benefits of short-duration rehabilitation programs before malignancy resection have not been assessed fully.

Smoking cessation

Pulmonary complications are decreased in thoracic surgical patients who are not smoking versus patients who continue to smoke up until the time of surgery [62]. Patients having cardiac surgery showed no decrease in the incidence of respiratory complications, however, unless smoking was discontinued for more than 8 weeks before surgery [63]. Carboxyhemoglobin concentrations decrease if smoking is stopped for more than 12 hours, which maximize tissue oxygen delivery and use [64]. It is extremely important for patients to avoid smoking postoperatively. Smoking leads to a prolonged period of tissue hypoxemia, and wound tissue oxygen tension

correlates with wound healing and resistance to infection [65].

Lung cancer

At the time of initial assessment, cancer patients should be assessed for the "4 M's" associated with malignancy—mass effects [66], metabolic abnormalities, metastases [67], and medications (Box 1). The prior use of medications that can exacerbate oxygen-induced pulmonary toxicity, such as bleomycin, should be considered [68–70]. The authors have seen several lung cancer patients who received preoperative chemotherapy with cisplatin, then developed an elevation of serum creatinine when they received NSAIDs postoperatively. For this reason, the authors do not administer NSAIDs routinely to patients who have been treated recently with cisplatin.

Postoperative analgesia

The strategy for postoperative analgesia should be developed and discussed with the patient during the initial preoperative assessment. Many techniques have been shown to be superior to the use of on-demand parenteral (intramuscular or intravenous) opioids alone in terms of pain control [71]. These include the addition of neuraxial blockade, intercostal/paravertebral blocks, interpleural local anesthetics, and NSAIDs to narcotic-based analgesia. Only

---

Box 1. Anesthetic considerations in lung cancer patients (the "4 M's")

1. *Mass effects:* obstructive pneumonia, lung abscess, superior vena cava syndrome, tracheobronchial distortion, Pancoast's syndrome, recurrent laryngeal nerve or phrenic nerve paresis, chest wall or mediastinal extension
2. *Metabolic effects:* Lambert-Eaton syndrome, hypercalcemia, hyponatremia, Cushing's syndrome
3. *Metastases:* particularly to brain, bone, liver, and adrenal
4. *Medications:* chemotherapy agents, pulmonary toxicity (bleomycin, mitomycin), cardiac toxicity (doxorubicin), renal toxicity (cisplatin)

epidural techniques have been shown consistently, however, to have the capability to decrease postthoracotomy respiratory complications [72,73]. It is becoming more evident that thoracic epidural analgesia is superior to lumbar epidural analgesia; this seems to be due to the synergy that local anesthetics have with opioids in producing neuraxial analgesia. Studies suggest that epidural local anesthetics increase segmental bioavailability of opioids in the cerebrospinal fluid [74] and that they increase the binding of opioids by spinal cord receptors [75]. Although lumbar epidural opioids can produce similar levels of postthoracotomy pain control at rest, only the segmental effects of thoracic epidural local anesthetic and opioid combinations reliably can produce increased analgesia with movement and increased respiratory function after a chest incision [76,77]. In patients with coronary artery disease, thoracic epidural local anesthetics seem to reduce myocardial oxygen demand and supply in proportion [78], in contrast to the effects of lumbar epidural local anesthetics, which can cause a decrease in myocardial perfusion and oxygen supply as diastolic pressure decreases, but heart rate and oxygen demand are unchanged. This has been shown to correlate with echocardiographic evidence of ischemia [79].

It is at the time of initial preanesthetic assessment that the risks and benefits of the various forms of postthoracotomy analgesia should be explained to the patient. Potential contraindications to specific methods of analgesia should be determined, such as coagulation problems, sepsis, or neurologic disorders. When it is not possible to place a thoracic epidural because of problems with patient consent or other contraindications, the authors' current second choice for analgesia is a paravertebral infusion of local anesthetic via a catheter placed intraoperatively in the open hemithorax by the surgeon; this is combined with intravenous patient-controlled opioid analgesia and NSAIDs [80].

If the patient is to receive prophylactic anticoagulants, and it is elected to use epidural analgesia, appropriate timing of anticoagulant administration and neuraxial catheter placement need to be arranged. Guidelines from the American Society of Regional Anesthesia suggest an interval of 2 to 4 hours before or 1 hour after catheter placement for prophylactic intravenous heparin administration [81]. There is no specific contraindication to neuraxial anesthesia with the use of subcutaneous unfractionated heparin. Low-molecular-weight heparin precautions are less clear; an interval of 12 to 24 hours before and 24 hours after catheter placement is recommended.

Premedication

Premedication should be discussed and ordered at the time of the initial preoperative visit. The most important aspect of preoperative medication is to avoid inadvertent withdrawal of the drugs that are taken for concurrent medical conditions (eg, bronchodilators, antihypertensives, β-blockers). For some types of thoracic surgery, such as esophageal reflux surgery, oral antacid and H_2-blockers are routinely ordered preoperatively. Although there is some theoretical concern in giving patients who may be prone to bronchospasm an H_2-blocker without an H_1-blocker, this has not been a clinical problem, and H_2-blockers are used frequently in patients who have asthmatic symptoms triggered by chronic reflux. The authors do not routinely order preoperative sedation or analgesia for pulmonary resection patients. Mild sedation, such as an intravenous short-acting benzodiazepine, is often given immediately before placement of invasive monitoring lines and catheters. In patients with copious secretions, an antisialagogue (eg, glycopyrrolate) is useful to facilitate fiberoptic bronchoscopy for positioning of a double-lumen tube or bronchial blocker. To avoid an intramuscular injection, this can be given orally or intravenously immediately after placement of the intravenous catheter.

Final preoperative assessment

The final preoperative anesthetic assessment for most thoracic surgical patients is performed immedi-

---

Box 2. Initial preanesthetic assessment for thoracic surgery

1. *All patients:* assess exercise tolerance, estimate ppoFEV$_{1\%}$, discuss postoperative analgesia, discontinue smoking
2. *Patients with ppoFEV$_1$ < 40%:* DLCO, V/Q scan, Vo$_2$max
3. *Cancer patients:* consider the ''4 M's''—mass effects, metabolic effects, metastases, medications
4. *COPD patients:* arterial blood gas, physiotherapy, bronchodilators
5. *Increased renal risk:* measure creatinine and blood urea nitrogen

> **Box 3. Final preanesthetic assessment for thoracic surgery**
>
> 1. Review initial assessment and test results
> 2. Assess difficulty of lung isolation: examine chest x-ray and CT scan
> 3. Assess risk of hypoxemia during one-lung ventilation

ately before admission of the patient to the operating room. At this time, it is important to review the data from the initial prethoracotomy assessment (Box 2) and the results of tests ordered at that time. In addition, two other specific areas affecting thoracic anesthesia need to be assessed: the potential for difficult lung isolation and the risk of desaturation during one-lung ventilation (OLV) (Box 3).

Difficult lung isolation

Anesthesiologists are familiar with the clinical assessment of the upper airway for ease of endotracheal intubation. In a similar fashion, each thoracic surgical patient must be assessed for the ease of endobronchial intubation. At the time of the preoperative visit, historical factors or physical findings may lead to suspicion of difficult endobronchial intubation (previous radiotherapy, infection, prior pulmonary or airway surgery). In addition, there may be a written bronchoscopy report with detailed description of anatomic features. Fiberoptic bronchoscopy is not totally reliable, however, for estimating potential problems with endobronchial tube positioning [82]. The most useful predictor of difficult endobronchial intubation is the plain chest x-ray (Fig. 5) [83].

The anesthesiologist should view the chest films before induction of anesthesia because neither the radiologist's nor the surgeon's report of the x-ray is made with the specific consideration of lung isolation in mind. A large portion of thoracic surgical patients also have a chest CT scan done preoperatively. As anesthesiologists have learned to assess x-rays for potential lung-isolation difficulties, it is also worthwhile to learn to examine the CT scan. Distal airway problems not detectable on the plain chest film sometimes can be visualized on the CT scan: An elongation of the distal trachea in its anterior-posterior dimension, the so-called saber-sheath trachea, can cause obstruction of the tracheal lumen of a left-sided, double-lumen tube during ventilation of the dependent lung for a left thoracotomy [84]. Similarly, extrinsic compression or intraluminal obstruction of a main stem bronchus, which can interfere with endobronchial tube placement, may be evident only on the CT scan. The major factors in successful lower airway management are anticipation and preparation based on the preoperative assessment.

Prediction of desaturation during one-lung ventilation

In most cases, it is possible to determine the patients who are most at risk of desaturation during

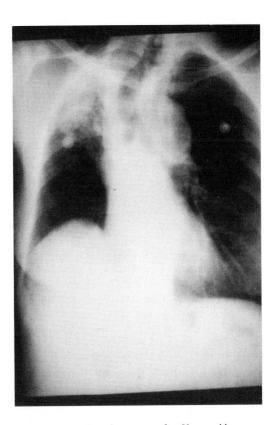

Fig. 5. Preoperative chest x-ray of a 50-year-old woman with a history of previous tuberculosis, right upper lobectomy, and recent hemoptysis presenting for right thoracotomy and possible completion pneumonectomy. The potential problems positioning a left-sided, double-lumen tube in this patient are easily appreciated by viewing the x-ray but are not mentioned in the radiologist's report. (*From* Slinger PD, Johnston MR. Preoperative evaluation of the thoracic surgery patient. In: Kaplan JA, Slinger PD, editors. Thoracic anesthesia. 3rd edition. Philadelphia: Churchill Livingstone; 2003. p. 1–23; with permission.)

OLV for thoracic surgery. The factors that correlate with desaturation during OLV are as follows:

1. High percentage of ventilation or perfusion to the operative lung on preoperative V/Q scan
2. Poor PaO_2 during two-lung ventilation, particularly in the lateral position intraoperatively
3. Right-sided surgery
4. *Good* preoperative spirometry (FEV_1 or FVC)

Identification of patients most likely to desaturate allows the anesthesiologist and surgeon to make a more informed decision about the use of OLV intraoperatively. In patients at high risk of desaturation, prophylactic measures can be used during OLV to decrease this risk. The most useful prophylactic measure is the use of CPAP, 2 to 5 cm H_2O of oxygen, to the nonventilated lung [85]. Because this measure often tends to make the surgical exposure more difficult, particularly during video-assisted thoracoscopic surgery, it is worthwhile to identify patients who require CPAP early so that it can be discussed with the surgeon and instituted at the start of OLV.

The most important predictor of PaO_2 during OLV is the PaO_2 during two-lung ventilation. Although the preoperative PaO_2 correlates with the intraoperative OLV PaO_2, the strongest correlation is with the intraoperative PaO_2 during two-lung ventilation in the lateral position before OLV [86,87]. The proportion of perfusion or ventilation to the nonoperated lung on preoperative V/Q scans also correlates with the PaO_2 during OLV [88]. If the operative lung has little perfusion preoperatively because of unilateral disease, the patient is unlikely to desaturate during OLV.

The side of the thoracotomy has an effect on PaO_2 during OLV. Because the left lung is 10% smaller than the right, there is less shunt when the left lung is collapsed. In a series of patients, the mean PaO_2 during left thoracotomy was approximately 70 mm Hg higher than during right thoracotomy [89].

Finally, the degree of obstructive lung disease correlates in an inverse fashion with PaO_2 during OLV. Other factors being equal, patients with more severe airflow limitation on preoperative spirometry tend to have a better PaO_2 during OLV than patients with normal spirometry [90]. The cause of this seemingly paradoxical finding seems to be related to the development of auto-PEEP during OLV in the obstructed patients [91]. Patients with normal healthy lungs with good elastic recoil and patients with increased elastic recoil, such as patients with restrictive lung diseases, tend to benefit from applied

PEEP during OLV, whereas patients with COPD do not [92].

Summary

Advances in anesthesia and surgery have made it so that almost any patient with a resectable lung malignancy is now an operative candidate given a full understanding of the risks and after appropriate investigation. This situation necessitates a change in the paradigm that anesthesiologists use for preoperative assessment. Understanding and stratifying the perioperative risks allows the anesthesiologist to develop a systematic focused approach to these patients at the time of the initial contact and immediately before induction, which can be used to guide anesthetic management.

References

[1] Slinger PD, Johnston MR. Preoperative evaluation of the thoracic surgery patient. In: Kaplan JA, Slinger PD, editors. Thoracic anesthesia. 3rd edition. Philadelphia: Churchill Livingstone; 2003. p. 1–23.

[2] Johnston MR. Curable lung cancer. Postgrad Med 1997;101:155–65.

[3] Brusasco V, Ratto GB, Crimi P, Sacco A, Motta G. Lung function after upper sleeve lobectomy for bronchogenic carcinoma. Scand J Thor Cardiovasc Surg 1988;22:73–8.

[4] Nakahara K, Ohno K, Hashimoto J, et al. Prediction of postoperative respiratory failure in patients undergoing lung resection for cancer. Ann Thorac Surg 1988;46:549–52.

[5] Reilly JJ. Evidence-based preoperative evaluation of candidates for thoracotomy. Chest 1999;116:474s–6s.

[6] Pierce RD, Copland JM, Sharpek K, Barter CE. Preoperative risk evaluation for lung cancer resection: predicted postoperative product as a predictor of surgical mortality. Am J Respir Crit Care Med 1994; 150:947–55.

[7] Epstein SK, Failing LJ, Daly BDT, Celli BR. Predicting complications after pulmonary resection. Chest 1993;104:694–700.

[8] Cerfolio RJ, Allen MS, Trastak VF, Deschamps C, Scanbon PD, Pairolero PC. Lung resection in patients with compromised pulmonary function. Ann Thorac Surg 1996;62:348–51.

[9] McKenna RJ, Fischel RJ, Brenner M, Gelb AF. Combined operations for lung volume reduction surgery and lung cancer. Chest 1996;110:885–8.

[10] Wang J, Olak J, Ferguson MK. Diffusing capacity predicts mortality but not long-term survival after resection for lung cancer. J Thorac Cardiovasc Surg 1999;17:581–5.

[11] Olsen GN, Bolton JWR, Weiman DS, Horning CA. Stair climbing as an exercise test to predict post-operative complications of lung resection. Chest 1991; 99:587–90.

[12] Walsh GL, Morice RC, Putnam JB, et al. Resection of lung cancer is justified in high risk patients selected by oxygen consumption. Ann Thorac Surg 1994; 58:704–10.

[13] Cahalin L, Pappagianopoulos P, Prevost S, Wain J, Ginns L. The relationship of the 6-min walk test to maximal oxygen consumption in transplant candidates with end-stage lung disease. Chest 1995;108:452–7.

[14] Rao V, Todd TRJ, Kuus A, Beth KJ, Pearson FG. Exercise oximetry versus spirometry in the assessment of risk prior to lung resection. Ann Thorac Surg 1995; 60:603–9.

[15] Ninan M, Sommers KE, Landranau RJ, et al. Standardized exercise oximetry predicts post pneumonectomy outcome. Ann Thorac Surg 1997;64:328–33.

[16] Bollinger CT, Wyser C, Roser H, et al. Lung scanning and exercise testing for the prediction of postoperative performance in lung resection candidates at increased risk for complications. Chest 1995;108:341–8.

[17] Reed CR, Dorman BH, Spinale FG. Mechanisms of right ventricular dysfunction after pulmonary resection. Ann Thorac Surg 1996;62:225–32.

[18] Van Miegham W, Demedts M. Cardiopulmonary function after lobectomy or pneumonectomy for pulmonary neoplasm. Respir Med 1989;83:199–206.

[19] Vesselle H. Functional imaging before pulmonary resection. Semin Thorac Cardiovasc Surg 2001;13: 126–35.

[20] Tisi GM. Preoperative evaluation of pulmonary function. Am Rev Respir Dis 1979;119:293–310.

[21] Lewis Jr JW, Bastanfar M, Gabriel F, Mascha E. Right heart function and prediction of respiratory morbidity in patients undergoing pneumonectomy with moderately severe cardiopulmonary dysfunction. J Thorac Cardiovasc Surg 1994;108:169–75.

[22] Amar D, Burt M, Roistacher N, Reinsel RA, Ginsberg RJ, Wilson R. Value of perioperative echocardiography in patients undergoing major lung resection. Ann Thorac Surg 1996;61:516–20.

[23] Neuman GG, Wiengarten AE, Abramowitz RM, et al. The anesthetic management of the patient with an anterior mediastinal mass. Anesthesiology 1984;60: 144–7.

[24] Pullerits J, Holzman R. Anaesthesia for patients with mediastinal masses. Can J Anaesth 1989;36:681–8.

[25] National Emphysema Treatment Trial Research Group. A randomized trial comparing lung-volume-reduction surgery with medical therapy for severe emphysema. N Engl J Med 2003;348:2059–73.

[26] Osaki T, Shirakusa T, Kodate M, et al. Surgical treatment of lung cancer in the octogenarian. Ann Thorac Surg 1994;57:188–93.

[27] Mizushima Y, Noto H, Sugiyama S, et al. Survival and prognosis after pneumonectomy in the elderly. Ann Thorac Surg 1997;64:193–8.

[28] Barry J, Mead K, Nadel EC, et al. Effect of smoking on the activity of ischemic heart disease. JAMA 1989;261:398–402.

[29] Eagle KA, Berger PB, Calkins H. ACC/AHA guideline update for perioperative cardiovascular examination for noncardiac surgery—executive summary. Anesth Analg 2002;94:1378–9.

[30] Von Knorring J, Leptantalo M, Lindgren L. Cardiac arrhythmias and myocardial ischemia after thoracotomy for lung cancer. Ann Thorac Surg 1992;53: 642–7.

[31] Ghent WS, Olsen GN, Hornung CA, et al. Routinely performed multigated blood pool imaging (MUGA) as a predictor of postoperative complication of lung resection. Chest 1994;105:1454–7.

[32] Miller JI. Thallium imaging in preoperative evaluation of the pulmonary resection candidate. Ann Thorac Surg 1992;54:249–52.

[33] Rao V, Todd TRS, Weisel RD, et al. Results of combined pulmonary resection and cardiac operation. Ann Thorac Surg 1996;62:342–7.

[34] Rao TKK, Jacob KH, El-Etr AA. Reinfarction following anesthesia in patients with myocardial infarction. Anesthesiology 1983;59:499–505.

[35] Ritchie AJ, Danton M, Gibbons JRP. Prophylactic digitalisation in pulmonary surgery. Thorax 1992;47: 41–3.

[36] Didolkar MS, Moore RH, Taiku J. Evaluation of the risk in pulmonary resection for bronchogenic carcinoma. Am J Surg 1974;127:700–5.

[37] Van Nostrand D, Ejelsberg MO, Humphrey EW. Preresectional evaluation of risk from pneumonectomy. Surg Gynecol Obstet 1968;127:306–12.

[38] Amar D, Roistacher N, Burt ME, et al. Effects of diltiazem versus digoxin on dysrhythmias and cardiac function after pneumonectomy. Ann Thorac Surg 1997;63:1374–81.

[39] Golledge J, Goldstraw P. Renal impairment after thoracotomy: incidence, risk factors and significance. Ann Thorac Surg 1994;58:524–8.

[40] Slinger PD. Post-pneumonectomy pulmonary edema: is anesthesia to blame? Curr Opin Anesthesiol 1999; 12:49–54.

[41] American Thoracic Society. Standards for the diagnosis and care of patients with chronic obstructive pulmonary disease. Am J Respir Critic Care Med 1995; 152:s78–121.

[42] Parot S, Saunier C, Gauthier H, Milic-Emile J, Sadoul P. Breathing pattern and hypercapnia in patients with obstructive pulmonary disease. Am Rev Respir Dis 1980;121:985–91.

[43] Hanson III CW, Marshall BE, Frasch HF, Marshall C. Causes of hypercarbia in patients with chronic obstructive pulmonary disease. Crit Care Med 1996;24: 23–8.

[44] Douglas NJ, Flenley DC. Breathing during sleep in patients with obstructive lung disease. Am Rev Respir Dis 1990;141:1055–70.

[45] Douglas NJ, Calverley PMA, Leggett RJE, Brash HM,

Flenley DC, Brezinova V. Transient hypoxaemia during sleep in chronic bronchitics and emphysema. Lancet 1979;1:1–4.

[46] Klinger JR, Hill NS. Right ventricular dysfunction in chronic obstructive pulmonary disease. Chest 1991;99: 715–23.

[47] Schulman DS, Mathony RA. The right ventricle in pulmonary disease. Cardiol Clin 1992;10:111–35.

[48] Myles PE, Madder H, Morgan EB. Intraoperative cardiac arrest after unrecognized dynamic hyperinflation. Br J Anaesth 1995;74:340–1.

[49] MacNee W. Pathophysiology of cor pulmonale in chronic obstructive pulmonary disease. Am J Respir Crit Care Med 1994;150:833–52.

[50] Cote TR, Stroup DF, Dwyer DM, Huron JM, Peterson DE. Chronic obstructive pulmonary disease mortality. Chest 1993;103:1194–7.

[51] DeMeester SR, Patterson GA, Sundareson RS, Cooper JD. Lobectomy combined with volume reduction for patients with lung cancer and advanced emphysema. J Thorac Cardiovasc Surg 1998;115:681–5.

[52] McKenna Jr RJ, Fischel RJ, Brennar M, Gelb AF. Combined operations for lung volume reduction and lung cancer. Chest 1996;110:885–8.

[53] Nguyen DM, Mulder DS, Shennib H. Altered cellular immune function in atelectatic lung. Ann Thorac Surg 1991;51:76–80.

[54] Huglitz UF, Shapiro JH. Atypical pulmonary patterns of congestive failure in chronic lung disease. Radiology 1969;93:995–1006.

[55] Susaki F, Ishizaki T, Mifune J, Fugimura M, Nishioku S, Miyabo S. Bronchial hyperresponsiveness in patients with chronic congestive heart failure. Chest 1990;97:534–8.

[56] Nisar M, Eoris JE, Pearson MG, Calverly PMA. Acute broncho-dilator trials in chronic obstructive pulmonary disease. Am Rev Respir Dis 1992;146:555–9.

[57] Warner DO. Preventing postoperative pulmonary complications. Anesthesiology 2000;92:1467–71.

[58] Stock MC, Downs JB, Gauer PK, Alster JM, Imreg PB. Prevention of postoperative pulmonary complications with CPAP, incentive spirometry and conservative therapy. Chest 1985;87:151–7.

[59] Niederman MS, Clemente P, Fein AM, et al. Benefits of a multidisciplinary pulmonary rehabilitation program. Chest 1991;99:798–804.

[60] Selsby D, Jones JG. Some physiological and clinical aspects of chest physiotherapy. Br J Anaesth 1990;64: 621–31.

[61] Kesten S. Pulmonary rehabilitation and surgery for end-stage lung disease. Clin Chest Med 1997;18: 174–81.

[62] Dales RE, Dionne G, Leech JA, et al. Preoperative prediction of pulmonary complications following thoracic surgery. Chest 1993;104:155–9.

[63] Warner MA, Diverti MB, Tinker JH. Preoperative cessation of smoking and pulmonary complications in coronary artery bypass surgery. Anesthesiology 1984; 60:383–90.

[64] Akrawi W, Benumof JL. A pathophysiological basis for informed preoperative smoking cessation counselling. J Cardiothorac Vasc Anesth 1997;11:629–40.

[65] Jonsson K, Hunt TK, Mathes SJ. Oxygen as an isolated variable influences resistance to infection. Ann Surg 1988;208:783–7.

[66] Gilron I, Scott WAC, Slinger P, Wilson JAS. Contralateral lung soiling following laser resection of a bronchial tumor. J Cardiothorac Vasc Anesth 1994;8: 567–9.

[67] Mueurs MF. Preoperative screening for metastases in lung cancer patients. Thorax 1994;49:1–3.

[68] Ingrassia III TS, Ryu JH, Trasek VF, Rosenow III EC. Oxygen-exacerbated bleomycin pulmonary toxicity. Mayo Clin Proc 1991;66:173–8.

[69] Thompson CC, Bailey MK, Conroy JM, Bromley HR. Postoperative pulmonary toxicity associated with mitomycin-C therapy. South Med J 1992;85:1257–9.

[70] Van Miegham W, Collen L, Malysse I, et al. Amiodarone and the development of ARDS after lung surgery. Chest 1994;105:1642.

[71] Kavanagh BP, Katz J, Sandler AN. Pain control after thoracic surgery: a review of current techniques. Anesthesiology 1994;81:737–59.

[72] Licker M, de Perrot M, Hohn L, et al. Perioperative mortality and major cardio-pulmonary complications after lung surgery for non-small call carcinoma. Eur J Cardiothorac Surg 1999;15:314–9.

[73] Ballantyne JC, Carr DB, deFerranti S, et al. The comparative effects of postoperative analgesic therapies on pulmonary outcome: cumulative meta-analysis of randomized, controlled trials. Anesth Analg 1998; 86:598–612.

[74] Hansdottir V, Woestenborghs R, Nordberg G. The pharmacokinestics of continous epidural sufentanil and bupivacaine infusion after thoracotomy. Anesth Analg 1996;83:401–6.

[75] Tejwani GA, Rattan AK, Mcdonald JS. Role of spinal opioid receptors in the antinociceptive interactions between intrathecal morphine and bupivacaine. Anesth Analg 1992;74:726–34.

[76] Hansdottir V, Bake B, Nordberg G. The analgesic efficiency and adverse effects of continuous epidural sufentanil and bupivacaine infusion after thoracotomy. Anesth Analg 1996;83:394–400.

[77] Mourisse J, Hasenbos MAWM, Gielen MJM, Moll JE, Cromheedse GJE. Epidural bupivacaine, sufentanil or the combination for post thoracotomy pain. Acta Anaesthesiol Scand 1992;36:70–4.

[78] Saada M, Catoire P, Bonnet F, et al. Effect of thoracic epidural anesthesia combined with general anesthesia on segmental wall motion assessed by trans-esophageal echocardiography. Anesth Analg 1992;75: 329–35.

[79] Saada M, Duval A-M, Bonnet F, et al. Abnormalities in myocardial wall motion during lumbar epidural anesthesia. Anesth Analg 1989;71:26–33.

[80] Karmakar MK. Thoracic paravertebral block. Anesthesiology 2001;95:771–80.

[81] Horlocker TT, Wedel DJ, Benzon H, et al. Regional anesthesia in the anticoagulated patient: defining the risks (the second ASRA Consensus Conference on Neuraxial Anesthesia and Anticoagulation). Reg Anesth 2003;28:172–97.

[82] Alliaume B, Coddens J, Deloof T. Reliability of auscultation in positioning of double-lumen endobronchial tubes. Can J Anaesth 1992;39:687–91.

[83] Saito S, Dohi S, Tajima K. Failure of double-lumen endobronchial tube placement: congenital tracheal stenosis in an adult. Anesthesiology 1987;66:83–5.

[84] Bayes J, Slater EM, Hadberg PS, Lawson D. Obstruction of a double-lumen tube by a saber-sheath trachea. Anesth Analg 1994;79:186–9.

[85] Slinger P, Triolet W, Wilson J. Improving arterial oxygenation during one-lung ventilation. Anesthesiology 1988;68:291–5.

[86] Slinger P, Suissa S, Triolet W. Predicting arterial oxygenation during one-lung anaesthesia. Can J Anaesth 1992;39:1030–5.

[87] Flacke JW, Thompson DS, Read RC. Influence of tidal volume and pulmonary artery occlusion on arterial oxygenation during endobronchial anesthesia. South Med J 1976;69:619–26.

[88] Hurford WE, Kokar AC, Strauss HW. The use of ventilation/perfusion lung scans to predict oxygenation during one-lung anesthesia. Anesthesiology 1987; 64:841–4.

[89] Lewis JW, Serwin JP, Gabriel FS, Bastaufar M, Jacobsen G. The utility of a double-lumen tube for one-lung ventilation in a variety of non-cardiac thoracic surgical procedures. J Cardiothorac Vasc Anesth 1992;6:705–10.

[90] Katz JA, Lavern RG, Fairley HB, et al. Pulmonary oxygen exchange during endobronchial anesthesia, effect of tidal volume and PEEP. Anesthesiology 1982; 56:164–70.

[91] Myles PS. Auto-PEEP may improve oxygenation during one-lung ventilation. Anesth Analg 1996;83: 1131–2.

[92] Slinger PD, Kruger M, McRae K, Winton T. The relation of the static compliance curve and positive end-expiratory pressure to oxygenation during one-lung ventilation. Anesthesiology 2001;95:1096–102.

ELSEVIER
SAUNDERS

Thorac Surg Clin 15 (2005) 27 – 38

THORACIC
SURGERY
CLINICS

New Anesthesia Techniques

Avery Tung, MD

Departments of Anesthesia and Critical Care and Critical Care Services, Burn Unit, University of Chicago,
5841 S. Maryland Avenue, MC4028, Chicago, IL 60637, USA

To a nonanesthesiologist, general anesthesia today may seem similar to anesthesia administered in the 1980s or 1990s. Refinements in techniques, equipment, and mechanistic understanding have improved significantly, however, the ability of anesthesiologists to induce and manage the states of general anesthesia and conscious sedation (Fig. 1). A greater understanding of the mechanisms underlying the effects of inhaled and intravenous anesthetics has allowed the development of novel anesthetic agents targeted toward specific aspects of brain function. In addition, the development of new monitors has allowed anesthesiologists to regulate more precisely the anesthetic state, allowing control of hemodynamics to be separated from management of consciousness. New anesthetics and anesthetic adjuncts have provided anesthesiologists with the flexibility to care for an increasingly wide spectrum of patients. Finally, refinements in anesthesia machine technologies and the intraoperative availability of two specialty gases have permitted many patients formerly considered "too sick for the operating room" to undergo difficult and invasive intraoperative procedures. This article discusses these relatively subtle "under the hood" improvements in anesthetic care, shows how they represent advances over previous approaches to anesthesia, and identifies how such advances can lead to improved care for patients undergoing thoracic surgery.

Advances in anesthetic care

Improved understanding of general anesthesia mechanisms

Background

Because different anesthetics can have differing clinical effects, general anesthesia traditionally has been defined not as a unitary state, but rather as an aggregate of four discrete clinical end points. These include hypnosis (loss of awareness of environment), amnesia (loss of memory), analgesia (blunting of pain sensation), and immobility in the face of surgical stimulation. Clinically, each of these end points seems to be dose dependent, with different thresholds for each end point and each agent. Anesthesiologists frequently use different agents for each end point. An anesthetic dose sufficient to cause hypnosis may not guarantee immobility, and patients rendered immobile by muscle relaxants may not be amnestic if insufficient anesthetic is given. Modern pharmacologic and genetic tools have combined to increase dramatically current understanding of how the hypnotic and amnestic components of the anesthetized state are generated and maintained.

New advances

Historically, two broad theories of anesthetic action have competed for acceptance. The first was the Meyer-Overton hypothesis, developed by the German biologists Overton and Meyer in 1939 [1]. This hypothesis was based on the strikingly linear relationship between an inhaled anesthetic's lipid solubility and its clinical potency [2] and suggested that anesthetics act by nonspecifically altering the

E-mail address: atung@airway.uchicago.edu

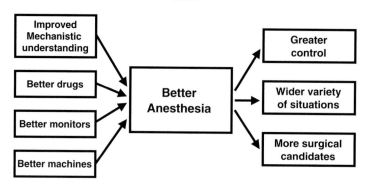

Fig. 1. Consequences of improved anesthetic care.

function of membrane bound proteins. Inconsistencies between theoretical predictions of the model and experimental observations have indicated, however, that this nonspecific mechanism is unlikely to account for the diverse effects of all inhaled anesthetics. The positive and negative enantiomers of isoflurane have similar lipid solubilities, but the positive enantiomer is 50% more potent [3]. In addition, some lipid-soluble compounds structurally similar to known inhaled anesthetics are convulsants instead of anesthetics [4]. Attempts to engineer new anesthetics have shown a cutoff effect, whereby elongating the carbon chains of known anesthetics beyond a certain limit results in a loss of anesthetic effect [5]. Finally, radiolabeling studies have indicated that anesthetics bind to different, specific areas of the cell membrane [6]. Taken together, these findings imply that structural specificity is required for anesthetic activity and suggest that anesthetics act via receptor-based mechanisms, with specific interactions at cellular receptors. More recent work not only has identified measurable effects of anesthetics on a large list of neuroregulators, including γ-aminobutyric acid (GABA)-A, glutamate, glycine, and N-methyl-D-asparate, but also genetically altered animals that differ in their response to inhaled anesthetics [7].

This modern theory of general anesthetics has changed the way anesthetics are viewed clinically. Historically the primary measure of potency for an inhaled anesthetic has been the minimal alveolar concentration (MAC) necessary to prevent movement in response to a painful stimulus, such as skin incision [8]. The realization that anesthesia is at least partly a receptor-based phenomenon suggested, however, that other end points of general anesthesia (amnesia, loss of awareness, cardiovascular stability) may be mediated by different mechanisms. The discovery in 1996 that analogs of inhaled anesthetics

may not prevent movement (and are technically not anesthetics), but still alter amnesia and impair learning confirmed this possibility [9]. Termed *non-immobilizers,* these compounds not only defy the Meyer-Overton correlation, but also show that immobility is an end point of anesthetic action distinctly different from loss of consciousness.

Different anesthetic end points may result not only from different receptors, but also different locations. Studies showing that MAC was not altered by destruction of the parietal cortex [10], high spinal transaction [11], or complete decerebration [12] implied that immobility was mediated in the spinal cord and not the brain. When delivered only to the brain (and not the spinal cord) of goats, twice the normal dosages of anesthetic were required to produce immobility [13]. Taken together, these observations suggested that full anesthetics acted in supraspinal and infraspinal locations to produce immobility and loss of consciousness, that anesthetics behave as nonimmobilizers when administered supraspinally, and that doses sufficient to produce loss of consciousness may not produce immobility.

Clinical consequences

The clinical consequences of the aforementioned model are twofold. First, realizing that immobility and consciousness (and cardiovascular control) are mediated by different mechanisms has allowed anesthesiologists to tailor their anesthetics better to patient needs. In addition to the four end points of anesthetic action described previously, anesthesiologists now strive also for control of unwanted autonomic responses, such as hypertension and tachycardia. In general, inhaled anesthetic requirements for loss of consciousness (dubbed *MAC-awake*) are lower than requirements to prevent mobility (MAC), which are lower still than requirements to prevent cardiovascular responses to surgical stimulation (MAC that "blocks adrenergic responsiveness," or *MAC BAR*) [14]. Although in the past anesthesiologists might use a single agent to anesthetize a patient, more current strategies might include anesthetic administration to obtund awareness, muscle relaxation to facilitate immobility, and β blockade to modulate cardiovascular responses to surgery. Today, patient movement during surgery, previously postulated to be a sign of "light anesthesia" or "waking up," may be interpreted otherwise as insufficient immobility, warranting additional muscle relaxant administration rather than increased anesthetic dosing. Similarly, cardiovascular responses to anesthetic administration today would prompt consideration of β blockade as much as that of increased anesthesia.

The second consequence of the observation that anesthetics act on specific areas of the brain was that anesthesia might be mediated by specific (as opposed to general) effects on the cortex and brainstem. More recent work has shown the existence of "sleep" circuits in the brain, suggesting that the brain is already hard-wired to enter an unconscious state [15]. In addition, c-Fos studies of neuronal activity during some types of anesthesia show changes in the activity of brain nuclei involved in the control of sleep and waking that simulate those occurring during sleep [16]. Behaviorally, animal work has shown that sleep deprivation increases anesthetic potency [17], and that during prolonged anesthesia, sleep debt does not accrue [18].

Similarities between the anesthetized state and sleep have clinical consequences for patients with sleep apnea. Anecdotally, these patients are known to be more susceptible to sedatives and narcotics and can be particularly difficult to care for in the postoperative period [19]. A mechanistic basis for this clinically observed relationship between sleep deprivation and anesthetic action may allow anesthesiologists to predict and facilitate the difficult postoperative care of these patients. In addition, the ability of propofol anesthesia to dissipate sleep debt introduces a potential new indication for sedation in the ICU, where sleep deprivation is common.

Anesthetic depth monitoring

Background

One reasonable consequence of the aforementioned model of anesthetic action is that unconsciousness represents an anesthetic end point different from immobility. Although patient movement can be readily detected, the end points of amnesia and loss of awareness are less easily assessed. Although

titrating an anesthetic to highly visible end points, such as movement or changes in blood pressure or heart rate, is relatively straightforward, no known monitor of awareness exists that allows anesthesiologists definitively to prevent awareness during anesthesia. Historically, anesthesiologists have focused on preventing movement, believing that for most agents, the threshold for movement during surgery is reliably higher than that for patient awareness. Some patients may be aware during surgery without moving [20], however, and critically ill or hemodynamically unstable patients, such as patients undergoing cardiopulmonary bypass, may tolerate only partial doses of anesthesia. For these patients, the incidence of awareness increases significantly [21].

New advances

The issue of intraoperative awareness has received significant media attention as a result of high-profile cases describing posttraumatic stress responses to the sensation of being aware during surgery [22]. Feeding this interest are advertising efforts from manufacturers of new monitors that digitally record and process the electroencephalogram (EEG) or electromyogram. These monitors scan the digitized EEG for clues of patient awareness and claim to provide the anesthesiologist with additional information regarding the likelihood of awareness in an anesthetized patient. The most widely known of these is the Bispectral index (BIS) monitor, manufactured by Aspect Medical Systems (Newton, MA); similar devices are made by Physiometrix (Billerica, MA).

This entirely new class of monitor uses computer-based analysis to seek clues in the EEG that suggest an awake and conscious brain. Although higher frequency, low-amplitude, desynchronized EEG patterns typically suggest wakefulness in unanesthetized patients, no definite EEG pattern has been discovered yet that detects awareness during anesthesia. Instead, these monitors process a series of measurements to arrive at a likelihood of awareness. The BIS is an amalgam of three separate components of the EEG waveform: the degree of burst suppression (EEG isoelectricity), the ratio of high-frequency to medium-frequency power, and phase synchrony between spatially separated EEG waveforms [23]. By empirically calibrating these values to a database of thousands of anesthetized patients, the device produces a number between 0 and 100, where *100* indicates the awake brain and *0* represents complete isoelectricity. In general, normal awake patients register BIS values between 93 and 99, whereas anesthetized patients register values between 30 and 85. Sleeping patients generate BIS values similar to values of anesthetized patients, and it is possible through relaxation for awake humans to lower their own BIS readings to the high 80s. Manufacturers of the device have argued that BIS values of 65 or lower rule out any meaningful likelihood of awareness [24].

Clinical consequences

It is unclear whether use of the BIS monitor or other processed EEG monitoring reduces the likelihood of intraoperative awareness. The real rate of awareness during surgery is difficult to assess with certainty in part because the incidence is so low and because complete detection requires extensive patient follow-up. One trial [25] studied 19,576 patients at six US medical centers and found a relatively consistent rate of awareness of 1 to 2 per 1000 patients. Another Scandinavian study [26] using historical controls found that use of the BIS device reduced awareness to 0.4 per 1000 patients. Currently a large-scale prospective trial is under way in Australia comparing patients monitored with the device with unmonitored controls. Although no definitive results are available yet, preliminary data from 2000 patients suggest a reduction in the incidence of awareness similar to the Scandinavian study [27]. Neither of these studies specified how many patients were hemodynamically unstable or had undergone cardiac surgery with cardiopulmonary bypass, two known risk factors for awareness [21].

While large-scale trials currently are being conducted to assess the value of the BIS monitor in preventing awareness, many potential issues in the perioperative use of the BIS monitor have been observed. First, BIS values seem to be anesthetic specific. Ketamine results in higher BIS values than inhaled anesthetics for the same depth of anesthesia [28]. This variability raises the question of what threshold to use when multiple anesthetics are administered during a single anesthetic. The proprietary nature of the specific algorithm used to calculate the BIS "value" has raised concern regarding its reproducibility with different iterations of the device. Second, similar to the pulse oximeter, the BIS monitor is extremely sensitive to movement, changes in muscle tone in the absence of movement, and cardiac rhythm generators. In a case report, ECG artifacts were responsible for altered BIS readings in a brain-dead patient due to cardiac activity [29]. Finally, BIS devices require approximately 15 to 30 seconds of processing time to produce a number and do not respond to rapid changes in stimulation or level of anesthesia. As a result, the BIS monitor was approved by the US Food and Drug Administration

(FDA) in 1996 as a monitor of brain state, but without proven ability to prevent awareness.

For these reasons, use of this monitor has spurred significant controversy among anesthesiologists. Current concepts of general anesthetic action suggest that because dose requirements for consciousness are less than those for hemodynamic stability, titrating anesthetics to awareness instead of hemodynamic variables would result in less anesthetic usage. Research with the BIS device confirms this possibility, showing reductions in anesthetic use and slightly more rapid emergence as a result in outpatient surgery [30]. Despite these potential uses, however, insufficient overall evidence currently exists to show the utility of perioperative processed EEG monitoring. As a result, such monitoring currently is used unevenly in the United States, and the American Society of Anesthesiologists has not formally taken a position on its intraoperative use. Nevertheless, sufficient potential has been shown by these devices to suggest that future versions of these monitors may play a role in clinical anesthesia care.

New anesthetic drugs

Background

Many more recently introduced anesthetic drugs also have improved the flexibility of anesthesia care and the ability of anesthesiologists to care for a wide spectrum of patients. These improvements have included *greater potency,* more *reliable action,* and *dramatically faster onset/offset of action*. In general, nearly every class of anesthetic agent now includes newer members that outperform their predecessors.

New advances

Although the most commonly used inhaled anesthetic in 1990 was isoflurane, in 2004 anesthesiologists also may choose desflurane and sevoflurane. These agents produce a similar state to that produced with isoflurane, but offer significant advantages. Desflurane is dramatically faster in onset and offset and allows a more rapid emergence [31]. Sevoflurane is much less pungent than other inhaled anesthetics, facilitating an inhaled induction in pediatric patients and patients for whom intravenous access is difficult. Reductions in airways resistance with sevoflurane use also have improved the ability to anesthetize patients with reactive airways disease [32]. Although these newer agents are not completely free of side effects (rapid upward titration of desflurane produces a hypertensive, tachycardic response), they have largely supplanted older anesthetics with known adverse effects, such as enflurane (renal failure) and halothane (hepatitis).

Improvements in intravenous agents also have increased the reliability and control of the anesthetized state. Because of a more rapid recovery profile, the intravenous sedative propofol has largely replaced sodium thiopental as an induction agent. Although propofol produces slightly more hypotension than thiopental at equipotent doses [33], its clearance is dramatically higher, and it produces little or no residual effect, even after prolonged infusions or multiple doses.

The increased reliability of intravenous anesthetics has allowed some anesthetics to be administered without the use of inhaled agents. Termed *TIVA* for "total intravenous anesthesia," this technique has found its greatest use in the outpatient setting, where its advantages (less nausea/vomiting, faster recovery) are more likely to outweigh its disadvantages (more expensive, harder to use). In inpatient settings, TIVA may be used during rigid bronchoscopy and other cases in which interrupted ventilation can make use of inhaled anesthetics difficult.

The design of modern neuromuscular blocking agents also has changed. Older drugs, such as metocurine and pancuronium, were cleared primarily by the kidney and had a prolonged effect in patients with renal failure. Most newer agents are cleared either via hepatic metabolism (vecuronium, rocuronium) or by spontaneous hydrolysis in the bloodstream (atracurium, cisatracurium). As a result, recovery of neuromuscular function after a dose of relaxant is increasingly reliable, reducing the likelihood of residual paralysis after emergence from anesthesia. Even today's more reliable agents, if given for prolonged periods in an ICU setting, can induce a syndrome of prolonged paralysis [34]. Modern narcotics, such as remifentanil, also exist with sufficiently rapid kinetics and potency that bolus doses can produce complete apnea, but allow normal respiratory function minutes later [35]. Overall, current agents are so effective for modern surgical procedures that the risk-to-reward ratio for further refinements may not be worth the effort, and future anesthetic drugs are likely to be members of an entirely new class.

One such drug is the α_2-adrenergic agonist, dexmedetomidine. This sedative acts via a mechanism different from nearly all of the other sedative/anesthetics currently available to anesthesiologists. Although agents such as propofol and thiopental act primarily on the GABA receptor, dexmedetomidine is pharmacologically related to the α_2-adrenergic agonist, clonidine. In contrast to clonidine, however,

dexmedetomidine has significantly (eight times) greater affinity for the α_2-receptor and faster onset and offset times [36]. The clinical properties of dexmedetomidine differ from those of older sedatives and may offer greater flexibility in sedating conscious adults in and out of the operating room.

α_2-Adrenoceptors are a subgroup of noradrenergic receptors that mediate the function of the sympathetic nervous system. Although several subtypes (a, b, and c) exist [37], dexmedetomidine acts primarily at the α_{2a}-receptor, which modulates arousal in the brain and mediates analgesia in the spinal cord. By binding to these receptors, dexmedetomidine reduces sympathetic sources of arousal and in particular blocks efferent output from the locus coeruleus, a brain nucleus involved in alertness and arousal.

This novel mechanism results in differences between dexmedetomidine-based sedation and sedation produced by propofol or thiopental with respect to the *"quality" of sedation, analgesia,* and *respiratory depression*. Although dexmedetomidine and propofol obtund consciousness and reduce responsiveness to external stimuli, studies in volunteers suggest better cognitive function during sedation with dexmedetomidine [38]. Clinical results have been mixed, however. One 2004 comparison of dexmedetomidine versus propofol/midazolam/fentanyl sedation for awake carotid endarterectomy [39] found only slightly improved arousability in the dexmedetomidine group. Another ICU study [40] comparing dexmedetomidine and propofol sedation found no difference in patient interactivity, although more patients sedated with dexmedetomidine were able to recall accurately the length of ICU stay. In contrast, a series of five patients sedated with dexmedetomidine for cerebral arteriovenous malformation embolization observed prolonged impairment of cognition compared with patients sedated with propofol [41]. One possibility for worsened outcome with neurovascular procedures is that dexmedetomidine acts as a mild cerebral vasoconstrictor [42] and may have altered regional blood flow adversely. Relative unfamiliarity with the nature of sedation produced by dexmedetomidine also may have contributed to these mixed observations.

Another difference between dexmedetomidine and more traditional sedatives is that dexmedetomidine has analgesic properties. When compared with propofol, which has no intrinsic analgesic properties and often must be used with analgesics such as morphine, use of dexmedetomidine for intraoperative sedation showed consistent analgesic sparing effects [43]. Dexmedetomidine also reduces the amount of inhaled anesthetic needed for immobility (MAC) [44].

Probably the greatest clinical difference between dexmedetomidine and sedatives such as midazolam or propofol is the lack of respiratory depression. In healthy volunteers, even large overdoses of dexmedetomidine had nearly no effect on respiratory drive, responsiveness to carbon dioxide, or incidence of airway obstruction [45]. In another study comparing dexmedetomidine with placebo in patients extubated after major surgery, no difference in respiratory rates, oxygen saturations, or partial pressure of carbon dioxide were observed [46]. Oxygenation was significantly better in the dexmedetomidine group. As a result, dexmedetomidine is the only ICU sedative approved by the FDA for continuous infusion in extubated patients.

Side effects of dexmedetomidine include bradycardia and hypotension resulting from the sympatholytic effect of α_2-adrenoceptor activation. In phase III trials, these side effects occurred at approximately twice the incidence in patients given dexmedetomidine as in patients given midazolam or propofol. In addition, high initial doses of dexmedetomidine may produce transient *hyper*tension secondary to dose-dependent vasoconstrictive effects on α_{2b}-receptors [47]. Finally, dexmedetomidine currently is approved only for 24 hours of continuous infusion, and few data exist to confirm its safety for more prolonged use. Unanswered issues in this regard include drug tolerance, withdrawal, and accumulation of drug or metabolites.

Clinical consequences

Because of its relative novelty, the role of dexmedetomidine in clinical practice is still evolving. Its most attractive properties are its minimal effect on respiratory drive and reduced need for supplemental analgesia. Dexmedetomidine has been used as a sedative during awake intubations and regional anesthetics, as an anesthetic for neurosurgical procedures, to reduce anxiety during weaning from mechanical ventilation, and as an ICU sedative. In light of current experience, dexmedetomidine is likely to remain an anesthetic adjunct, used in situations when more familiar, first-line agents fail.

New anesthesia ventilators

Background

One area in which anesthesia technology has evolved is in the design and function of anesthesia machines. The anesthesia machine performs three fundamental functions: (1) the regulation and delivery of precise gas mixtures, (2) monitoring, and (3) mechanical ventilation. Of these, advances in the

performance and flexibility of anesthesia ventilators have facilitated the intraoperative care of critically ill patients significantly. These improvements have included more robust flow delivery under high airway pressures, greater flexibility in ventilator mode, and more comprehensive monitoring of ventilation. Although relatively invisible to nonanesthesiologist observers, these refinements have allowed anesthesiologists to duplicate more closely the performance of ICU ventilators, enabling intraoperative care for patients previously believed to be too sick.

New advances

Ventilator performance.   Ventilator performance is described most effectively by two parameters. The first is the maximal rate at which gas can be delivered to the lungs. Higher flow rates increase the range of possible ventilator settings, by permitting similar tidal volume delivery at shorter inspiratory times. Patients with significant expiratory airflow obstruction who require a prolonged expiratory phase or with a high minute ventilatory requirement are typical of those who may require shorter inspiratory times. In general, most anesthesia machines deliver 20 to 50 L/min of inspiratory flow, whereas ICU ventilators reliably can deliver 100 L/min in a fixed flow mode (eg, volume control) and 180 L/min in a variable flow mode (eg, pressure control). Because patients rarely require inspiratory flow rates greater than 50 L/min under normal conditions, these differences in flow delivery do not affect most patients.

The second important parameter is the stability of gas flow rates with increasing airway pressure. When airway pressures increase, the ability of anesthesia ventilators to deliver inspiratory flow decreases, whereas flow delivery by ICU ventilators remains relatively unchanged [48]. In patients with increased airway pressures, whether from narrow or partially occluded endotracheal tubes, lung injury, or chest wall stiffness, this difference can result in inadequate tidal volume delivery, hypercarbia, respiratory acidosis, and atelectasis.

The reason for this difference between anesthesia and ICU ventilators lies in the basic design of the two ventilator types. In contrast to ICU ventilators, anesthesia ventilators must carefully regulate, then deliver a precise gas mixture containing a mixture of oxygen, nitrogen, nitrous oxide, and anesthetic agent. To promote stability of the inhaled gas mixture, anesthesia machines filter exhaled gases to remove carbon dioxide and recirculate the resulting gas mixture. In contrast, exhaled gases from the ICU ventilator are vented directly into the atmosphere.

The need for anesthesia ventilators to recirculate exhaled gases into the inspiratory limb requires the ventilator circuit to contain a carbon dioxide "absorber" and a bellows to deliver the inspired/expired gas mixture back to the patient. These components add a significant amount of volume to the circuit. In contrast, most modern ICU ventilators deliver positive-pressure ventilation by gating gas directly from the wall outlet. The internal "circuit" volume of a typical ICU ventilator is less than 100 mL, whereas the internal volume of an anesthesia ventilator can be greater than 2 L (and is usually closer to 5 L). When the ventilator must deliver a tidal volume in the presence of high airway pressures, much of the tidal volume is compressed into the ventilator circuit and fails to reach the patient. The result of reduced tidal volume delivery is decreased minute ventilation, hypercapnia, respiratory acidosis, and atelectasis from inadequate lung expansion.

The twin risk factors for anesthesia ventilator failure are high airway pressures and high minute ventilatory requirements. As a rule of thumb, with standard anesthesia machines, the "50-50" rule prevails: If airway pressures of 50 cm H_2O and inspiratory flow rates of 50 L/min are required, the anesthesia machine is operating at the outer edge of its performance curve. Any further increase in inspiratory flow requirements or airway pressures would result in an inability to deliver the desired tidal volumes and potential ventilator failure. For this reason, anesthesiologists providing intraoperative care for critically ill patients with lung injury often have opted to use a "critical care" type of ventilator instead.

Newer anesthesia machines from the three major manufacturers of anesthesia machines in the United States (Datex-Ohmeda, Drager North America, and Siemens) have approached the twin problems of limited inspiratory flow and instability of flow delivery with high airway pressure in three ways. First, these newer ventilators are designed with smaller bellows and smaller carbon dioxide absorbers. By reducing the internal volume of the circuit, the volume lost by gas compression in the circuit during inspiration is decreased. Second, some ventilators have better flow generators. Finally, many newer machines have an electronic compensation system, which monitors airway pressures and delivered tidal volumes and augments tidal volume delivery to compensate for effects of gas compression.

As a result of these changes, some modern anesthesia ventilators are able to maintain stable gas flow of 75 L/min up to airway pressures of 75 cm H_2O. This relatively modest improvement in flow stability allows nearly all critically ill patients to be ventilated in an intraoperative setting. Although elective surgery generally is contraindicated in patients with acute lung injury, burn patients with inhalation injury or trauma patients with lung contusions may require operative intervention during the acute phase of lung injury. Although these patients may exceed the 50/50 threshold (50 L/min gas flow and 50 mm Hg inspiratory airway pressure), patients exceeding a hypothetical 70/70 threshold are likely to be too unstable to travel to the operating room regardless of the ventilator type. Some criteria for intraoperative use of a critical care ventilator are listed in Table 1.

Pressure control mode. Another feature increasingly available on modern anesthesia machines is a choice of ventilator modes that modify the delivery of gas flow or allow the patient to control partly ventilator activity. One of these is pressure control mode, which uses inspiratory pressure instead of tidal volume as a target. In volume control mode (standard in nearly all anesthesia machines), the ventilator is set to deliver a set volume at a set rate. Flow rates are fixed at a constant value during inspiration. In pressure control mode, the ventilator continuously modulates gas flow to sustain a set pressure during the inspiratory phase. The result is a tidal volume that can vary with changes in lung compliance or airways resistance.

Pressure control mode does not improve outcomes when used long-term in the ICU, but may have some short-term advantages. In adult respiratory distress

Table 1
Indications for use of a critical care–type ventilator in the operating room

Indication	Reason
Preoperative pressure control ventilation	Occult ETT obstruction Oxygenation
High airway pressures (PIP >50 cm H_2O) and high inspiratory flows (>50 L/min)	Anesthesia ventilator failure at high flow rates and airway pressures
High preoperative PEEP values or increased A-a gradient (PaO_2/FIO_2 <100)	Inability to tolerate intraoperative fluid shifts Inability to monitor PEEP Potential anesthesia ventilator failure
Coexisting expiratory obstruction (auto-PEEP)	Inability to monitor auto-PEEP Inadequate inspiratory flow rates
Large fluid shifts	Potential anesthesia ventilator failure

syndrome (ARDS), use of pressure control ventilation may improve oxygenation and reduce respiratory work [49]. In addition, under conditions of partial endotracheal tube obstruction, use of volume control mode may result in dangerous elevations in airway pressure (see earlier). In pressure control mode, delivery of tidal volume is preserved with progressive endotracheal tube occlusion until the obstruction is severe [50]. As a result, when ventilating patients using narrow or partially obstructed endotracheal tubes, use of pressure control mode may allow adequate ventilation without potentially harmful increases in airway pressure. This benefit of pressure control mode may be useful for thoracic surgery patients. During one-lung ventilation, use of pressure control mode improves oxygenation compared with volume control mode [51]. The ability of pressure control ventilation to deliver better tidal volumes at similar airway pressures to volume control ventilation also may play a role in patients with tracheal or bronchial suture lines, in whom excessive airway pressures may exacerbate leaks.

Improved monitoring.   Most newer anesthesia machines (machines produced after approximately 1997) have improved monitoring capabilities. Historically, anesthesia machines have provided only rudimentary information about mechanical ventilation, monitoring tidal volume, respiratory rate, and peak airway pressure. Newer machines are capable, however, of monitoring positive end-expiratory pressure (PEEP), inspiratory flow, inspiratory plateau pressures, and delivered tidal volumes. These additional capabilities allow anesthesiologists to customize ventilation better for individual patients and detect abnormalities in ventilation that may lead to intraoperative morbidity.

Of these new capabilities, perhaps the most important is the comparison between delivered and set tidal volumes. Older anesthesia machines monitor tidal volumes, but do not alert anesthesiologists when tidal volume delivery falls below set levels. A decrease in tidal volume delivery owing to ongoing increases in airway pressure (see earlier for explanation) may not be detected until its consequences (inadequate ventilation, hypercapnia, and respiratory acidosis) become evident. Newer anesthesia machines not only alarm when detected tidal volumes fall below set levels, but also compensate automatically by delivering additional volume.

For thoracic surgery patients, many of whom have chronic expiratory airflow disease, the ability of newer machines to measure inspiratory peak and pause pressures and end-expiratory pressures also facilitates intraoperative ventilation. Many thoracic

surgery patients have obstructive airways disease and are at risk for bronchospasm and auto-PEEP. In these patients, diagnosing auto-PEEP may be important in avoiding adverse respiratory and circulatory consequences. In contrast to older machines, which do not monitor end-expiratory pressure, newer machines provide this information continuously to the anesthesiologist, allowing him or her to arrive at a diagnosis and begin therapy more rapidly. Finally, older anesthesia machines lack any intrinsic ability to provide PEEP, forcing the anesthesiologist to use an external device with fixed PEEP values of either 5 or 10 cm H_2O. Most newer machines now are able to generate their own PEEP and can do so for any value between 2 and 20 cm H_2O. Such flexibility may be particularly valuable in patients undergoing one-lung ventilation or patients with ARDS who often are subjected to deliberate hypoventilation and concomitant PEEP.

Specialty gases: heliox and nitric oxide

Background
In thoracic surgery patients with intrinsic lung disease, two gases that have potential utility are heliox (helium/oxygen mixtures) and nitric oxide (NO). This section discusses important technical issues involved in the intraoperative administration of both of these agents.

New advances
Heliox.   During quiet breathing in humans, gas flow in the lung is generally laminar until the second-generation bronchi, where a transition to turbulent flow occurs [52]. In patients with airways obstruction, however, turbulent flow can occur more frequently [53]. Because resistance to turbulent flow is greater than resistance to laminar flow, an increase in turbulent flow in the lung can increase the overall resistance to gas flow and the work of breathing. The resistance to turbulent flow depends on gas density, however, forming the basis for the use of heliox for obstructive airways disease. Because heliox is much less dense than nitrogen and oxygen, turbulent flow generates less resistance. As a result, it has been investigated for use in patients with increased turbulent flow resulting from upper airway obstructions or compressive lesions of the trachea [54] and in patients with chronic obstructive pulmonary disease (COPD) or asthma [55].

The clinical utility of heliox is unclear. Although a 2001 meta-analysis in patients with asthma found no outcome benefit [56], several studies of patients with severe asthma have found reductions in pulsus paradoxus and improved oxygenation with heliox use [57]. In small trials of intubated COPD patients, heliox reduces intrinsic PEEP and reduces work of breathing during spontaneous breathing [58]. The prevalence of airway obstruction in thoracic surgery patients raises the possibility that use of this gas also may assist intraoperative ventilation for thoracic surgery.

Few data exist to document or evaluate the efficacy of perioperative heliox use. This lack of data is due partly to technical difficulties in the delivery of heliox via anesthesia machine. For an anesthesia machine, which is precisely calibrated for each of the gases it typically uses, the introduction of heliox requires that it take the place of one of the other gases. For maximal flexibility, heliox usually is connected to the air inlet. Connected in this way, however, heliox introduces two errors in the monitoring of ventilation. The first is that because of its reduced density, heliox causes the air flowmeter to read erroneously low compared with air flowing at the same rate. The second is that excess gas flow into the breathing circuit, by the design of the anesthesia machine, increases delivered tidal volumes above expected levels and alters the fraction of inspired oxygen (FIO_2) [59]. Although some newer anesthesia machines are designed to deliver heliox routinely, these are not available in most anesthetizing locations. For most anesthesiologists, the best approach is to bring a critical care ventilator, outfitted with the ability to deliver heliox, to the operating room if such therapy is required.

Nitric oxide. The rationale for use of NO in thoracic surgery is discussed more thoroughly elsewhere in this issue. This section addresses technical issues surrounding its intraoperative use. NO has two potential uses in thoracic surgery patients. The first is to facilitate oxygenation, and the second is as a pulmonary vasodilator for patients with pulmonary hypertension. Dosage ranges for these two applications differ widely. Although NO improves oxygenation at doses ranging from 5 to 15 parts per million (ppm), its effect as a pulmonary vasodilator begins at 15 ppm and seems to have benefit in a dose-dependent fashion up to 80 ppm [60].

NO has two important toxicities. The first is that in susceptible patients, NO can induce methemoglobinemia, altering oxygen carrying capacity and the accuracy of the pulse oximeter. Intraoperative use of this drug mandates a means for monitoring for methemoglobin formation. The second is the production of the toxic gas and ozone precursor, nitrogen dioxide (NO_2). A yellowish brown gas, NO_2 forms spontaneously from NO and oxygen and is a direct-acting airway irritant. Prolonged inhalation of concentrations of 10 ppm can produce coughing, bronchospasm, and shortness of breath; inhalation of higher concentrations (50–100 ppm) can induce pulmonary edema, hemoptysis, bronchiolitis obliterans, and frank ARDS [61]. Because the formation of NO_2 is promoted by high concentrations of NO and oxygen, it may be present in the ventilator circuit when NO levels and the FIO_2 are high. As a result, use of NO, particularly at the high levels needed for pulmonary hypertension, requires that a means for measuring NO_2 also be available. National industrial health standards recommend threshold limits for NO_2 exposure to 1 ppm [62]. Because anesthesia machines can recirculate exhaled gases, prolonged contact between NO and oxygen is possible, increasing the risk of toxic NO_2 production.

The most important concern regarding the intraoperative use of NO is a physiologic "rebound" response that occurs with abrupt withdrawal of the drug. This rebound can occur in 25% of patients receiving NO and entails immediate decreases in cardiac output of greater than 20% and oxygen saturation [63]. Although the mechanism of this effect is unknown, it is postulated to be due to rebound pulmonary hypertension after NO withdrawal. For anesthesiologists preparing to transport and anesthetize a patient in the ICU on NO (or to begin NO in the operating room), the implication of such a rebound response is that NO should not be turned off for transport or for moving the patient onto or off the transport gurney. In general, because of the specialized requirements for dosing of NO, it is best to consult with the respiratory therapy department when initiating NO in the operating room or when transporting a patient who is receiving NO. Table 2 lists complications with use of heliox and NO.

Table 2
Complications of intraoperative heliox and nitric oxide use

Heliox	Nitric oxide
Limited FIO_2	Methemoglobinemia
Difficult to deliver using anesthesia machine (machine not calibrated for heliox use)	NO_2 formation (worse in anesthesia machines)
Requires ICU ventilator	Rebound hypoxemia/hypotension

Conclusion

As when anesthesia was first demonstrated in 1846, an anesthetized patient today appears motionless and insensate, calmly breathing a carefully composed mixture of gases to maintain the unconscious state. Then as now, the fundamental mechanism by which general anesthesia is generated and maintained is unknown. Nevertheless, understanding of anesthesia mechanisms and the ability to control and manage the conduct of general anesthesia continue to evolve. Although more recent advances in anesthesia techniques are subtle and difficult to detect for the nonanesthesiologist, they have added dramatically to the ability of the anesthesiologist to predict, understand, monitor, and control sources of variability in anesthetic action among individuals. Newer drugs, developed with an improved understanding of anesthesia mechanisms, and newer equipment, designed for lung-injured patients, also have expanded the definition of patients who are "cleared for surgery" to include patients who would have been too sick 10 years ago. Taken together, these changes have produced a modern anesthetic that looks identical to anesthetics of an earlier time, but significantly and dramatically changed.

Summary

- Advances in anesthesia involve refinements in understanding, technique, and technology. These refinements have led to better control of the anesthetic state, effective anesthesia for a wider variety of situations, and the ability to bring sicker patients to the operating room.
- Although the molecular mechanisms underlying the general anesthetic state are unknown, evidence suggests a specific, receptor-based effect. This concept has allowed anesthesiologists to treat anesthetic end points of immobility, lack of awareness, and autonomic control separately.
- It is likely that anesthesia and naturally occurring sleep interact physiologically.
- New, processed EEG monitors may allow anesthesiologists to titrate more finely anesthetic dose, with possible benefits in terms of speed of recovery and detection of intraoperative awareness.
- Since the 1990s, new anesthetic drugs (propofol, desflurane/sevoflurane, cisatracurium) have enhanced greatly control of the anesthetic state.
- The new intravenous anesthetic agent dexmedetomidine offers sedation with preserved respiration and cognitive function. Although its role has yet to be defined fully, it currently plays a role in ICU sedation and monitored anesthesia care.
- New anesthesia ventilators have better monitoring and better flow delivery at high airway pressures. These improvements significantly narrow the performance gap between anesthesia and ICU ventilators.
- In patients with COPD, pulmonary hypertension, or severe hypoxemia, heliox may improve gas flow, and NO may reduce pulmonary vascular resistance and improve oxygenation.

References

[1] Overton CE. Studien über die Narkose zugleich ein Beitrag zur Allgemeinen Pharmakologie. Jena, G Fischer, 1901.
[2] Koblin DD. Mechanisms of anesthetic action. In: Miller RD, editor. Anesthesia. 5th edition. Philadelphia: Churchill Livingstone; 2000. p. 48–73.
[3] Lysko GS, Robinson JL, Casto R, Ferrone RA. The stereospecific effects of isoflurane isomers in vivo. Eur J Pharmacol 1994;263:25–9.
[4] Fang Z, Laster MJ, Gong D, Ionescu P, Koblin DD, Sonner J, et al. Convulsant activity of nonanesthetic gas combinations. Anesth Analg 1997;84:634–40.
[5] Liu J, Laster MJ, Koblin DD, Eger 2nd EI, Halsey MJ, Taheri S, et al. A cutoff in potency exists in the perfluoroalkanes. Anesth Analg 1994;79:238–44.
[6] North C, Cafiso DS. Contrasting membrane localization and behavior of halogenated cyclobutanes that follow or violate the Meyer-Overton hypothesis of general anesthetic potency. Biophys J 1997;72:1754–61.
[7] Campagna JA, Miller KW, Forman SA. Drug therapy: mechanisms of actions of inhaled anesthetics. N Engl J Med 2003;348:2110–24.
[8] Quasha AL, Eger 2nd EI, Tinker JH. Determination and applications of MAC. Anesthesiology 1980;53:315–34.
[9] Kandel L, Chortkoff BS, Sonner J, Laster MJ, Eger 2nd EI. Nonanesthetics can suppress learning. Anesth Analg 1996;82:321–6.
[10] Todd MM, Weeks JB, Warner DS. A focal cryogenic brain lesion does not reduce the minimum alveolar concentration for halothane in rats. Anesthesiology 1993;79:139–43.
[11] Rampil IJ. Anesthetic potency is not altered after hypothermic spinal cord transection in rats. Anesthesiology 1994;80:606–10.
[12] Rampil IJ, Mason P, Singh H. Anesthetic potency (MAC) is independent of forebrain structures in the rat. Anesthesiology 1993;78:707–12.
[13] Antognini JF, Schwartz K. Exaggerated anesthetic requirements in the preferentially anesthetized brain. Anesthesiology 1993;79:1244–9.

[14] Eger 2nd EI. Age, minimum alveolar anesthetic concentration, and minimum alveolar anesthetic con-centration-awake. Anesth Analg 2001;93:947–53.

[15] Saper CB, Chou TC, Scammell TE. The sleep switch: hypothalamic control of sleep and wakefulness. Trends Neurosci 2001;24:726–31.

[16] Nelson LE, Guo TZ, Lu J, Saper CB, Franks NP, Maze M. The sedative component of anesthesia is mediated by GABA(A) receptors in an endogenous sleep pathway. Nat Neurosci 2002;5:979–84.

[17] Tung A, Szafran MJ, Bluhm B, Mendelson WB. Sleep deprivation potentiates the onset and duration of loss of righting reflex induced by propofol and isoflurane. Anesthesiology 2002;97:906–11.

[18] Tung A, Lynch JP, Mendelson WB. Prolonged sedation with propofol in the rat does not result in sleep deprivation. Anesth Analg 2001;92:1232–6.

[19] Ostermeier AM, Roizen MF, Hautkappe M, Klock PA, Klafta JM. Three sudden postoperative respiratory arrests associated with epidural opioids in patients with sleep apnea. Anesth Analg 1997;85:452–60.

[20] Bogetz MS, Katz JA. Recall of surgery for major trauma. Anesthesiology 1984;61:6–9.

[21] Ghoneim MM. Awareness during anesthesia. Anes-thesiology 2000;92:597–602.

[22] Associated Press. Waking up during surgery. Accessed at: http://www.cbsnews.com/stories/2003/11/24/eveningnews/main585347.shtml on June 21, 2004.

[23] Rampil IJ. A primer for EEG signal processing in anesthesia. Anesthesiology 1998;89:980–1002.

[24] Kelly S. OR manual. Aspect Newton, MA: Medical Systems, Inc; 2002.

[25] Sandin RH, Enlund G, Samuelsson P, Lennmarken C. Awareness during anaesthesia: a prospective case study. Lancet 2000;355:707–11.

[26] Ekman A, Lindholm ML, Lennmarken C, Sandin R. Reduction in the incidence of awareness using BIS monitoring. Acta Anaesthesiol Scand 2004;48:20–6.

[27] Myles PS, Leslie K, McNeil J, Forbes A, Chan MT. Bispectral index monitoring to prevent awareness during anaesthesia: the B-Aware randomised control trial. Lancet 2004;363:1757–63.

[28] Vereecke HE, Struys MM, Mortier EP. A comparison of bispectral index and ARX-derived auditory evoked potential index in measuring the clinical interaction between ketamine and propofol anaesthesia. Anaes-thesia 2003;58:957–61.

[29] Myles PS, Cairo S. Artifact in the bispectral index in a patient with severe ischemic brain injury. Anesth Analg 2004;98:706–7.

[30] Gan TJ, Glass PS, Windsor A, Payne F, Rosow C, Sebel P, et al, and the BIS Utility Study Group. Bispectral Index monitoring allows faster emergence and improved recovery from propofol, alfentanil, and nitrous oxide anesthesia. Anesthesiology 1997;87:808–15.

[31] Jones RM, Cashman JN, Eger 2nd EI, Damask MC, Johnson BH. Related articles, links kinetics and potency of desflurance (I-653) in volunteers. Anesth Analg 1990;70:3–7.

[32] Rooke GA, Choi JH, Bishop MJ. The effect of iso-flurane, halothane, sevoflurane, and thiopental/nitrous oxide on respiratory system resistance after tracheal intubation. Anesthesiology 1997;86:1294–9.

[33] McCollum JS, Dundee JW. Comparison of induction characteristics of four intravenous anaesthetic agents. Anaesthesia 1986;41:995–1000.

[34] Murphy GS, Vender JS. Neuromuscular-blocking drugs: use and misuse in the intensive care unit. Crit Care Clin 2001;17:925–42.

[35] Glass PS, Hardman D, Kamiyama Y, Quill TJ, Marton G, Donn KH, et al. Preliminary pharmacokinetics and pharmacodynamics of an ultra-short-acting opioid: remifentanil (GI87084B). Anesth Analg 1993;77:1031–40.

[36] Coursin DB, Coursin DB, Maccioli GA. Dexmedeto-midine. Curr Opin Crit Care 2001;7:221–6.

[37] MacDonald E, Scheinin M. Distribution and pharma-cology of alpha 2-adrenoceptors in the central nervous system. J Physiol Pharmacol 1995;46:241–58.

[38] Hindmarch I. Instrumental assessment of psychomotor functions and the effects of psychotropic drugs. Acta Psychiatr Scand Suppl 1994;380:49–52.

[39] Bekker AY, Basile J, Gold M, Riles T, Adelman M, Cuff G, et al. Dexmedetomidine for awake carotid endarterectomy: efficacy, hemodynamic profile, and side effects. J Neurosurg Anesthesiol 2004;16:126–35.

[40] Venn RM, Grounds RM. Comparison between dexme-detomidine and propofol for sedation in the intensive care unit: patient and clinician perceptions. Br J Anaesth 2001;87:684–90.

[41] Bustillo MA, Lazar RM, Finck AD, Fitzsimmons B, Berman MF, Pile-Spellman J, et al. Dexmedetomidine may impair cognitive testing during endovascular embolization of cerebral arteriovenous malformations: a retrospective case report series. J Neurosurg Anes-thesiol 2002;14:209–12.

[42] Karlsson BR, Forsman M, Roald OK, Heier MS, Steen PA. Effect of dexmedetomidine, a selective and potent alpha 2-agonist, on cerebral blood flow and oxygen consumption during halothane anesthesia in dogs. Anesth Analg 1990;71:125–9.

[43] Hall JE, Uhrich TD, Barney JA, Arain SR, Ebert TJ. Sedative, amnestic, and analgesic properties of small-dose dexmedetomidine infusions. Anesth Analg 2000;90:699–705.

[44] Aantaa R, Jaakola ML, Kallio A, Kanto J. Reduc-tion of the minimum alveolar concentration of iso-flurane by dexmedetomidine. Anesthesiology 1997;86:1055–60.

[45] Ebert TJ, Hall JE, Barney JA, Uhrich TD, Colinco MD. The effects of increasing plasma concentrations of dexmedetomidine in humans. Anesthesiology 2000;93:382–94.

[46] Venn RM, Hell J, Grounds RM. Respiratory effects of dexmedetomidine in the surgical patient requiring intensive care. Crit Care 2000;4:302–8.

[47] Jorden V, Tung A. Dexmedetomidine: clinical update. Semin Anesth 2002;21:265–74.

[48] Marks JD, Schapera A, Kraemer RW, Katz JA. Pressure and flow limitations of anesthesia ventilators. Anesthesiology 1989;71:403–8.

[49] Kallet RH, Campbell AR, Alonso JA, et al. The effects of pressure control versus volume control assisted ventilation on patient work of breathing in acute lung injury and acute respiratory distress syndrome. Respir Care 2000;45:1085–96.

[50] Tung A, Morgan SE. Modeling the effect of progressive endotracheal tube occlusion on tidal volume in pressure-control mode. Anesth Analg 2002;95:192–7.

[51] Tugrul M, Camci E, Karadeniz H, et al. Comparison of volume controlled with pressure controlled ventilation during one-lung anaesthesia. Br J Anaesth 1997;79:306–10.

[52] Olson DE, Dart GA, Filley GF. Pressure drop and fluid flow regime of air inspired into the human lung. J Appl Physiol 1970;28:482–94.

[53] Otis A, Bembower W. Effect of gas density on resistance to respiratory gas flow in man. J Appl Physiol 1949;2:300–6.

[54] Ho AM, Dion PW, Karmakar MK, Chung DC, Tay BA. Use of heliox in critical upper airway obstruction: physical and physiologic considerations in choosing the optimal helium:oxygen mix. Resuscitation 2002;52:297–300.

[55] Ho AM, Lee A, Karmakar MK, Dion PW, Chung DC, Contardi LH. Heliox vs air-oxygen mixtures for the treatment of patients with acute asthma: a systematic overview. Chest 2003;123:882–90.

[56] Rodrigo G, Rodrigo C, Pollack C, Travers A. Helium-oxygen mixture for nonintubated acute asthma patients. Cochrane Database Syst Rev 2001;1:CD002884.

[57] Manthous CA, Hall JB, Caputo MA, Walter J, Klocksieben JM, Schmidt GA, et al. Heliox improves pulsus paradoxus and peak expiratory flow in nonintubated patients with severe asthma. Am J Respir Crit Care Med 1995;151(2 Pt 1):310–4.

[58] Jolliet P, Watremez C, Roeseler J, Ngengiyumva JC, de Kock M, Clerbaux T, et al. Comparative effects of helium-oxygen and external positive end-expiratory pressure on respiratory mechanics, gas exchange, and ventilation-perfusion relationships in mechanically ventilated patients with chronic obstructive pulmonary disease. Intensive Care Med 2003;29:1442–50.

[59] Tung A, Morgan S. Delivery of heliox by anesthesia machine produces error in fresh gas flow and tidal volume measurements. Anesthesiology 2000;93:A576.

[60] Gerlach H, Rossaint R, Pappert D, et al. Time-course and dose-response of nitric oxide inhalation for systemic oxygenation and pulmonary hypertension in patients with adult respiratory distress syndrome. Eur J Clin Invest 1993;23:499–502.

[61] Weinberger B, Laskin DL, Heck DE, Laskin JD. The toxicology of inhaled nitric oxide. Toxicol Sci 2001;59:5–16.

[62] National Institute for Occupational Safety and Health Guide to Occupational Hazards. Accessed online on May 27, 2004 at: http://www.cdc.gov/niosh/npg/npgd0454.html.

[63] Christenson J, Lavoie A, O'Connor M, Bhorade S, Pohlman A, Hall JB. The incidence and pathogenesis of cardiopulmonary deterioration after abrupt withdrawal of inhaled nitric oxide. Am J Respir Crit Care Med 2000;161:1443–9.

ELSEVIER
SAUNDERS

Thorac Surg Clin 15 (2005) 39–53

THORACIC
SURGERY
CLINICS

Developments in General Airway Management

David Ferson, MD[a],*, T. Linda Chi, MD[b]

[a]Department of Anesthesiology and Pain Medicine, The University of Texas M.D. Anderson Cancer Center,
1515 Holcombe Boulevard, Unit 42, Houston, TX 77030-4590, USA
[b]Department of Diagnostic Imaging, The University of Texas M.D. Anderson Cancer Center, 1515 Holcombe Boulevard,
Houston, TX 77030-4590, USA

One of the most important functions of an anesthesiologist is to secure and maintain a patent airway. This function is especially important for patients with respiratory disease, who cannot tolerate even short periods of apnea. Many pathologic processes often produce anatomic changes in the patient's airway that require specialized techniques for ventilation and tracheal intubation. During procedures involving the respiratory tract, the surgeon and anesthesiologist often share access to the patient's airway; is essential that they work collaboratively to ensure patient safety and the success of the procedure. This article describes the impact of modern imaging techniques on preoperative airway evaluation, discusses airway-related morbidity and mortality and the American Society of Anesthesiologists' Difficult Airway Guidelines, and reviews developments in airway management that have significantly improved the quality and safety of anesthesia in patients with respiratory problems. Because lung separation techniques are discussed in another article in this issue, the focus here is on the tremendous impact of the laryngeal mask airway (LMA) and the flexible fiberscope in clinical practice.

Airway imaging

Although ordering and interpreting radiologic studies are not in the usual domain of anesthesiologists, imaging techniques such as MRI, CT, and

helical CT provide a wealth of information about the airway that can be instrumental in identifying pathology and in formulating an anesthetic plan. Studies using radiologic imaging have contributed greatly to the general understanding of airway anatomy and physiology and to the critical examination of old and new techniques of airway management.

The airway, defined as a continuum from the nose and mouth to the lungs, traverses anatomic landmarks arbitrarily divided into the head, neck, and chest. With modern imaging modalities (CT and MRI), anesthesiologists have an unparalleled opportunity to visualize and evaluate airway structures for anesthetic planning and management. A basic understanding of how the anatomic airway structures appear in the various imaging techniques is essential to comprehend how different pathologic processes affect airway anatomy and function. This understanding is especially important when considering different techniques for intubating the trachea.

Computed tomography

Practically speaking, CT scans have become "routine." The spatial resolution of CT is the best of all imaging modalities currently available. Another advantage of CT technology is that it can depict accurately any pathology involving bones. Data acquisition using CT is quick, and images can be produced in all three planes (Figs. 1–3) for surface rendering, three-dimensional reformation, and display of different organs in an anatomic format that can be recognized easily by clinicians. CT has become the gold standard for ruling out fractures of the cervical

* Corresponding author.
E-mail address: dferson@mdanderson.org (D. Ferson).

1547-4127/05/$ – see front matter © 2005 Elsevier Inc. All rights reserved.
doi:10.1016/j.thorsurg.2004.10.002

thoracic.theclinics.com

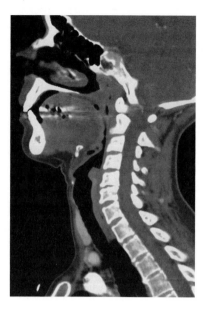

Fig. 1. CT scan of the airway, sagittal view, depicts bones and soft tissues of the airway.

spine because the bony structures of patients with such pathologies can be displayed accurately on CT.

Magnetic resonance imaging

Airway structures displayed by MRI offer detailed information on soft tissues but not bony structures (Fig. 4). In patients with neck pathologies, such as tumors, MRI can be useful in assessing the impact of the pathologic processes on airway patency. This information can help the anesthesiologist determine the best method for intubation of the patient's trachea or the feasibility of orotracheal or nasotracheal intubation.

Airway-related morbidity and mortality

The first comprehensive analysis of adverse airway outcomes was published in 1990 with data from the American Society of Anesthesiologists (ASA) Closed Claims Study [1]. Thirty-four percent of the adverse outcomes were caused by respiratory events, and 85% of these events resulted in brain damage or death [1]. It has been estimated that of all deaths from causes directly attributable to anesthesia, 30% are associated with the inability to secure the airway and ventilate the lungs in a timely fashion [1–3]. Although many of the cases in the Closed Claims database occurred before the adoption of the ASA

monitoring standards in 1987, adverse airway and respiratory events continue to occur.

Practice guidelines for management of the difficult airway

To help guide clinicians in the process of airway management, the ASA developed practice guidelines for patients with difficult-to-manage airways and published the ASA Difficult Airway Algorithm [4] in 1993. The guidelines and algorithm were based on a review of published literature, the opinions of consultant anesthesiologists, and the consensus of the community of practitioners likely to be affected by them. These guidelines were revised and updated in 2003 to include techniques that were developed and studied after the original guidelines were published [5] and specifically address evaluation of the airway (including an 11-point airway physical examination), strategy for intubation of the difficult airway, strategy for extubation of the difficult airway, and follow-up care. The guidelines highlight the importance of an initial consideration of the merits and feasibility of three fundamental management choices: (1) a non-surgical versus surgical technique for initial approach to intubation, (2) awake intubation versus intubation after induction of general anesthesia, and (3) preservation versus ablation of spontaneous ventilation. The laryngeal mask airway (LMA) as an example of a supralaryngeal device was incorporated into the emergency airway management arm of the algorithm (see LMA description later).

The new ASA practice guidelines define the difficult-to-manage airway as a clinical situation in which a conventionally trained anesthesiologist experiences difficulty with facemask ventilation of the upper airway, tracheal intubation, or both. Difficult facemask ventilation is defined as inadequate mask seal, excessive gas leak, or excessive resistance to ingress or egress of gas or inadequate ventilation as reflected by absent or inadequate chest movement, absent or inadequate breath sounds, auscultatory signs of severe obstruction, gastric air entry, poor carbon dioxide return, and decreasing oxygen saturation as measured by pulse oximetry. Several factors may contribute to difficulties in ventilating the lungs with a facemask. Langeron et al [6] prospectively studied 1502 patients to determine physical characteristics that could predict difficulty in facemask ventilation. They concluded that the presence of one or more of the following patient characteristics should alert clinicians to the possibility of difficult

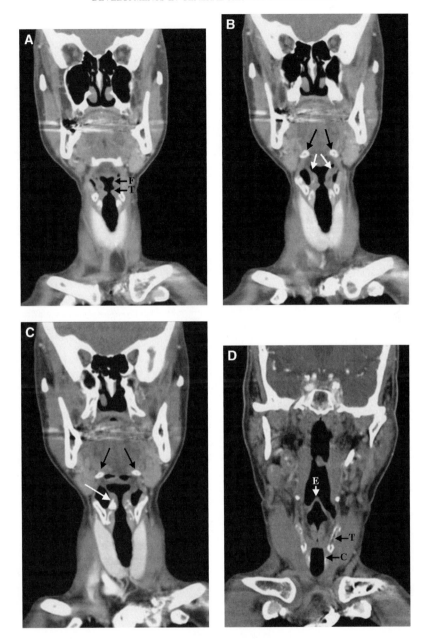

Fig. 2. CT scan of the airway, coronal view, allows visualization of airway structures in the anteroposterior direction. (*A*) Position of the true vocal cords (T) and false vocal cords (F). (*B*) Aryepiglottic folds (*white arrows*) and hyoid bone (*black arrows*). (*C*) Arytenoid cartilage (*white arrow*) and hyoid bone (*black arrows*) at the level of epiglottis. (*D*) Epiglottis (E), thyroid cartilage (T), and cricoid cartilage (C).

facemask ventilation: (1) age 55 years or older, (2) body mass index >26 kg/m², (3) lack of teeth, (4) snoring, (5) macroglossia, and (6) presence of a beard.

The ASA Difficult Airway Algorithm characterizes difficult laryngoscopy, difficult intubation, and failed intubation. *Difficult laryngoscopy* is defined as the inability to visualize any portion of the vocal cords after multiple attempts at conventional laryngoscopy. *Difficult intubation* describes tracheal intubation that requires multiple attempts and frequently multiple operators in the presence or absence of

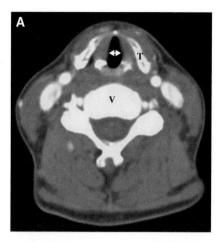
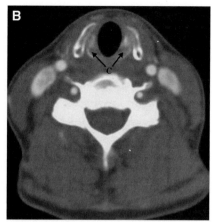

Fig. 3. CT scan of the airway, axial view, depicts the airway anatomy in the craniocaudal direction. (*A*) Thyroid cartilage (T), vocal cords (*double-headed arrow*), and vertebral body (V). (*B*) View of the larynx below the vocal cords provides a good image of the cricoid cartilage (C) (*arrows*).

tracheal pathology. *Failed intubation* is defined as failure to place the tracheal tube after multiple attempts. Several factors may contribute to difficult laryngoscopy and difficult or failed intubation. No single test reliably predicts which patient will be difficult to intubate. Careful evaluation of each patient's airway before general anesthesia is an absolute necessity. Evaluation includes obtaining an airway history from the patient and performing a physical examination, which should include the assessment of multiple features that are associated with difficult laryngoscopy and difficult intubation [7–10].

Although the algorithm is not a foolproof system, it increases the awareness that respiratory problems remain the major contributor to serious morbidity and mortality directly attributed to anesthesia, and it provides a useful framework for the clinical management of patients with anticipated or unexpected airway problems. Introduction of the ASA Difficult Airway Algorithm in 1993 stimulated interest in the development of different tools and techniques for patients with difficult-to-manage airways. Anesthesia practitioners are not required to master all the techniques in the algorithm, but rather to be aware that different airway management techniques have

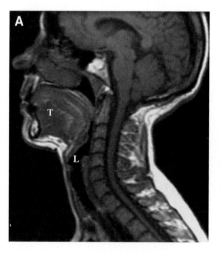
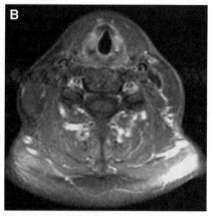

Fig. 4. MRI of the airway. (*A*) Sagittal view shows in detail the soft tissues of the human airway but no bony detail; cervical vertebrae are visualized only because of the marrow signal. L, larynx; T, thyroid cartilage. (*B*) MRI axial view of the larynx at the level of the vocal cords.

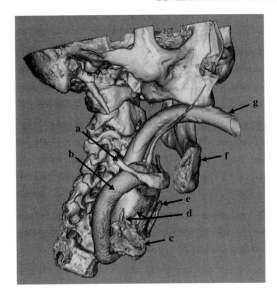

Fig. 5. LMA forms a seal with the periglottic tissues without crossing the vocal cords; the LMA is a supraglottic airway. Structures outlined include the hyoid bone (*a*), LMA cuff (*b*), cricoid cartilage (*c*), arytenoid cartilages (*d*), thyroid cartilage (partially removed for better visualization) (*e*), mandible (partially removed for better visualization) (*f*), and LMA shaft (*g*).

unique advantages and disadvantages, depending on the clinical situation.

Before the introduction of the LMA, percutanous transtracheal jet ventilation (≤50 lb per square inch), using a large-bore (16G) intravenous catheter placed through the cricothyroid membrane, was a primary method for emergency airway management in a "cannot-ventilate-cannot-intubate" scenario [11]. Effective transtracheal jet ventilation relies on the egress of air through a patent upper airway, however, and should not be used in patients with obstruction of the upper airway because it can lead to significant barotrauma.

Some techniques and devices that are described in the algorithm are rarely used in clinical practice. A study by Combes et al [12] showed that most anesthesiologists chose either the gum elastic bougie (a semirigid stylet that is passed blindly underneath the epiglottis into the trachea, over which an endotracheal tube [ETT] is passed) or an intubating LMA-Fastrach (LMA, NA, San Diego, California) to intubate patients with a grade 3 or 4 laryngoscopic view (only the epiglottis or soft palate can be seen)—even though the ASA Difficult Airway Algorithm recommends many other options and techniques. The discrepancy between the algorithm guidelines and

clinical practice stems from the fact that the algorithm is based on collective evidence from the scientific literature (ranging from individual case reports to prospective studies) and does not specify which techniques are used most often in clinical practice.

Laryngeal mask airway

The LMA is a supraglottic airway device developed by Brain in England and introduced into clinical practice in 1988. The LMA is a minimally invasive device designed for the management of the airway in an unconscious patient. It consists of an inflatable mask fitted with a tube that exits the mouth to permit ventilation of the lungs (Fig. 5). The mask fits against the periglottic tissues, occupying the hypopharyngeal space and forming a seal above the glottis instead of within the trachea. The LMA is a *supraglottic* airway management device that connects the natural and artificial airways at the level of the larynx. This unique arrangement permits easy access to the larynx through the LMA (Fig. 6). In the first article on the LMA, published in 1983 [13], Brain described his new airway device as "an alternative to either the endotracheal tube or the face-mask with either spontaneous or positive pressure ventilation." During the past 20 years, however, the LMA's role has evolved beyond routine airway management, and now the LMA has many specialized applications for different surgical and diagnostic procedures involving the airway, including pulmonary medicine, critical care, and resuscitation.

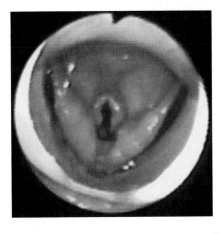

Fig. 6. View of the larynx through a fiberoptic scope placed coaxially through the LMA.

Difficult intubation or mask ventilation

The success of the LMA in patients who are difficult to intubate by conventional laryngoscopy and difficult to ventilate with a facemask is due to its design. The LMA fits into the potential space of the pharynx similar to the way a hand fits into a glove. In contrast to rigid laryngoscopy, insertion of the LMA does not rely on direct visualization of the larynx. Many factors that are associated with difficult rigid laryngoscopy (poor visualization of laryngeal structures during laryngoscopy) do not affect the insertion of and ventilation through the LMA [7–10]. The potential of the LMA for the emergency and nonemergency management of patients with difficult airways was appreciated shortly after its invention. In February 1983, an early prototype was used successfully Brain in a 114-kg man undergoing laparotomy who could not be intubated. The first publication describing the LMA as a possible solution to airway management problems in emergency situations appeared in the scientific literature in 1984 [14]. By 1985, the LMA had been used successfully in five adults in whom difficult intubation was anticipated, and in October 1987, it was used for the first time in cases of failed pediatric intubation [15]. In 1989, Allison and McCrory [16] used fiberoptic guidance through the LMA for tracheal intubations, and in 1991, McCririck and Pracilio [17] first reported an awake intubation via the LMA. Numerous case reports appeared, describing airway management with the LMA in several clinical situations, including, but not limited to, adult and pediatric patients with (1) cervical spine pathology or instability [17–21], (2) morbid obesity [22], (3) micrognathia and macrognathia [23,24], (4) Klippel-Feil syndrome [25], (5) Treacher Collins syndrome [26], (6) Pierre Robin syndrome [27], (7) Goldenhar's syndrome [28], (8) Hurler's syndrome [29], (9) Down syndrome [30], and (10) unexpected failed intubation associated with difficult facemask ventilation [31].

Airway evaluation, neck surgery, and laser surgery of the larynx

One of the unique advantages of the LMA in patients with pathologic processes involving the airway is that it offers access to the larynx and tracheobronchial tree (Fig. 6). Access is particularly useful for diagnostic evaluation of the larynx and trachea. The LMA also is useful during neodymium: yttrium-aluminum-garnet (Nd:YAG) laser surgery. It is difficult to manage the airway using an ETT in patients who require Nd:YAG laser treatment of

lesions in the larynx, the vocal cords, or the proximal part of the trachea because the presence of the ETT limits access to the lesions. Laser-induced airway fire is a high risk when an ETT is used. In contrast, the LMA provides an unobstructed view of the surgical field and virtually eliminates the risk of airway fire (Fig. 7).

Head and neck surgery is associated with the risk of bruising or otherwise traumatizing nerves that control the motor functions of the larynx. The LMA can be useful in evaluating the function of the vocal cords at the conclusion of neck dissection and thyroid and parathyroid surgery [32]. While the patient is still under general anesthesia, the LMA is inserted behind the ETT and inflated. The anesthesiologist removes the ETT so that the patient can breathe spontaneously. As the patient emerges from general anesthesia, a fiberscope is inserted through the lumen of the LMA to observe the function of the vocal cords. At the University of Texas M.D. Anderson Cancer Center, this technique has become an important diagnostic tool to determine the functional status of the nerves providing motor function to the larynx, which enables anesthesiologists and surgeons to make informed decisions about the postoperative airway management of patients. Similarly, patients undergoing brainstem surgery in the area that involves the lower cranial nerves, which control the pharynx and larynx, can be evaluated fiberoptically via the LMA in the ICU. Evaluation helps the intensivist and the surgeon determine whether patients would be able to maintain an airway postoperatively.

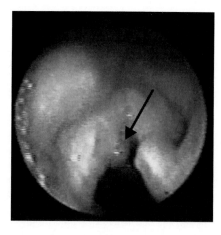

Fig. 7. Left vocal cord polyp (*arrow*) as seen through a fiberoptic scope placed via the LMA. This lesion can be treated easily with Nd:YAG laser surgery delivered through the fiberoptic scope, while continuous ventilation is maintained with the LMA.

Thoracic surgeons and pulmonary medicine physicians have shown interest in the LMA because of the unique access it provides to the larynx and respiratory tree. Diagnostic fiberoptic laryngoscopy and fiberoptic bronchoscopy (FOB) can be performed readily through the LMA in children and adults under general anesthesia or under topical anesthesia with sedation [33–35].

In infants, an appropriately sized LMA offers the following advantages as a conduit for FOB: (1) The LMA tube is much larger (5-mm internal diameter) than the corresponding ETT, permitting the use of a larger bronchoscope, which gives a better view than through the 2- to 2.5-mm bronchoscope normally required to fit through the ETT in this age group; (2) with the LMA, the larynx can be examined, including vocal cord movement and the part of the trachea normally occupied by the ETT; (3) with a larger diameter LMA airway tube, ventilation is easy, and observation is uninterrupted; and (4) an ETT is not needed for cases of laryngeal or tracheal stenosis, which might be made worse by its passage [36]. Theroux et al [37] described the use of a No. 1 size LMA as a conduit for intubation in a 2.5-kg infant with Schwartz-Jampel syndrome who could not be intubated by other means. The uncuffed ETT was advanced over a 2.2-mm bronchoscope, which was passed easily into the trachea through the LMA. In 1997, Mizikov et al [38] reported their experience of using FOB via the LMA in 45 children: 15 diagnostic cases, 22 cases of lavage, 7 cases of foreign-body removal, and 1 case of electrocoagulation of an adenoma.

Laser surgery of the trachea

In 1992, Slinger et al [39] provided a detailed account of a difficult case of palliative laser resection of a severely obstructing distal tracheal mass. The airway initially was managed using a No. 4 size LMA, through which a 6-mm Olympus FOB was passed via a swivel connector to apply the laser. Ventilation was spontaneous with propofol/isoflurane anesthesia. After 120 minutes, 50% of the tracheal lumen had been restored, at which point it was decided to convert to rigid bronchoscopy so that the surgeon could remove larger pieces of tissue using forceps, speeding the procedure. This method was repeated in two other, less severe cases without complications. The authors pointed out that the laser is not likely to burn the silicone LMA tube if it is switched on only when in the trachea. Although the rigid bronchoscope is still considered the gold standard for such cases, the LMA offers an excellent

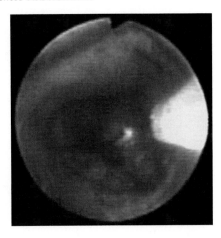

Fig. 8. Lesions located in the trachea can be accessed easily and treated with Nd:YAG laser. The LMA allows for safe and effective ventilation of the patient during laser surgery of the trachea because the LMA has a large shaft.

alternative, and in patients presenting a difficult laryngoscopic view (Cormack-Lehane grade 3 or 4), the LMA might be the technique of choice for the laser treatment of tracheal tumors (Fig. 8).

Tracheobronchial stent placement

Another advantage of using the LMA in patients with pathology involving the tracheobronchial tree is found during stent placement under fiberoptic guidance [40]. With the LMA and a 6-mm FOB, a bigger cross-sectional area is provided than with a 9-mm ETT, which typically is used during stent placement. With the LMA, ventilation is better during stent placement than with an ETT in patients who already have compromised respiratory function [39]. In patients who have an obstruction high in the trachea, the LMA also is better than an ETT because the LMA forms a connection with the natural airway at the level of the larynx for unencumbered access to the area below the glottis during stent placement. In contrast, when an ETT is used, the tip of the tube and the cuff are in the trachea; to place the stent successfully, the ETT must be partially withdrawn, which increases the risk of accidental extubation and inability to ventilate the lungs at the crucial point of the procedure (Fig. 9).

New variations of the laryngeal mask airway

In addition to the LMA-Classic, other LMA models have been developed and introduced into

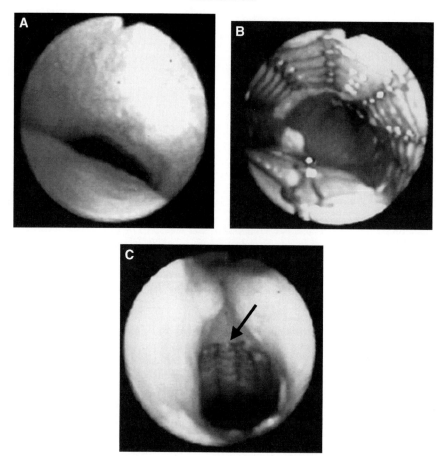

Fig. 9. View of the trachea through a fiberoptic bronchoscope placed coaxially through the LMA. (*A*) Severe narrowing of the upper trachea caused by lung cancer. (*B*) Restoration of the narrowed lumen by a tracheal stent. (*C*) Location of the upper portion of the stent (*arrow*) in close proximity to the vocal cords; such high placement of the stent would be impossible using the endotracheal tube.

clinical practice, including the LMA-Flexible (Fig. 10), the intubating LMA-Fastrach (Fig. 11), and the LMA-ProSeal (Fig. 12).

LMA-Flexible

The LMA-Flexible, which was introduced into clinical practice in 1994, is designed specifically for procedures performed on the head and neck that require the anesthesiologist and surgeon to share access to the airway (Fig. 13). Traditionally, surgeons have used special ETTs with a spiral coil built into them to increase the flexibility of the tube and to prevent kinking when manipulated during surgery for access to the operating field. To make an LMA specifically for head and neck procedures, a similar spiral coil was incorporated into the LMA's shaft, creating the LMA-Flexible.

Intubating LMA-Fastrach

The intubating LMA-Fastrach was introduced in 1997 in response to clinicians' demands for a device with the ventilatory properties of the LMA-Classic that would serve as a better conduit for intubation. The LMA-Fastrach is designed to facilitate blind or fiberoptically guided tracheal intubations without the need to move the cervical spine during intubation. Available only in adult sizes, the LMA-Fastrach consists of an anatomically curved stainless steel tube 13 mm in internal diameter that is connected firmly at its distal end to the laryngeal mask. The angle of the metal shaft was carefully designed, using measurements from sagittal MRI, to fit well into the oral and pharyngeal space while the head and neck are kept in a neutral position. Proximally the metal shaft forms a standard 15-mm connector for the anesthesia circuit,

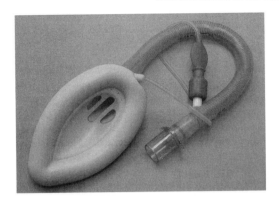

Fig. 10. The flexible LMA, which was introduced into clinical practice in 1994, has a spiral coil built into the shaft to increase the flexibility of the tube and to prevent kinking. Because of the flexibility, the surgeon can manipulate the flexible LMA's shaft during the procedure and improve access to the operating field. The flexible LMA has been used successfully in patients undergoing a variety of head and neck, eye, and oral surgeries. (Courtesy of LMA North America, Inc., San Diego, California.)

attempts or fewer in all patients. The overall success rates for blind and fiberoptically guided intubations were 97% and 100%. This study represents the largest analysis to date examining the use of the LMA-Fastrach in patients with difficult-to-manage airways. It shows that the LMA-Fastrach may be a particularly valuable tool in the emergency or elective airway management of patients in whom other techniques have failed and in the treatment of patients with immobilized cervical spines. The LMA-Fastrach also can be used as an intubating tool in patients with normal airways. In studies conducted by Brain et al [42] in 1997 and more recently by Kahl et al [43], the hemodynamic response to the LMA-Fastrach was similar to the response to the LMA-Classic; in patients with compromised cardiovascular systems, the LMA-Fastrach could be a less stimulating alternative to rigid laryngoscopy for intubation of the trachea. If the LMA-Fastrach is used in patients with normal airways, clinicians can develop their skill and familiarity with the device before using it in emergency situations.

LMA-ProSeal

The LMA-ProSeal was designed with the principal objective of providing a separate conduit for gastric fluids to bypass the glottis. The adult models of the LMA-ProSeal contain a second cuff attached to the dorsal surface of the device that improves the seal by pressing the ventral cuff into the periglottic tissue. The seal is better than that with the LMA-Classic, making positive-pressure ventilation more reliable.

Currently, data on the LMA-ProSeal in patients with difficult-to-manage airways are meager [44–47]. It is difficult to intubate the patient through the LMA-ProSeal because the airway tube is narrow and located off-center in relation to the laryngeal inlet. The LMA-ProSeal has been shown to be effective,

and a rigid guiding handle serves to insert the device and to stabilize and direct the device during intubation attempts. This shaft can accommodate an ETT 9 mm in diameter. The shaft of the LMA-Fastrach is shorter than that of the LMA-Classic, eliminating the need for longer ETTs in patients with long necks. The LMA-Fastrach is particularly useful for the ventilation and intubation of patients with difficult-to-manage airways (Fig. 14).

A study assessed the effectiveness of the LMA-Fastrach in 254 patients, including patients with Cormack-Lehane grade 4 views; patients with immobilized cervical spines;, patients with airways distorted by tumors, surgery, or radiation therapy; and patients wearing stereotactic frames [41]. Insertion of the LMA-Fastrach was accomplished in three

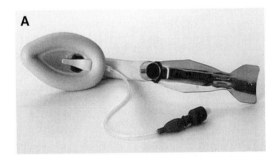

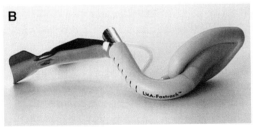

Fig. 11. The intubating LMA (LMA-Fastrach) consists of (*A*) the mask, which has the same shape as the LMA-Classic, and (*B*) a 13-mm internal diameter stainless steel shaft, which can accommodate an ETT 9 mm in internal diameter. (Courtesy of LMA North America, Inc., San Diego, California.)

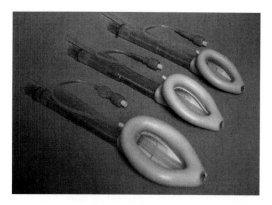

Fig. 12. The LMA-ProSeal was designed to achieve two objectives: to separate the respiratory and gastrointestinal tracts and, also, to provide a better seal around the glottis and allow positive-pressure ventilation in a more reliable manner than the LMA-Classic. (Courtesy of LMA North America, Inc., San Diego, California.)

however, for ventilation and oxygenation in morbidly obese patients [48].

Although LMAs in general (and the LMA-ProSeal in particular) have many advantages, they do not provide as secure an airway as translaryngeal intubation with an ETT. Risk for aspiration, dislodgment of the device during patient movement, laryngospasm, and reduced ability to deliver positive-pressure ventilation in some settings remain limitations.

Fiberoptic endoscopy in airway management

In 1954, Hopkins [49] first introduced the technology of using optically arranged glass fiber bundles in a flexible instrument to visualize the gastrointestinal tract internally. Commercial fiberoptic gastroscopes became available shortly thereafter and were incorporated quickly into clinical practice. It was not until 1966, however, that the fiberscope concept first was applied to examine the respiratory tract. The first flexible bronchofiberscope was manufactured according to specifications and characteristics developed by Ikeda [50]. Ovassapian [51] was one of the first anesthesiologists to use the flexible bronchofiberscope to guide elective and emergency intubations in patients with difficult-to-manage airways. Ovassapian [52] also was the first to develop a systematic approach to teaching anesthesiologists the correct technique of flexible fiberoptic intubation, popularizing the use of the instrument in modern anesthetic practice.

Several improvements have been made in fiberoptic technology, making fiberscopes more affordable, efficacious, and popular in anesthesia and critical care. Advances in microchip designs have led to the development of a new generation of high-quality bronchoscopes, called *videobronchoscopes,* which no longer rely on transmitting images through coherent fiberoptic bundles. Instead, videobronchoscopes employ the charge-coupled device (CCD), a microcamera chip that uses the single-plate red, green, and blue surface-scanning method to create images. The CCD camera is positioned behind the lens at the distal tip of the videobronchoscope. The colors red, green, and blue are transmitted sequentially from the light source to the object. The red, green, and blue light reflected by the object is received in sequence by the CCD and transmitted electronically to the image processor as black-and-white images. These images are reconstructed and displayed in color on the monitor. Videobronchoscopes are lightweight and have a larger working channel, a much wider optical angle, and better image resolution than traditional fiberscopes. These qualities are particularly important in the smaller fiberoptic bronchoscopes, which must be used to place and position double-lumen tubes and bronchial blockers, when the necessarily small working channel limits the suctioning capabilities.

Ancillary airway equipment

Over the years, ancillary devices, such as oral airways and endoscopy masks (intubating masks), have been developed to aid fiberoptic intubation. Oral airways, such as the Berman intubating pharyngeal

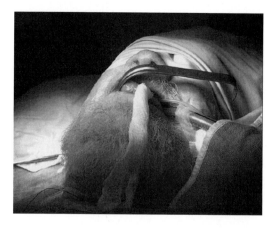

Fig. 13. The use of the flexible LMA in a patient undergoing oral surgery.

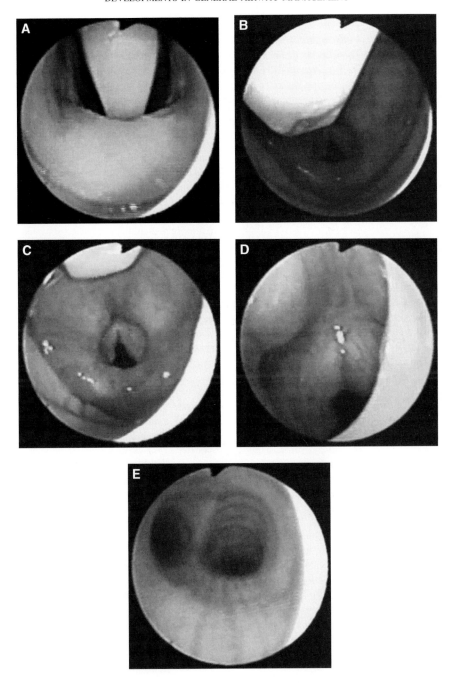

Fig. 14. Fiberoptic view of intubation through the LMA-Fastrach. (*A*) Epiglottic elevating bar (EEB), as seen from inside the shaft. (*B*) The tip of the ETT, as it advances through the LMA-Fastrach, pushes the EEB upward. (*C–D*) This movement of the EEB lifts the epiglottis out of the way (*C*) and provides a clear passage for the ETT through the vocal cords (*D*) and into the middle of the trachea (*E*).

airway, Ovassapian fiberoptic intubating airway, Patil-Syracuse endoscopic airway, and Williams airway intubator, help the endoscopist keep the fiberscope in midline and protect the instrument from being damaged should the patient bite on the cord accidentally [53–57]. Oral airways aid ventilation by facilitating the patient's ability to maintain spontaneous respiration. In contrast, with endoscopy masks, assisted or controlled ventilation is possible during intubation with the fiberscope inserted through a separate port/diaphragm in the mask [56,57].

Topical anesthesia for awake intubation

An awake fiberoptic orotracheal or nasotracheal intubation is frequently the first choice in patients considered difficult to mask ventilate and intubate with conventional laryngoscopy. The preoperative preparation is crucial to gain the patient's trust, reduce anxiety, and ensure optimal cooperation during this procedure. During the preanesthetic visit, the anesthesiologist explains the procedure and reassures the patient that appropriate medications will be administered for comfort and sedation. To decrease secretions and enhance the action of local anesthetics, an antisialagogue agent is given intravenously at least 20 minutes before airway instrumentation [58]. Whether the bronchoscopy is performed by a pulmonologist, thoracic surgeon, or anesthesiologist, topical anesthesia should be applied to attenuate or abolish protective airway reflexes and to prevent coughing and laryngeal spasm. The larynx, in its entirety, receives motor and sensory innervation from the vagus nerve, although some elements of the glossopharyngeal nerve may be present from the vagus nucleus in the hindbrain [59]. Topical anesthesia of the airway can be accomplished easily because of the superficial submucosal location of the sensory nerve endings. Lidocaine is the most widely used medicine for topical anesthesia of the respiratory tract during bronchoscopy and awake tracheal intubation [60]. The drug can be delivered to the airway using several methods and is available in different preparations (ie, 0.5%, 1%, 2%, and 4% solutions; 2.5% viscous gels; 10% aerosol preparation; and 2.5% and 5% ointment). Other medications used for airway topicalization include cocaine, tetracaine, and benzocaine. Topical cocaine is particularly useful in minimizing the risk of bleeding during nasal intubation because cocaine causes vasoconstriction in addition to local anesthesia [61]. Tetracaine, which is a derivative of para-aminobenzoic acid, has a longer duration of action than lidocaine or cocaine.

Tetracaine has a narrow therapeutic margin, however, and serious complications, including sudden death as the first sign of local anesthetic toxicity, have been reported [62]. Tetracaine no longer is recommended for tracheobronchial topical anesthesia. Benzocaine, another local anesthetic, has a rapid onset of action (15–30 seconds) and a short duration of action (5–10 minutes). Benzocaine can produce methemoglobinemia, however, especially in neonates, who are more susceptible to benzocaine because fetal hemoglobin is oxidized more easily than adult hemoglobin [63,64].

Local anesthetics can be applied to the mucous membranes by spraying the mucosa directly or using cotton-tipped applicators or aerosol inhalation. In the "spray as you go" technique, described and popularized by Ovassapian [58], anesthetic is applied to specific parts of the airway. This technique is useful in anesthetizing the larynx and trachea. During "spray as you go," the clinician positions the tip of the fiberscope directly above the structures that need to be anesthetized. Local anesthetic is administered in small increments directly through the small suction channel (0.5–1 mm diameter) of the fiberoptic scope. In scopes with a larger suction channel (2–2.5 mm diameter), the stream of the local anesthetic can be controlled easily, first by passing a long angiocath or epidural catheter (0.5–1 mm internal diameter) through the suction channel, then by connecting the catheter to the syringe via a three-way stopcock for suctioning during the procedure. When used correctly, the "spray as you go" technique seems to be optimal for most awake intubations, including in patients who are at risk for aspiration because the airway is anesthetized sequentially, keeping patients' protective reflexes intact until the last few moments before intubation.

In patients with increased intracranial pressure or an open eye injury, coughing can be detrimental. In patients with severe coronary disease, stimulation of the airway associated with awake fiberscopy could lead to tachycardia and hypertension, increasing the risk of myocardial ischemia. To avoid this risk, an aerosolized topical anesthetic can be delivered safely with a nebulizer in these patients. The patient is instructed to breathe slowly and deeply while 4 to 6 mL of 4% lidocaine is administered via a nebulizer using 8 to 10 L/min of oxygen to achieve the optimal aerosolization. The advantages of aerosol inhalation include ease and simplicity of application and safety. Nebulization causes little, if any, discomfort and is well tolerated and accepted by patients. The risk of coughing is minimized. This technique is time-consuming, however, and in some patients may result in suboptimal anesthesia to the larynx [65,66].

Another method of providing anesthesia to the airway during fiberoptic intubation is to use a variety of nerve blocks in combination with translaryngeal instillation of local anesthetic. In anesthetic practice, the superior laryngeal nerve frequently is blocked during awake fiberoptic intubation. The nerve is anesthetized by injecting 2 to 3 mL of 1% lidocaine bilaterally between the superior horn of the thyroid cartilage and the hyoid bone. Alternatively, as described by Labat [67], the needle is inserted at the thyroid notch and directed upward and backward toward the thyrohyoid membrane. Because the superior laryngeal nerve block provides anesthesia above the vocal cords only, the portion of the larynx located below the vocal cords and trachea is anesthetized by translaryngeal instillation of a local anesthetic. Percutaneous injection of a local anesthetic into the transcricothyroid membrane first was described by the French anesthesiologist Canuyt [68] and subsequently adopted for bronchoscopy and tracheal intubation [69,70]. The patient is asked to refrain from talking, swallowing, or coughing during the injection. The skin above the cricothyroid membrane is anesthetized by local infiltration of 1% lidocaine through a 25G needle. Subsequently a 20G over-the-needle catheter connected to a 5-mL syringe filled with 3 mL of 4% lidocaine is inserted perpendicularly through the cricothyroid membrane and into the trachea. Aspiration of air into the syringe confirms the correct placement of the catheter in the airway. The needle is removed from the catheter, the syringe is reattached to the catheter, and aspiration is repeated to confirm the position of the catheter in the trachea. The patient is asked to take a deep breath. With the catheter firmly secured by one hand, lidocaine is injected rapidly. As the patient coughs, the local anesthetic is sprayed from the trachea to the oropharynx, anesthetizing the lower portion of the larynx. A more detailed description of the fiberoptic technique is provided by Ovassapian in his textbook [71,72]. One of the best centers for teaching excellence in fiberoptic intubation has been established by Ovassapian at the University of Chicago. This center offers basic and advanced clinical training in the use of fiberoptic intubation and bronchoscopy.

Indirect rigid laryngoscopes

Many indirect rigid laryngocopes have been designed to facilitate tracheal intubation in patients with the same kind of difficulties as patients for whom flexible fiberoptic intubation is useful. These laryngocopes combine fiberoptic visualization with the mechanics involved in direct laryngoscopy. These devices, which include the Bullard laryngoscope [73], the UpsherScope [74], and the WuScope [75], are generally more portable, less costly, and better for displacement of supraglottic soft tissue and control of blood or secretions than the flexible fiberoptic bronchoscope. Mastering these devices entails a learning curve, and one laryngoscope has not been shown to be superior to another.

Summary

Since the 1970s, improvements in airway management have been significant. New imaging modalities such as CT and MRI can display airway structures with unparalleled detail, which improves preoperative planning and the treatment of patients with pathologic processes involving the respiratory tract or with difficult-to-manage airways. Because of the introduction of flexible fiberscopes, pulmonologists and thoracic surgeons can diagnose diseases of the respiratory tract effectively and treat patients with these diseases safely. The use of flexible fiberscopes has expanded rapidly into other medical specialties, including anesthesia and critical care. Modern anesthesiologists now use flexible fiberscopes daily to intubate patients safely, especially when traditional intubating techniques fail. The cost of fiberscopes has decreased dramatically, and their optical systems have improved. Several centers of excellence have been developed where clinicians can learn basic and advanced techniques of fiberoptic intubation. The LMA has shown that the supraglottic airway approach is not only feasible, but also in many situations superior to tracheal intubation. Although the LMA initially was recommended as an alternative to the facemask, its use has expanded, benefiting many children and adults undergoing a variety of diagnostic and therapeutic procedures. Use of an LMA in combination with a flexible fiberscope has opened up new possibilities for treating patients safely and effectively while providing optimal comfort during a procedure and has been particularly beneficial in thoracic surgery. The most recent iteration of the ASA Difficult Airway Algorithm has revised further a systematic approach to the clinical care of patients with different types of difficult-to-manage airways.

References

[1] Caplan RA, Posner KL, Ward RJ, et al. Adverse respiratory events in anesthesia: a closed claims analysis. Anesthesiology 1990;72:828–33.

[2] Benumof JL, Scheller MS. The importance of transtracheal jet ventilation in the management of the difficult airway. Anesthesiology 1989;71:769.

[3] Bellhouse CP, Dore C. Criteria for estimating likelihood of difficulty of endotracheal intubation with Macintosh laryngoscope. Anaesth Intensive Care 1987; 42:487.

[4] American Society of Anesthesiologists Task Force on Management of the Difficult Airway. Practice guidelines for management of the difficult airway: a report. Anesthesiology 1993;78:597.

[5] Practice guidelines for management of the difficult airway: an updated report by the American Society of Anesthesiologists Task Force on Management of the Difficult Airway. Anesthesiology 2003;98:1269.

[6] Langeron O, Masso E, Huraux C, et al. Prediction of difficult mask ventilation. Anesthesiology 2000;92:1229.

[7] Mallampati SR. Clinical sign to predict difficult tracheal intubation (hypothesis). Can J Anaesth 1983;30:316.

[8] Mallampati SR, Gatt SP, Gugino LD, et al. A clinical sign to predict difficult tracheal intubation: a prospective study. Can J Anaesth 1985;32:429.

[9] Cormak RS, Lehane J. Difficult tracheal intubation in obstetrics. Anaesthesia 1984;39:1105–11.

[10] El-Ganzouri AR, Mc Carthy RJ, Tuman KJ, et al. Preoperative airway assessment: predictive value of a multivariate risk index. Anesth Analg 1996;82:1197.

[11] Jacobs HB. Needle catheter brings oxygen to the trachea. JAMA 1972;222:1231.

[12] Combes X, Le Roux B, Suen P, et al. Unanticipated difficult airway in anesthetized patients: prospective validation of a management algorithm. Anesthesiology 2004;5:1146.

[13] Brain AIJ. The laryngeal mask—a new concept in airway management. Br J Anaesth 1983;55:801–5.

[14] Brain AIJ. The laryngeal mask airway: a possible new solution to airway problems in the emergency situation. Arch Emerg Med 1984;1:229–32.

[15] Brain AIJ. The development of the laryngeal mask—a brief history of the invention, early clinical studies and experimental work from which the laryngeal mask evolved. Eur J Anaesthesiol 1991;4:5–17.

[16] Allison A, McCrory J. Tracheal placement of a gum elastic bougie using the laryngeal mask airway. Anaesthesia 1990;45:419–20.

[17] McCririck A, Pracilio JA. Awake intubation: a new technique. Anaesthesia 1991;46:661–3.

[18] Smith BL. Brain airway in anesthesia for patients with juvenile chronic arthritis. Anaesthesia 1988;43:421.

[19] Silk JM, Hill HM, Calder I. Difficult intubation and the laryngeal mask. Eur J Anaesthesiol 1991;4:47–51.

[20] Asai T. Fiberoptic tracheal intubation through the laryngeal mask airway in an awake patient with cervical spine instability. Anesth Analg 1993;77:404.

[21] Logan A. Use of the laryngeal mask in a patient with an unstable fracture of the cervical spine. Anaesthesia 1991;46:987.

[22] Godley M, Ramachandra AR. Use of LMA for awake intubation for Caesarian section. Can J Anaesth 1996;43:299–302.

[23] Aye T, Milne B. Use of the laryngeal mask prior to definitive intubation in a difficult airway: a case report. J Emerg Med 1995;13:711–4.

[24] Thomason KD. A blind nasal intubation using a laryngeal mask airway. Anaesthesia 1993;48:785–7.

[25] Adejumo SWA, Davies MW. The laryngeal mask airway—another trick. Anaesthesia 1996;51:604.

[26] Fuchs K, Kukule I, Knoch M, Wiegand W. The laryngeal mask versus intubation in difficult intubation conditions in the Franceschetti-Zwahlen-Klein syndrome (Treacher-Collins syndrome). Anasthesiol Intensivmed Noftallmed Schmerzther 1993;28:190–2.

[27] Baraka A. Laryngeal mask airway for resuscitation of a newborn with Pierre Robin syndrome. Anesthesiology 1995;83:645–6.

[28] Johnson CM, Sims C. Awake fiberoptic intubation via a laryngeal mask in an infant with Goldenhar's syndrome. Anaesth Intensive Care 1994;22:194–7.

[29] Goldie AS, Hudson I. Fiberoptic tracheal intubation through a modified laryngeal mask. Paediatr Anaesth 1992;2:344.

[30] Gronert BJ. Laryngeal mask airway for management of airway and extracorporeal shock wave lithotripsy. Paediatr Anaesth 1996;6:147–50.

[31] McClune S, Regain M, Moore J. Laryngeal mask airway for Caesarean section. Anaesthesia 1990;45:2278.

[32] Eltzschig HK, Posner M, Moore Jr FD. The use of readily available equipment in a simple method for intraoperative monitoring of recurrent laryngeal nerve function during thyroid surgery: initial experience with more than 300 cases. Arch Surg 2002;137:452–6.

[33] Brimacombe J, Tucker P, Simmons S. The laryngeal mask airway for awake diagnostic bronchoscopy: a retrospective study of 200 consecutive patients. Eur J Anaesthesiol 1995;12:1017–23.

[34] Du Plessis M, Marshall Barr A, Verghese C, et al. Fiberoptic bronchoscopy under general anesthesia using the laryngeal mask airway. Eur J Anaesthesiol 1993;10:363–5.

[35] Ferson DZ, Nesbitt JC, Nesbitt K, et al. The laryngeal mask airway: a new standard for airway evaluation in thoracic surgery. Ann Thorac Surg 1997;63:768–72.

[36] Maekawa H, Mikawa K, Tanaka O, Goto R, Obara H. The laryngeal mask may be a useful device for fiberoptic airway endoscopy in pediatric anesthesia. Anesthesiology 1991;75:169–70.

[37] Theroux MC, Kettrick RG, Khine HH. Laryngeal mask airway and fiberoptic endoscopy in an infant with Schwartz-Jampel syndrome. Anesthesiology 1995; 82:605.

[38] Mizikov VM, Variushina TV, Kirimov I. Fiberoptic bronchoscopy via laryngeal mask in children. Anesteziol Reanimatol 1997;5:78–80.

[39] Slinger P, Robinson R, Shennib H, Benumof JL, Eisenkraft JB. Alternative technique for laser resection of a carinal obstruction. J Cardiothorac Vasc Anesth 1992;6:749–55.

[40] Catala JC, Garcia-Pedrajas F, Carrera J, Monedero P. Placement of an endotracheal device via the laryngeal mask airway in a patient with tracheal stenosis. Anesthesiology 1996;84:239–40.

[41] Ferson DZ, Rosenblatt WH, Johansen MJ, Osborn I, Ovassapian A. Use of the intubating LMA-Fastrach in 254 patients with difficult-to-manage airways. Anesthesiology 2000;95:1175–81.

[42] Brain AIJ, Verghese C, Addy EV, Kapila A, Brimacombe J. The intubating laryngeal mask II: a preliminary clinical report of a new means of intubating the trachea. Br J Anaesth 1997;79:704–9.

[43] Kahl M, Eberhart LHJ, Behnke H, et al. Stress response to tracheal intubation in patients undergoing coronary artery surgery: direct laryngoscopy versus an intubating laryngeal mask airway. J Cardiothorac Vasc Anesth 2004;18:275–80.

[44] Twigg SJ, Cook TM. Anaesthesia in an adult with Rubenstein-Taybi syndrome using the ProSeal laryngeal mask airway. Br J Anaesth 2002;89:786–7.

[45] Nixon T, Brimacombe J, Goldrick P, McManus S. Airway rescue with the ProSeal laryngeal mask airway in the intensive care unit. Anaesth Intensive Care 2003; 31:475–6.

[46] Rosenblatt WH. The use of the LMA-ProSeal in airway resuscitation. Anesth Analg 2003;97:1773–5.

[47] Brown NI, Mack PF, Mitera DM, Dhar P. Use of the ProSeal laryngeal mask airway in a pregnant patient with a difficult airway during electroconvulsive therapy. Br J Anaesth 2003;91:752–4.

[48] Keller C, Brimacombe J, Kleisasser A, Brimacombe L. The laryngeal mask airway ProSeal as a temporary ventilatory device in grossly and morbidly obese patients before laryngoscope-guided tracheal intubation. Anesth Analg 2002;94:737–40.

[49] Hopkins HH. The physics of the fiberoptic endoscope. In: Berci G, editor. Endoscopy. New York: Appleton-Century-Crofts; 1976. p. 27–63.

[50] Ikeda S. Atlas of flexible bronchofiberscopy. Baltimore: University Park Press; 1974.

[51] Ovassapian A. Management of the difficult airway. In: Ovassapian A, editor. Fiberoptic endoscopy and the difficult airway. 2nd edition. Philadelphia: Raven Press; 1996. p. 201–30.

[52] Ovassapian A. Learning fiberoptic intubation. In: Ovassapian A, editor. Fiberoptic endoscopy and the difficult airway. 2nd edition. Philadelphia: Raven Press; 1996. p. 263–71.

[53] Berman RA. A method for blind intubation of the trachea or esophagus. Anesth Analg 1977;56:866–7.

[54] Ovassapian A. A new fiberoptic intubating airway. Anesth Analg 1987;66(Suppl):S132.

[55] Patil V, Stehling LC, Zauder HL. Mechanical aids for fiberoptic endoscopy. Anesthesiology 1982;57:69–70.

[56] Williams RT, Harrison RE. Prone tracheal intubation simplified using an airway intubator. Can Anaesth Soc J 1981;28:288–9.

[57] Mallios C. A modification of the Laerdal anaesthesia mask for nasotracheal intubation with the fiberoptic laryngoscope. Anaesthesia 1980;35:599–600.

[58] Ovassapian A. Flexible bronchoscopic intubation of awake patients. J Bronchol 1994;1:240–5.

[59] Widdicombe JG. Sensory innervation of the lungs and airways. In: Cervero F, Morrison JFB, editors. Progress in brain research, vol. 67. Amsterdam: Elsevier Science; 1986. p. 49–64.

[60] Ovassapian A. Topical anesthesia of the airway. In: Ovassapian A, editor. Fiberoptic endoscopy and the difficult airway. 2nd edition. Philadelphia: Raven Press; 1996. p. 47–60.

[61] Schenck NL. Local anesthesia in otolaryngology. Ann Otol 1975;84:65–72.

[62] Weisel W, Tella RA. Reaction to tetracaine used as topical anesthetic in bronchoscopy. JAMA 1951;147: 218–22.

[63] Severinghouse JW, Xu-F-D, Spellman MJ. Benzocaine and methemoglobin: recommended actions. Anesthesiology 1991;74:385–6.

[64] Rodriguez LF, Smolik LM, Zbehlik AJ. Benzocaine-induced methemoglobinemia: report of a severe reaction and review of the literature. Ann Pharmacother 1994;28:643–9.

[65] Bourke DL, Katz J, Tonneson A. Nebulized anesthesia for awake endotracheal intubation. Anesthesiology 1985;63:690–2.

[66] Faber LP. Flexible fiberoptic bronchoscopy. In: Berri G, editor. Endoscopy. New York: Appleton-Century-Crofts; 1976. p. 571–86.

[67] Labat G. In: Regional anesthesa: its technical and clinical application. 2nd edition. Philadelphia: WB Saunders; 1928. p. 143.

[68] Canuyt G. Les injections intratracheales par la voie intercricothyroidienne. Soc Med Chir Bordeau 1920; 249–59.

[69] Harken DE, Salzberg AM. Transtracheal anesthesia for bronchoscopy. N Engl J Med 1948;239:383–5.

[70] Bonica JJ. Transtracheal anesthesia for tracheal intubation. Anesthesiology 1948;10:736–8.

[71] Ovassapian A. Fiberoptic tracheal intubation in adults. In: Ovassapian A, editor. Fiberoptic endoscopy and the difficult airway. 2nd edition. Philadelphia: Raven Press; 1996. p. 71–103.

[72] Ovassapian A. Fiberoptic tracheal intubation in children. In: Ovassapian A, editor. Fiberoptic endoscopy and the difficult airway. 2nd edition. Philadelphia: Raven Press; 1996. p. 105–15.

[73] Bjoraker DG. The Bullard intubating laryngoscopes. Anesthesiol Rev 1990;17:64–70.

[74] Pearce AC, Shaw S, Macklin S. Evaluation of the Upsherscope: a new rigid fibrescope. Anaesthesia 1996;51:561–4.

[75] Wu TL, Chou HC. A new laryngoscope: the combination intubating device. Anesthesiology 1994;81: 1085–7.

ELSEVIER
SAUNDERS

Thorac Surg Clin 15 (2005) 55 – 70

THORACIC
SURGERY
CLINICS

Advances and New Insights in Monitoring

John P. Lawrence, MD

Department of Anesthesia, University of Cincinnati, 231 Albert Sabin Way, PO Box 670531, Cincinnati, OH 45267-0531, USA

The field of anesthesiology has been at the forefront of advancing the standards and science of patient monitoring. New innovations and guidelines in patient monitoring and evaluation have helped make new surgical techniques possible and better health care a reality. Although it has not been proved that monitoring affects outcome, circumstantial evidence suggests that basic cardiorespiratory monitoring decreases the incidence of serious accidents [1]. In the Australian Incident Study, 52% of incidents related to anesthesia were detected by a monitor first [2]. After the introduction of basic cardiorespiratory monitoring in the Harvard hospitals during the 1980s, the numbers of serious accidents and deaths were substantially reduced [1]. Before the 1960s, patient monitoring during anesthesia consisted primarily of observation, palpation, auscultation, and assessment of vital signs [3]. In 1986, the American Society of Anesthesiologists (ASA) first published the Standards for Basic Anesthesia Monitoring [4].

As health care continues to overcome challenging ailments, the need for new techniques of patient monitoring has never been greater. Although there have been some important advances in monitoring technology, a thorough understanding of the application of available technology is just as important to safe, state-of-the-art patient care. This article summarizes basic principles of patient monitoring as they relate to technologic advances, reviews pitfalls of commonly used patient monitors, and describes advances in monitoring technology that promise to improve patient care.

Standards of monitoring

The ASA Standards for Basic Anesthetic Monitoring first were published in 1986 and later reaffirmed in 2003 [4]. *Standards* are defined by the ASA as "rules" (eg, minimal requirements for sound practice). The first of the two monitoring standards states that "qualified anesthesia personnel shall be present throughout the conduct of all general anesthetics and monitored anesthesia care." The presence of a trained and experienced anesthetist is the main determinant of patient safety during anesthesia [1]. No piece of electronic equipment can replace a trained, vigilant clinician capable of intervening on behalf of the patient. The modern instruments of monitoring technology available for use today have little value unless (1) used consistently, (2) operated properly, (3) interpreted correctly, and (4) applied appropriately. It cannot be overemphasized that if the monitors are not used properly, they simply have no value and may endanger the patient because their use can lead to a false sense of security or misguided treatment. The electronic circuitry of monitoring technology is not capable of ensuring adequate oxygenation, ventilation, and circulation. Only a clinician trained in the use of monitoring technology and medicine is capable of assimilating all of the information and ensuring patient safety.

Standard 2 states that during all anesthetics, the patient's oxygenation, ventilation, circulation, and temperature shall be evaluated continually [4]. The document further elaborates on the methods by which these physiologic parameters must be monitored, including oxygen concentration of the inspired gas, blood oxygenation, presence of expired carbon dioxide, volume of expired gas, electrocardiogram, peripheral pulse, and blood pressure.

E-mail address: lawrenjp@ucmail.uc.edu

1547-4127/05/$ – see front matter © 2005 Elsevier Inc. All rights reserved.
doi:10.1016/j.thorsurg.2004.09.002

Oxygenation

Pulse oximetry

It has long been known that the presence of peripheral cyanosis is a late and unreliable method to detect arterial hypoxemia, and, when present, it usually indicates a significant problem that could result in full cardiovascular collapse. Between the mid-1980s and early 1990s, the pulse oximeter went from experimental technology to one of the most ubiquitous pieces of medical equipment in use today [5]. The use of a pulse oximeter and a monitor of the inspired oxygen concentration are required according to Standard 2 of the ASA Standards of Basic Anesthetic Monitoring [4].

Principles

The pulse oximeter permits measurement of the arterial oxygen saturation by detecting differences in absorption of oxygenated and deoxygenated hemoglobin. Two light-emitting diodes, red (660 nm) and near infrared (940 nm), are used. Oxygenated hemoglobin has been found to absorb light best at the 940-nm wavelength, whereas deoxygenated hemoglobin has been found to absorb light best at the 660-nm wavelength. When the relative ratio of the transmission of the two wavelengths of light is compared with the standard, a percentage of oxygenated hemoglobin can be obtained. The oxygen saturation must be interpreted in the context of the oxyhemoglobin dissociation curve, with leftward or rightward shifts of this curve invalidating the rule of thumb, which is that when the oxygen saturation is 90%, the PaO_2 is approximately 60 mm Hg (Fig. 1). As the PaO_2 decreases to less than 60 mm Hg, the pulse oximeter becomes a poor indicator of the actual oxygen saturation, especially when the oxygen saturation reading is less than 80%.

Limitations

One limitation of the pulse oximeter (and all commercially available monitors) is the nature of the display. Pulse oximeters do not display the real-time instantaneous oxygen saturation. Pulse oximeters (and other monitors) display a time-weighted average: The number displayed on the monitor is the average oxygen saturation level over the previous 8 to 12 seconds, depending on the brand and setting of the monitor. Some devices change (increase) this time averaging as a way to reduce the artifact of patient movement or low perfusion states [6]. It is reassuring to see a normal saturation, but it is important to appreciate that when the oxygen saturation

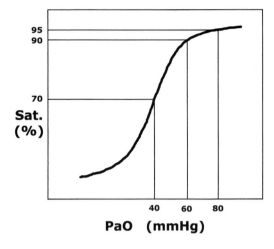

Fig. 1. Oxyhemoglobin dissociation curve. (*From:* Dionne RA, Becker D, Phero JC. Management of pain and anxiety in the dental office. Philadelphia: WB Saunders; with permission.)

decreases acutely on the monitor, the patient's actual saturation declined 12 seconds prior (or longer). Similarly, improvement of the oxygen saturation reading when adequate oxygenation is restored takes equally as long. Not recognizing this inherent delay in the recovery of the oxygen saturation reading can lead the clinician to believe that interventions or procedures (eg, intubation) are unsuccessful and erroneously discontinue them (eg, remove a properly placed endotracheal tube). The clinician may need to use information from more than one monitor (pulse oximeter and capnograph) to assess the same situation. Although the pulse oximeter is reliable in reporting the oxygen saturation and facilitating correction of hypoxemia, there are few data that have shown that the use of the pulse oximeter alters duration of hospital stay or mortality [7].

Innovations

Pulse oximeter technology has undergone some innovations to overcome two of the most frequently encountered artifacts, patient movement and low perfusion states. Box 1 contains a complete list of

---

Box 1. Factors leading to malfunction or misleading information

- Motion artifact
- Low perfusion states
- Ambient light interference
- Electromechanical interference
- Abnormal hemoglobin species

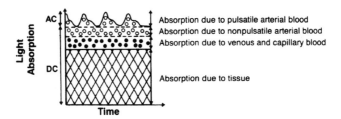

Fig. 2. Principle of pulse oximetry.

factors leading to malfunction or misleading information. In 1989, the Masimo Corporation (Irvine, California) developed a way to overcome these artifacts [8–10]. This new technology employs a concept called *Signal Extraction Pulse Oximetry* [6]. The basic concept of Signal Extraction Pulse Oximetry revises an original assumption of pulse oximetry *that the absorbance due to venous and capillary blood remained constant*. To understand, one needs to review one of the basic concepts of conventional pulse oximetry.

The conventional pulse oximeter probe transilluminates the patient's tissues (usually a finger) with red and infrared light. When the probe transilluminates a finger, a portion of the light is absorbed by the tissues between the light source and sensor, but this is not constant over time. The blood volume in the sample tissue changes with each heart beat. If it is assumed that the absorption due to tissue, venous and capillary blood, and nonpulsatile arterial blood is constant (denoted DC), the only absorption that is of interest is the absorption due to pulsatile arterial blood (Fig. 2). Conventional pulse oximeters measure the absorbance at two wavelengths (660 nm and 940 nm) as stated before, but the pulse oximeter evaluates the absorbance at these two wavelengths and separates out the absorbance due to the AC and the DC portions. The different absorbance values of AC and DC at the two wavelengths are inserted into the formula $R = (AC_{660}/DC_{660})/(AC_{940}/DC_{940})$. The calculated R value is compared with an internal nomogram and generates an oxygen saturation number that is displayed on the monitor [11].

Masimo Corporation revised the basic concept by assuming that when a patient's hand moved, the absorbance due to venous and capillary blood changes and creates signal noise (or artifact) that masks the true physiologic signal. The Masimo system uses adaptive filters to filter out the venous signal (nonarterial noise) from the arterial signal by making the assumption that the higher signal is the actual arterial saturation (Fig. 3). In clinical trials, Masimo has proved to report oxygen saturation more reliably in the settings of patient motion and low perfusion states [12,13].

If the Masimo pulse oximeter is unavailable, the clinician can verify the quality of information from the conventional pulse oximeter by verifying the

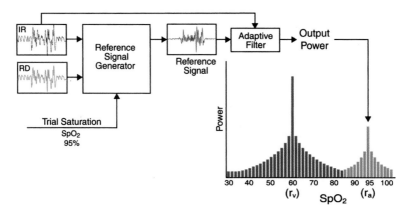

Fig. 3. Discrete Saturation Transform (DST) algorithm. (Courtesy of Masimo Corporation, Irvine, California; with permission. Copyright 2004 Masimo Corporation. All rights reserved.)

presence of a pulsatile waveform. Without a pulsatile waveform, any information that is displayed must be viewed with skepticism.

Abnormal hemoglobin species can lead to misinterpretation of pulse oximetry data [14]. Carbon monoxide poisoning can lead to the development of carboxyhemoglobin, the absorption pattern of which is similar to oxygenated hemoglobin (Fig. 4). This similar pattern causes the pulse oximeter to include carboxyhemoglobin mistakenly with oxygenated hemoglobin in the R value calculation, leading to artifactually high oxygen saturation. Additionally the plethoric appearance of the patient further misleads the clinician into a false sense of security. Withholding oxygen therapy in this setting is especially deleterious because the most effective treatment of carbon monoxide poisoning is supplemental oxygen therapy [11].

Methemoglobinemia leads to an erroneously low oxygen saturation reading. Methemoglobin absorbs red and infrared light equivalently at 940 nm and 660 nm. The pulse oximeter calculates an R value that is meaningless because it fails to reflect the actual ratio of oxygenated hemoglobin to deoxygenated hemoglobin. When the resulting R value is calculated and the R value is compared with the internal nomogram, a lower saturation is generated. As the amount of methemoglobin increases, the oxygen saturation reading approaches 85% [11]. This 85% saturation does not reflect oxygenated hemoglobin, however, only the methemoglobin. The patient's cyanotic

appearance further confuses the situation and leads to the mistaken impression that the patient is unresponsive to standard therapies. The patient is at risk of complications from overly aggressive attempts at correcting a misleading pulse oximeter reading.

Cerebral oximetry

One of the newest variations on the traditional pulse oximeter is the cerebral oximeter. The published uses of this device include adult and pediatric cardiovascular surgery [15], carotid endarterectomy [16], general anesthesia [17], neurosurgery and delayed ischemic neurologic deficit [18], implantable cardioverter-defibrillator implants [19], interventional cardiology procedures [20], trauma [21], and septic shock [22]. There are two commercially available noninvasive monitors of cerebral oxygenation, the INVOS (In-Vivo Optical Spectroscopy) cerebral oximeter made by Somanetics and the NIRO-300 made by Hamamatsu. The INVOS and the NIRO-300 use near-infrared spectrophotometry to detect and monitor the cerebral oxygen saturation.

Principles

The theory behind the INVOS device is that it transmits near-infrared light photons (730 nm and 810 nm) into the skin, skull, and brain over the forehead. The monitor displays an average level of

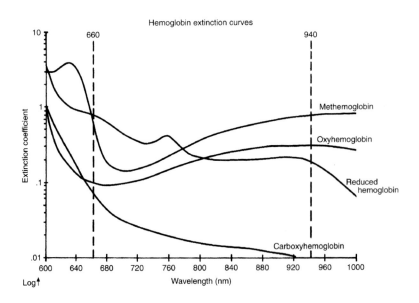

Fig. 4. Hemoglobin extinction curves.

tissue oxygenation based on the quantity of returned photons of light as a function of the wavelength [23–25]. This theory and application of near-infrared light technology is similar to that used by the traditional pulse oximeter except that the INVOS monitor analyzes the average oxygenation of all tissues under the probe (skin, skull, and brain) without analyzing the pulsatile nature of the underlying tissues. To eliminate the absorbance data due to scalp and skull tissue, which are of little interest, there is a signal subtraction algorithm that uses one transmitting light source and two sensor locations (30 mm and 40 mm) within the same self-adhesive electrode (Fig. 5). (The signal detected at the 30-mm sensor [largely due to scalp and skull tissue] is subtracted from the signal at the 40-mm sensor [due to scalp, skull, and brain], which reduces the interference from the scalp and skull.) The manufacturer reports that the subtraction algorithm reduces the artifact from scalp and skull to about 15% of the reported saturation value [25].

The NIRO-300 (Hamamatsu Photonics) uses a single self-adhesive probe that transmits four wavelengths of near-infrared light (775 nm, 825 nm, 850 nm, 904 nm) [25]. The light is detected about 50 mm away from the transmitter by three closely mounted detectors (Fig. 6). The photodiode chip is able to calculate the quantitative tissue oxygenation index, which represents the ratio of oxyhemoglobin to total hemoglobin oxygenation (oxygenated hemoglobin + deoxygenated hemoglobin) [25].

Use

Early evidence suggests that when cerebral oximetry is used in cardiac surgery patients, there is a reduction in ICU stay [26], neurologic injuries, renal failure, and length of stay [27,28]. A prospective analysis of the use of the INVOS system in pediatric patients undergoing repair of congenital heart lesions reported a 6% to 7% incidence of obvious neurologic sequelae (ie, seizure, movement, vision, or speech disorder) in patients who either did not show a change in the cerebral oximeter reading or in whom an intervention was performed to improve the cerebral oxygenation compared with a 26% incidence in neurologic events when an intervention was indicated but not performed [29].

The INVOS and NIRO systems have been compared with each other in healthy pediatric patients undergoing uncomplicated noncardiac operations, and in this study little agreement was found between the two devices. The authors concluded that there was a large range in reported saturation index and tissue oxygenation index values in healthy children, making it difficult to define a normal range, and that these monitors probably were not going to be useful for routine general anesthetics [25].

The setting where the INVOS 5100 and NIRO-300 likely will be most useful is in clinical situations in which the cerebral blood flow or cerebral oxygen saturation are anticipated to fluctuate to the degree that an adverse neurologic outcome may occur or be worsened unless an intervention is made to opti-

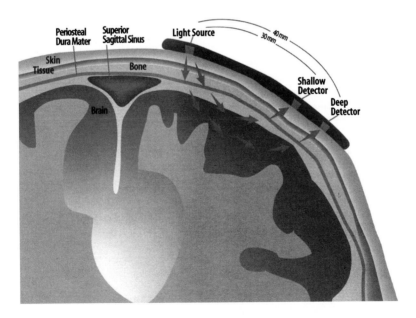

Fig. 5. INVOS electrode. (Courtesy of Somanetics Corporation, Troy, Michigan; with permission.)

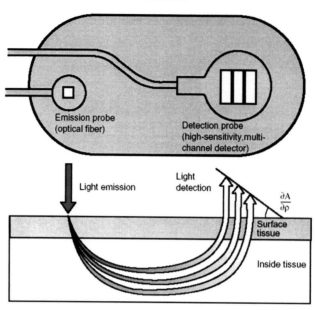

Fig. 6. NIRO-300 electrode. (Courtesy of Hamamatsu Corporation; with permission.)

mize the blood flow or oxygen delivery. It seems reasonable that critically ill patients and patients undergoing cardiac and neurologic operations would be in this group.

Ventilation

Standard 2 of the ASA Standards for Basic Anesthetic Monitoring states that the adequacy of ventilation is to be monitored during all anesthetics [4]. Although a great deal of information can be obtained by observation and auscultation, subtle and possibly hazardous situations can go unnoticed. For this reason, monitoring of exhaled tidal volume, airway pressure, and respiratory gases is required to provide anesthesia safely. Modern anesthesia machines have monitors of tidal volume and airway pressure built in to monitor exhaled tidal volume and minute ventilation. These monitors alert the clinician when the minute ventilation falls below a set minimum or if the patient is exposed to either excessive or inadequate airway pressure. These monitors also are an integral part of all modern ventilators found in ICUs.

Capnometry

One of the most significant advances in anesthesiology came in the early 1980s when capnography became an integral monitor of the adequacy of

intubation and ventilation. Capnometry is the detection and quantification of exhaled carbon dioxide, and *capnography* is the display of the carbon dioxide waveform as a function of time. Three types of monitors can detect and quantify carbon dioxide: mass spectrophotometer, Raman scattering, and infrared detectors. Most monitors used today are of the infrared variety. A sample of exhaled gas is drawn from the breathing circuit (close to the endotracheal tube). The sample of gas is transilluminated with infrared light, and the absorbance pattern is analyzed and displayed as a function of time (Fig. 7). The

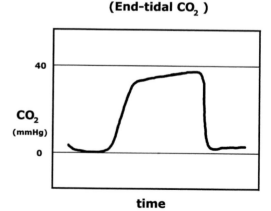

Fig. 7. Normal capnograph waveform. (Dionne RA, Becker D, Phero JC. Management of pain and anxiety in the dental office. Philadelphia: WB Saunders; with permission.)

capnograph has had a tremendous impact on reducing the complications associated with intubation and mechanical ventilation [30]. The original purpose of the capnograph was to confirm endotracheal intubation and limit the risk of esophageal intubation, but the capnograph can provide a wealth of additional information about the quantity of carbon dioxide production, pattern of breathing, quality of airflow in the lungs, level of cardiac output, and degree of alveolar dead space [11,31].

Although capnography is used routinely in the operating room, it is used rarely in the ICU; perhaps this is due to unfamiliarity with the potential value of the technology to clinical practice in the ICU. Capnography is useful in providing a general assessment of the cardiac output, and in severe states when invasive blood pressure monitoring is not available, it may provide the only evidence of cardiac output [31,32]. The clinician can determine the patient's respiratory drive and level of narcosis easily by noting the apneic threshold, which is the carbon dioxide level at which the patient initiates spontaneous breathing efforts [11]. Analysis of the character of the end-tidal carbon dioxide (ETCO$_2$) tracing can yield the presence of reduced airflow on expiration caused by either foreign-body obstruction or intrinsic lung diseases, such as emphysema or asthma, by noting a slow up-sloping of the curve rather than a flat horizontal line. Additionally, emergency department physicians are recognizing the value of capnography as a real-time bedside monitor for evaluating the responsiveness of intubated asthmatics to bronchodilator therapy [33]. The detection of hypercarbia by the capnograph has long been known to be a sensitive indicator of malignant hyperthermia [34], but the usefulness in this manner is not limited to malignant hyperthermia; it can be a nonspecific indicator for any hypermetabolic state.

Capnography usually is used to measure the exhaled carbon dioxide of both lungs simultaneously. When a double-lumen endotracheal tube is used for thoracic operations, however, dual capnography can be used to monitor separately the exhaled carbon dioxide of each lung. This technique was used to detect a critical perfusion defect in an individual lung due to an embolus and facilitated prompt therapy to alleviate the problem [35]. Additionally, in the unique situation of independent ventilation for unilateral lung injuries, ETCO$_2$ has been shown to assist the clinician in optimizing the ventilatory settings [36].

Finally, the capnograph can be used to evaluate a relatively difficult quantity to determine alveolar dead space. Ordinarily the ETCO$_2$ closely approximates the plasma PaCO$_2$, with the ETCO$_2$ about 2 to 5 mm Hg less than the PaCO$_2$. Clinically, anesthesiologists have noticed for some time that this gradient does not remain constant, and the change in the gradient can be used to estimate the amount of alveolar dead space. Pulmonary embolism even in the absence of hemodynamic compromise increases the dead space, which manifests as an abrupt decrease in the ETCO$_2$. Additionally an increase in the gradient indicates a worsening of the dead space (worsening of the clinical situation), and a decrease in the gradient suggests a decrease in the gradient (improvement in the clinical situation) [37].

In thoracic surgery, the transcutaneous carbon dioxide monitor may reflect the PaCO$_2$ more accurately [38]. Radiometer (Copenhagen, Denmark) manufactures a device that uses a probe to heat an area of the skin to 42°C. The device reports the average tissue level of carbon dioxide at the site of probe application. One drawback is that these types of devices require about 20 minutes to obtain a reading, and the probe may cause a thermal burn [38]. Also the responsiveness of the monitor in the setting of acute changes in ventilation makes the device unreliable as a detector of esophageal intubation or endobronchial intubation.

Spirometry

Many sophisticated ICU ventilators today have the capability of displaying not only traditionally measured parameters, such as peak airway pressure and tidal volume, but also expiratory flow rates and auto–positive end-expiratory pressure (PEEP). The ventilators on most anesthesia machines do not have this capability, however, and additional monitors, such as side-stream spirometers, are used. To monitor ventilation comprehensively, one must evaluate lung compliance using pressure waveforms and expiratory spirometry [11].

The two types of compliance that can be obtained from airway pressure waveforms are dynamic compliance (Cdyn), and static compliance (Cstat):

$$Cdyn = V_T / (P_{pk} - PEEP) \text{ and}$$

$$Cstat = V_T / (P_{plat} - PEEP)$$

By analyzing lung compliance, it is possible to determine the degree of thoracic compliance and the presence of endobronchial intubation. Spirometry has been used for years in the outpatient setting to monitor severity of reversible airway disease, such as asthma, and for preoperative evaluation for thoracic surgery. It can be used intraoperatively to detect

A

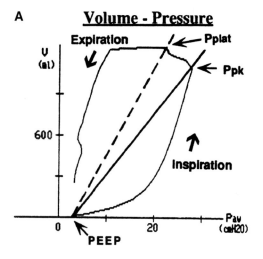

B

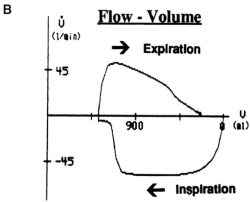

Fig. 8. (*A* and *B*) Side-stream spirometry.

mechanical airway obstruction, endobronchial intubation, and air leaks and to evaluate the response to bronchodilator therapy (Fig. 8).

Displacement of the double-lumen endotracheal tube occurs frequently and often can be identified by fiberoptic inspection before it manifests clinically as failure of lung isolation or hypoxemia. Continuous spirometry also can be used to identify the malposition of the double-lumen tube. The flow-volume pattern of ventilation is largely the same for one-lung or two-lung ventilation as long as the double-lumen tube is positioned correctly, but when the double-lumen tube is malpositioned, expiratory flow, inspiratory flow, or both can be restricted [39]. Lastly, side-stream spirometry has been used to assess the degree of air leak during lung volume reduction surgery by identifying early termination of the expiratory flow pattern indicative of lost lung volume [40].

Circulation

Standard 2 of the ASA Standards for Basic Anesthetic Monitoring requires that the adequacy of circulation be monitored during all anesthetics. The standards require the use of an electrocardiogram, measurement of the blood pressure, and "at least one of the following: palpation of a pulse, auscultation of heart sounds, monitoring of a tracing of intra-arterial pressure, ultrasound peripheral pulse monitoring, or pulse plethysmography or oximetry" [4].

Noninvasive blood pressure

Although noninvasive blood pressure measurement has been available for decades, automated devices are relatively new. The automated devices have simplified and standardized the measurement of blood pressure, but the method for blood pressure measurement is different for automated devices than for the traditional auscultatory method, and this difference can lead to misinterpretation. The standard auscultatory method is not reviewed here.

The automated blood pressure cuff inflates and deflates automatically detecting the presence and amplitude of pulsations in the arm (oscillometric method) [41]. The peak amplitude of pulsations in the arm is designated the *mean arterial blood pressure,* and the systolic and diastolic blood pressures are calculated from an analysis of the peak amplitude of pulsations and the rate of increase and decline of the pulsations. The mean arterial pressure is measured, and the systolic and diastolic pressures are calculated (Fig. 9); this may surprise many individuals and is one of the many reasons to explain the difference between the blood pressure reported by the noninvasive cuff and arterial line. The blood pressure reported from an arterial line directly measures the systolic and diastolic pressures and calculates the mean pressure.

Limitations

Although the automated blood pressure device is reliable, is easy to use, and keeps the clinician's hands free to care for the patient, a few things can happen that can lead to a false sense of security. The artifacts that the clinician should be aware of are those due to improper cuff size and measuring the pressure at the wrong location. The width of the cuff should be 20% to 30% of the circumference of the arm. If the cuff is too small, the blood pressure is measured as artificially high. If the blood pressure cuff is too large, the blood pressure is measured as artificially low. Some commercially available dispos-

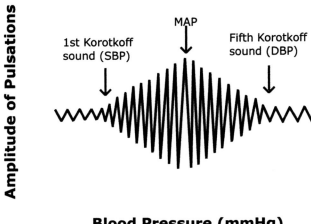

Fig. 9. Oscillometric method of noninvasive blood pressure measurement. (Dionne RA, Becker D, Phero JC. Management of pain and anxiety in the dental office. Philadelphia: WB Saunders; with permission.)

able cuffs have a colored line that provides an indicator of the proper fit. Additionally, if the blood pressure cuff is placed on the nondependent arm in the lateral decubitus position, the reading is lower than if it is placed on the dependent arm by an amount proportional to the vertical distance from the heart.

Invasive arterial blood pressure

When beat-to-beat monitoring of blood pressure is required or when noninvasive measurement is technically difficult, an invasive monitor of blood pressure (arterial line) is used. The arterial line can provide erroneous information, however, and lead to misguided diagnosis and therapy.

Consideration of the technical requirements for invasive monitoring provides some insight into the sources of error in this type of measurement. The standard arterial line system requires four things: mechanical coupling (intravascular catheter), a pressure transducer (strain gauge that converts mechanical motion of fluid to electrical signals), an amplifier and processing unit, and display monitor. The arterial line system measures the pressure wave that is propagated down the aorta and vascular system. The velocity of the wave is much faster than the actual movement of blood. The transmission velocity of the pressure waveform varies inversely with the capacitance of the vessels. As the wave travels to the periphery, it becomes progressively more distorted. Distortion occurs with (1) damping of high-frequency components secondary to the viscoelastic properties of the arterial walls and (2) augmentation and narrowing of the systolic portion of the wave caused

by reflection of waves at branching points, tapering of arteries, resonance, and changes in transmission velocity. The systolic pressure in a large peripheral artery (radial artery) is commonly 10 mm Hg higher than in the aorta, and the diastolic pressure is lower. The mean pressure is usually slightly lower in the periphery because of loss of pressure across the arterial resistance and is least sensitive to artifacts.

Limitations

Several factors can lead to erroneous reporting of blood pressure, and this may mislead the clinician. The most important is the concept of "damping." Every system has a resonant frequency that is directly proportional to the stiffness of the tubing, diaphragm, and cross-sectional area of the catheter. The resonant frequency is inversely proportional to the catheter length and fluid density. As the frequency of the blood pressure waves approaches the resonant frequency of the system, the system starts to resonate and distort the measurement, which can be 25% on the systolic and 10% on the diastolic pressure. The mean pressure is not affected as much [42]. A system that is overresonant is considered to be "underdamped," whereas a system that is "overdamped" is considered "dampened." The underdamped system yields systolic pressures that exceed the actual systolic pressure. This can be identified easily as a sharp peaking to the systolic pressure waveform often with extra nonphysiologic components. When most people say that "there is a lot of whip in the line," they actually are saying that the system is underdamped. The common practice of introducing an air bubble into the system to provide additional damping is *not* recommended because, in addition to the risk of air embolus, this decreases the resonant frequency of the system and leads to further distortion of the waveform. Conversely, when the system is over-damped, the waveform underrepresents the true systolic pressure and overrepresents the true diastolic pressure. There is damping to the mean. The system is said to be dampened.

Methods to change the resonance in an arterial line system include changing the length, diameter, or type of tubing that connects the arterial cannula to the transducer, but these often are not clinically practical. The degree of damping increases as the diameter or length of tubing is increased, or a softer type of tubing is used. In the ICU, it is common to see long lengths of tubing connecting the monitor catheters to the transducers. The ideal connection is short and stiff tubing, although this may be clinically inconvenient.

Innovations

One of the newest innovations is a continuous, noninvasive blood pressure monitor called the Med-wave Vasotrac (Danvers, Massachusetts) system. This system uses a wrist module that is strapped to the patient's wrist and compresses the radial artery against the radius, analyzing the pulsations. Every 15 heart beats, the monitor updates. The monitor collects 250 data points in the process of performing a measurement. A computerized algorithm is used to determine the patient's systolic, diastolic, and mean arterial pressures [43,44]. In clinical trials, it has been found to be accurate and reliable in reporting blood pressures in surgical and critical care patients [45]. The only published limitation to the system is the requirement that the patient's wrist diameter must be less than 11 cm, and the patient's blood pressure needs to be between 40 mm Hg and 240 mm Hg [44]. This device is likely to be most useful in patients who need frequent determinations of blood pressure but do not require arterial blood gas analysis.

Central venous pressure

The central venous pressure (CVP) monitor has been used for many years as an invasive monitor of preload and blood volume [41]. Focusing only on the number that is reported on the monitor rather than evaluating waveform morphology invites erroneous interpretation and misses the opportunity to glean additional information.

Principles

Proper interpretation of the information from the central line begins with first ensuring that the central

line is properly placed at the junction of the superior vena cava and right atrium and that the transducer is appropriately zeroed and leveled at the patient's heart. Second, the clinician must bear in mind that the intrathoracic pressure and respiration erroneously can increase and decrease the CVP reported on the monitor. The proper time to measure the CVP is at end expiration. If the patient is breathing sponta-neously (intubated or not), the negative intrathoracic pressure is superimposed on the right atrial pressure causing the CVP to be artificially low. During positive-pressure ventilation, the CVP is elevated erroneously owing to PEEP and the delivery of the positive-pressure breath. The pressure needs to be measured at end expiration while on zero PEEP. If it would be harmful to discontinue PEEP briefly, the PEEP can be mathematically subtracted from the accurate end-expiratory CVP.

A complete and accurate understanding of the CVP waveform can provide additional information. The normal CVP waveform consists of three peaks and two descents (Box 2; Fig. 10). Finally, a considerable amount of information regarding com-mon disease states can be identified by careful inspection of the CVP waveform (Box 3).

Pulmonary artery catheter

The pulmonary artery catheter (PAC) previously was thought to be a lifesaving device [46,47], but in

---

Box 2. Elements of the central venous pressure waveform

Peaks

    a—atrial contraction (after the P wave)
    c—isovolumic contraction of the right ventricle and closing of the tricuspid valve (after QRS complex)
    v—venous filling of the right atrium through the inferior vena cava/supe-rior vena cava (after the T wave)

Descents

    x—systolic collapse of the atrial pres-sure (probably mostly from the retraction of the tricuspid valve)
    y—opening of the tricuspid valve to allow blood to flow into the ventricle

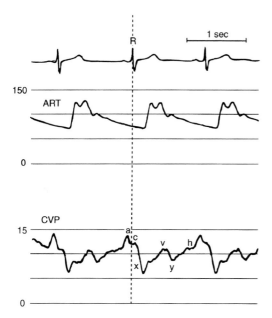

Fig. 10. Normal central venous pressure (CVP) waveform. *Abbreviation:* ART, arterial pressure waveform.

recent years the safety and usefulness of the PAC have been questioned [48]. PACs are rarely used during thoracic surgery, but when used one might think that thermodilution cardiac output would be unreliable in the setting of lateral decubitus position and one-lung ventilation. Although any information gained from the PAC when the patient is in the lateral decubitus position under one-lung ventilation should be viewed with considerable skepticism, two articles in the animal literature suggest that the lateral position and one-lung ventilation have a minimal effect on the reliability of thermodilution cardiac output [49,50]. Clinical judgment should be used when considering the validity of information from the PAC during thoracic procedures.

Innovations

The oximetric PAC previously was thought to be a major innovation, but its clinical use and assessment in the literature have declined over the last several years. Continuous end-diastolic volume (CEDV) measurement could be the next generation of PAC technology. CEDV monitoring is a variation on the continuous cardiac output monitor that was introduced in the early 1990s. CEDV is a new computerized algorithm that allows continuous calculation of right ventricular ejection fraction and continuous right ventricular end diastolic volume index (CEDVI) using a continuous cardiac output catheter. Early studies have shown that CEDVI is a better indicator

---

Box 3. Effect of disease states on central venous pressure waveform

1. *Atrial fibrillation:* The a wave disappears and the c wave becomes more prominent as a result of the greater atrial volume at the beginning of systole.
2. *Junctional rhythm:* A cannon a wave is seen as a result of atrial contraction during ventricular systole when the tricuspid valve is closed.
3. *Tricuspid regurgitation:* There is a large fusion of the C-V waves (sometimes called a giant v wave) that obliterates the x descent. The right atrium is said to be ventricularized.
4. *Tricuspid stenosis:* The gradient from the right atrium to right ventricle produces a prominent a wave and slurred y descent.
5. *Increased right ventricle stiffness:* Increased right ventricle stiffness (due to right ventricular infarct, pericardial constriction, or pulmonary hypertension) may produce a prominent a wave but overall a normal waveform.
6. *Right ventricular infarcts:* Right ventricular infarcts may elevate CVP markedly, and it may exceed the pulmonary capillary wedge pressure. The waveform may look like an M or W due to prominent a and v waves. The prominent a wave results from atrial contraction into a stiff right ventricle, and the prominent v wave suggests tricuspid regurgitation.
7. *Pericardial constriction:* An elevated CVP is seen, and the trace is similar to the right ventricular infarct (M or W waves). A short y descent also may be seen followed by a plateau, which is called the *square root sign*.
8. *Cardiac tampanade:* The CVP is artificially elevated, and the y descent is obliterated creating a monophasic waveform. Blunted a and c waves also are seen.

of preload in critically ill patients than the pulmonary artery occlusion pressure, and there is excellent correlation between the CEDVI and the cardiac index [51,52].

A new variation on the pulmonary artery thermodilution technique has been developed called *transpulmonary thermodilution cardiac output*. This technique uses a central venous line and an arterial line in either the aorta or the axillary artery to detect the change in temperature that can be used to correlate with cardiac output. Animal studies suggest that this method of cardiac output detection is equivalent to thermodilution cardiac output [53].

Additionally, LiDCO Group Plc has developed and marketed a device that measures the cardiac output by analyzing the lithium concentrations at an arterial line after the lithium has been introduced into the patient's circulation through a peripheral or central line [54]. The LiDCO system is a bolus indicator method of determination of the cardiac output and serves to calibrate the PulseCO system. The PulseCO System calculates the continuous beat-to-beat stroke volume, stroke volume variation, and cardiac output by analysis of the arterial line waveform [55]. The patient must have only an arterial line and either a peripheral or central venous line for introduction of the lithium bolus (Fig. 11). This device is an advance in monitoring because it eliminates the need and risk posed by the insertion and use of a PAC. To date, there is little in the human literature evaluating its usefulness.

Transesophageal echocardiography

Echocardiography was introduced into the operating room in the 1970s, and the first published use of intraoperative transesophageal echocardiography (TEE) was in 1980. TEE was rarely used, however, until Doppler technology became available in the mid-1980s. TEE since has become commonplace [56]. In 1993, the ASA and Society of Cardiovascular Anesthesiologists established a 12-member Ad Hoc Task Force on Practice Parameters for Transesophageal Echocardiography. The detailed report was

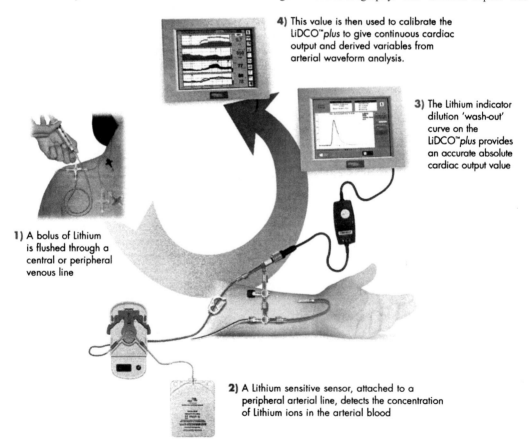

4) This value is then used to calibrate the LiDCO™*plus* to give continuous cardiac output and derived variables from arterial waveform analysis.

3) The Lithium indicator dilution 'wash-out' curve on the LiDCO™*plus* provides an accurate absolute cardiac output value

1) A bolus of Lithium is flushed through a central or peripheral venous line

2) A Lithium sensitive sensor, attached to a peripheral arterial line, detects the concentration of Lithium ions in the arterial blood

Fig. 11. LiDCO system. (Courtesy of LiDCO Ltd., Cambridge, United Kingdom; with permission.)

Table 1
Indications for transesophageal echocardiography use

Category I	Category II	Category III
Preoperative	Preoperative	Preoperative: None
1. Unstable patients with suspected aortic aneurysm, dissection, or transection	1. Stable patients with suspected aortic aneurysm, dissection, or transection	
Intraoperative	Intraoperative	Intraoperative
1. Any valve repair	1. Any valve replacement	1. Evaluation of myocardial perfusion, coronary artery anatomy, or graft patency
2. Most congental heart surgery requiring cardiopulmonary bypass	2. Repair of cardiac aneurysms	2. Repair of cardiomyopathy other than hypertrophic obstructive cardiomyopathy
3. Repair of hypertrophic obstructive cardiomyopathy	3. Removal of cardiac tumors	3. Uncomplicated endocarditis
4. Repair of aortic dissection with possible aortic valve involvement	4. Detection of foreign bodies	4. Monitoring for emboli during orthopedic surgery
5. Acute, persistent, and life-threatening hemodynamic disturbance unresponsive to treatment	5. Air detection	5. Repair of thoracic aortic injuries
6. Pericardial window procedure	6. Intracardiac thrombectomy	6. Uncomplicated pericarditis
7. Unstable patients in the ICU	7. Pulmonary embolectomy	7. Pleuropulmonary disease
8. Endocarditis	8. Cardiac trauma	8. Placement of balloon pumps, AICDs, or PACs
	9. Aortic embolus or atherosclerosis	9. Cardioplegia administration
	10. Thoracic aortic dissections without aortic valve involvement	
	11. Pericardiectomy, pericardial, effusion, or surgery	
	12. Heart or lung transplant	
	13. Use of Ventricular assist devises	
Perioperative: None	Perioperative	Perioperative: None
	1. Patients at risk for hemodynamic disturbances	
	2. Patients at increased risk of myocardial ischemia or infarction	

Abbreviations: AICDs, automatic implantable cardioverter defibrillators; PACs, pulmonary artery catheters.
From, Report by the American Society of Anesthesiologists and the Society of Cardiovascular Anesthesiologists Task Force on Transesophageal Echocardiography. Practice guidelines for perioperative transesophageal echocardiography. Anesthesiology 1996;84:986–1006; with permission.

published in the journal *Anesthesiology* in 1996. The committee established three categories of indications for TEE use (Table 1). Category I indications are supported by the strongest evidence or opinion of task force members. Category II indications are supported by weaker evidence and expert consensus. Category III indications have little evidence or support by scientific literature or expert opinion.

Principles

The TEE machine combines the two imaging modes (M mode and two-dimensional mode) with Doppler technologies (color Doppler, continuous wave Doppler, pulse wave Doppler, and tissue Doppler) to provide the clinician with the ability to assess the structure and function of the heart in real time. TEE can assist the surgeon in correcting inadequate repairs before leaving the operating room. TEE reduces the need for reoperation and has facilitated the prevention of perioperative complications [56].

Limitations

TEE monitoring has some limitations. It provides information only at specific points in time, it requires an operator skilled in its use, it is a costly technology to acquire and maintain, and it is cumbersome to transport. There have been case reports of intraoperative deaths attributed to inaccurate interpretation of the TEE information resulting in improper clinical decisions [56]. Insertion and manipulation of the TEE probe can cause dental, pharyngeal, esophageal, and laryngeal trauma [56]. TEE is used infrequently for thoracic surgery. Image acquisition may be more difficult in the lateral decubitus position; however, in skilled hands, this rarely nullifies the value of this monitoring and diagnostic tool [57].

Innovation

A new device called HemoSonic has arisen from echocardiography technology; and it provides the clinician with real-time, longitudinal information regarding cardiac output, contractility, stroke volume, vascular resistance, and aortic diameter [58,59]. The HemoSonic (Arrow International, Reading, Pennsylvania) probe is a flexible cable less than 7mm in diameter that is placed orally or nasally with the tip positioned in the midesophageal region. The probe is connected to a relatively small and portable console that easily sits at the bedside. The console interprets the Doppler flow pattern of blood flow in the descending thoracic aorta and displays information regarding stroke volume, cardiac output, heart rate, left ventricular ejection time indexed to heart rate, acceleration and peak velocity (of blood flow), aortic diameter, and total systemic vascular resistance. It has several advantages: It is easily inserted, requires minimal technical skills, is not associated with major complications, and can be left in place for prolonged periods (2 weeks) [59]. In clinical studies, it was found that in addition to good correlation with cardiac output, a good correlation was found with the corrected flow times and preload. Even more compelling, in a study by Sinclair et al [60], prospective use of the device to optimize intraoperative volume management resulted in a higher cardiac index at the end of surgery and a significantly shorter hospital stay in patients undergoing proximal femur fracture repair.

Summary

It cannot be overemphasized that a piece of electrical equipment is not capable of replacing a vigilant, well-trained clinician. As monitoring devices become more sophisticated, the potential for artifact or misinterpretation increases. When applied appropriately, operated properly, and interpreted correctly, however, the monitors afford the patient the best possible outcome.

References

[1] Buhre W, Rossaint R. Perioperative management and monitoring in anesthesia. Lancet 2003;362:1839–46.

[2] Webb RK, Van der Walt JH, Runciman WB, et al. The Australian Incident Monitoring Study: which monitor? An analysis of 2000 incident reports. Anaesth Intensive Care 1993;21:529–42.

[3] Vandam LD. History of anesthetic practice. In: Miller RD, editor. Anesthesia. 5th edition. Philadelphia: Churchill Livingstone; 2000. p. 1–11.

[4] American Society of Anesthesiologists House of Delegates. Standards for basic anesthetic monitoring. Approved 1986, 2003. Available at: http://www.asahq.org/publicationsAndServices/standards/02.pdf#2.

[5] Barker SJ, Tremper KK. Pulse oximetry: applications and limitations. Int Anesthesiol Clin 1987;25:155–75.

[6] Technical Bulletin. Masimo—signal extraction technology. Irvine (CA): Masimo Corporation (HeadQuarters). Available at: http://www.masimo.com/IMAGES/technology/lab1035.pdf.

[7] Pedersen T, Moller AM, Pedersen BD. Pulse oximetry for perioperative monitoring: systematic review of randomized, controlled trials. Anesth Analg 2003;96:426–31.

[8] Elfadel IM, Weber WM, Barker SJ. Motion-resistant pulse oximetry. J Clin Monit 1995;11:262.

[9] Weber WM, et al. Low perfusion-resistant pulse oximetry. J Clin Monit 1995;11:284.

[10] Dumas C, Wahr J, Tremper KK, et al. Clinical evaluation of a prototype motion-artifact-resistant pulse oximeter in the recovery room. Anesth Analg 1996;83:269–72.

[11] Moon RE, Camporesi EM. Respiratory monitoring. In: Miller RD, editor. Anesthesia. 5th edition. Philadelphia: Churchill Livingstone; 2000. p. 1255–95.

[12] Elfadel IM, Weber WM, Barker SJ. Motion-resistant pulse oximetry. J Clin Monit 1995;11:262.

[13] Weber WM, Elfadel IM, Barker SJ. Low perfusion-resistant pulse oximeter. J Clin Monit 1995;11:284.

[14] Michaelis G, Biscoping J, Salzer A, Hempelmann G. Effect of dyshemoglobinemia (methemoglobinemia and carboxyhemoglobinemia) on accuracy of measurement in pulse oximetry in operations of long duration. Anaesth Intensivther Notfallmed 1988;23:102–8.

[15] Bar-Yosef S, Sanders EG, Grocott HP. Asymmetric cerebral near infra-red oximetric measurements during cardiac surgery. J Cardiothorac Vasc Anesth 2003;6:773–4.

[16] Cuadra SA, Zwerling JS, Feuerman M, et al. Cerebral oximetry monitoring during carotid endarterectomy: effect of carotid clamping and shunting. Vasc Endovasc Surg 2003;37:407–13.

[17] Casati A, Fanelli G, Pietropaoli P, et al. In a population of elderly patients undergoing elective non-cardiac surgery cerebral oxygen saturation is associated with prolongued length of stay. Anesthesiology 2003;99:A551.

[18] Armonda RA, McGee B, Veznadaraglu E, et al. Near-infrared spectroscopy (NIRS) measurements of cere-

bral oximetry in the neurovascular ICU. Crit Care Med 1999;27:173.

[19] deVries JW, Visser GH, Bakker PE. Neuro-monitoring in defibrillation threshold testing: a comparison between EEG, near-infrared spectroscopy and jugular bulb oximetry. J Clin Monit 1997;13:303–7.

[20] deVries JW, Haanschoten MC. Resuscitation in pediatric balloon valvuloplasty: effects on cerebral perfusion and oxygenation. J Cardiothorac Vasc Anesth 2000; 14:581.

[21] Dunham CM, Sosnowski C, Porter JM, et al. Correlation of noninvasive cerebral oximetry with cerebral perfusion in the severe head injured patient: a pilot study. J Trauma 2002;52:40–6.

[22] Bailey H, Sanrota T, Trooskin S, et al. Hyperdynamic cardiac performance may fail to support cerebral oxygen consumption during sepsis. Crit Care Med 1999; 27:A85.

[23] INVOS Cerebral Oximeter. Principles of operation technical bulletin. Troy (MI): Somanetics. Available at: www.somanetics.com/invos_principles.htm.

[24] NIRO-300, Infrared radiation oxygen monitor unit. Product information brochure. Middle Cove (NSW, Australia): SDR Clinical Technology. Available at: http:// www.hpk.co.jp/Eng/products/Syse/Niro300E.htm.

[25] Dullenkopf A, Frey B, Baenziger O, et al. Measurement of cerebral oxygenation state in anaesthetized children using the INVOS 5100 cerebral oximeter. Paediatr Anaesth 2003;13:384–91.

[26] Yao FSF, Levin SK, Wu D, et al. Maintaining cerebral oxygen saturation during cardiac surgery shortened ICU and hospital stays. Anesth Analg 2001;92:SCA86.

[27] Alexander HC, Kronenefeld MA, Dance GR. Reduced postoperative length of stay may result from using cerebral oximetry monitoring to guide treatment. Presented at Outcomes 2001, The Key West Meeting, May 23–26, 2001. Ann Thorac Surg 2002;73:373.

[28] Iglesias I, Murkin JM, Bainbridge D, et al. Monitoring cerebral oxygen saturation significantly decreases postoperative length of stay: a prospective randomized study. Presented at Outcomes 2003: The Key West Meeting, Florida. Available at: http://outcomeskeywest. com/Pdfs/2003/7-1.pdf.

[29] Austin 3rd EH, Edmonds Jr HL, Auden SM, et al. Benefit of neurophysiological monitoring for pediatric cardiac surgery. J Thorac Cardiovasc Surg 1997;114: 707–17.

[30] Tinker JH, Dull DL, Caplan RA, et al. Role of monitoring devices in prevention of anesthetic mishaps: a closed claims analysis. Anesthesiology 1998;71:541–6.

[31] Dubin A, Murias G, Estenssoro E, et al. End-tidal CO2 pressure determinants during hemorrhagic shock. Intensive Care Med 2000;26:1619–23.

[32] Jin X, Weil MH, Tang W, et al. End-tidal carbon dioxide as a noninvasive indicator of cardiac index during circulatory shock. Crit Care Med 2000;28:2415–9.

[33] Ward KR, Yealy DM. End-tidal carbon dioxide monitoring in emergency medicine: Part 2. clinical applications. Acad Emerg Med 1998;5:637–46.

[34] Martin i Lopez MA, Perez i Garcia A, Sanchez i Pallares M, Oferil i Riera F. Importance of capnography in the early clinical diagnosis of malignant hyperthermia syndrome. Rev Esp Anestesiol Reanim 1999;46:177–8.

[35] Shankar KB, Russell R, Aklog L, Mushlin PS. Dual capnography facilitates detection of a critical perfusion defect in an individual lung—a case report. Anesthesiology 1999;90:302–4.

[36] Cinnella G, Dambrosio M, Brienza N, et al. Compliance and capnography monitoring during independent lung ventilation: report of two cases. Anesthesiology 2000;93:275–8.

[37] Hardman JG, Aitkenhead AR. Estimating alveolar dead space from the arterial to end-tidal CO(2) gradient: a modeling analysis. Anesth Analg 2003; 97:1846–51.

[38] Oshibuchi M, Cho S, Hara T, et al. A comparative evaluation of transcutaneous and end-tidal measurements of CO_2 in thoracic anesthesia. Anesth Analg 2003;97:776–9.

[39] Bardoczky GI, Levarlet M, Engelman E, DeFranscquen P. Continuous spirometry for detection of double-lumen endobronchial tube placement. Br J Anaesth 1993;70:499–502.

[40] Robinson R. The use of side-stream spirometry to assess air leak during and after lung volume reduction surgery. Anesthesiology 1999;91:571–3.

[41] Mark JB, Slaughter TF, Reves GJ. Cardiovascular monitoring. In: Miller RD, editor. Anesthesia. 5th edition. Philadelphia: Churchill Livingstone; 2000. p. 1117–206.

[42] Reich DL, Moskowitz DM, Kaplan JA. Hemodynamic monitoring. In: Kaplan J, et al, editor. Cardiac anesthesia. 4th edition. Philadelphia: WB Saunders; 1999. p. 321–58.

[43] Vasotrac APM 205A. System features and specifications. Danvers (MA): Medwave, Inc. Available at: http://vasotrac.com/TRACTECH.HTM.

[44] Vasotrac APM 205A. Product brochure. Danvers (MA): Medwave, Inc. Available at: http://www.vasotrac.com/ TRACBROC.HTM.

[45] Belani K, Ozaki M, Hynson J, et al. A new noninvasive method to measure blood pressure: results of a multicenter trial. Anesthesiology 1999;91:686–92.

[46] Shah KB, Rao TL, Laughlin S, El-Etr AA. A review of pulmonary artery catheterization in 6,245 patients. Anesthesiology 1984;61:271–5.

[47] Swan HJ, Ganz W, Forrester JS, et al. Catheterization of the heart in man with use of a flow-directed balloon tipped catheter. N Engl J Med 1970;283:447–51.

[48] Connors A, Speroff T, Dawson N, et al. The effectiveness of right heart catheterization in the initial care of critically ill patients. JAMA 1996;276:889–97.

[49] Landais A, Morin JP, Roche A, et al. Measurement of cardiac output by the thermodilution method during left thoracotomy in the lateral position in the dog. Acta Anaesthesiol Scand 1990;34:158–61.

[50] Boucek C, Klain M, Obuchowski N, et al. Pulmonary

artery catheter monitoring during single-lung ventilation in dogs. J Clin Monit 1992;8:209–15.

[51] Durham R, Neunaber K, Vogler G, et al. Right ventricular end-diastolic volume as a measure of preload. J Trauma 1995;39:218–23.

[52] Dennis JW, Menawat SS, Sobowalc OO, et al. Superiority of end-diastolic volume and ejection fraction measurements over wedge pressures in evaluating cardiac function during aortic reconstruction. J Vasc Surg 1992;16:372–7.

[53] Huter L, Schwarzkopf K, Preussler NP, et al. Measuring cardiac output in one-lung ventilation: a comparison of pulmonary artery and transpulmonary aortic measurements in pigs. J Cardiothorac Vasc Anesth 2004;18:190–3.

[54] Linton R, Band D, O'Brien T, Jonas M, Leach R. Lithium dilution cardiac output measurement: a comparison with thermodilution. Crit Care Med 1997;25: 1796–800.

[55] LiDCOplus. Frequently asked questions and features and benefits. Cambridge (UK): LiDCO Ltd. Available at: http://www.pulseco.com/faqs.asp.

[56] Thys D, Abel M, Bollen B, et al. A report by the American Society of Anesthesiologists and the Society of Cardiovascular Anesthesiologists Task Force on Transesophageal Echocardiography. Practice guidelines for perioperative transesophageal echocardiography. Anesthesiology 1996;84:986–1006.

[57] Izumi C, Iga K, Himura Y, Gen H, Konishi T. Influence of gravity on pulmonary venous flow velocity patterns: analysis of left and right pulmonary venous flow velocities in left and right decubitus positions. Am Heart J 1999;137:419–26.

[58] HemoSonic. Product information. Arrow International. Available at: http://www.hemosonic100.com/technology/procedure.htm.

[59] Marik PE. Pulmonary artery catheterization and esophageal doppler monitoring in the ICU. Chest 1999;116:1085–91.

[60] Sinclair S, James S, Singer M. Intraoperative intravascular volume optimization and length of hospital stay after repair of proximal femoral fracture: a randomized controlled trial. BMJ 1997;315:909–12.

ELSEVIER
SAUNDERS

Thorac Surg Clin 15 (2005) 71 – 83

THORACIC
SURGERY
CLINICS

Progress in Lung Separation

Javier H. Campos, MD

Department of Anesthesia, University of Iowa Health Care, 200 Hawkins Drive, Iowa City, IA 52242-1079, USA

Methods to achieve lung separation have been available since the introduction of the red rubber Robert-Shaw double-lumen endotracheal tube (DLT) more than 60 years ago [1]. Ever since, new technology and alternative methods have been used to separate the lungs either partially (selective lobar collapse) or totally (whole one-lung collapse). This article focuses on the current methods used to achieve lung separation in the intraoperative period in a surgical patient undergoing thoracic, esophageal, vascular, or robotic chest surgery, with a special emphasis on the latest technology. Specific considerations are given to the current use of the disposable polyvinyl chloride DLT, including a left-sided or right-sided DLT, and alternative methods to achieve lung separation with the use of bronchial blockade technology.

Techniques for one-lung ventilation (OLV) can be accomplished with two different methods. The first involves a bifurcated DLT that independently can block either the right or the left lung. The second method involves blockade of a main stem bronchus with bronchial blockers to allow lung collapse distal to the occlusion [2,3].

The disposable DLT, made of polyvinyl chloride material, is the most commonly used device for lung separation in North America. The left-sided DLT is used more commonly [4] than the right-sided DLT [5,6]. Each DLT has advantages and disadvantages in the practice of thoracic anesthesia. In practice, the most common indications for lung separation are (1) for surgical exposure, (2) for prevention of contamination to the contralateral lung from bleeding or

pus material, and (3) during differential lung ventilation or for continuity of the airway gas exchange such as with bronchopleural fistula.

Double-lumen endotracheal tubes

Size selection

Regarding selection of the proper size of a DLT, all studies have focused on the left-sided DLT, in part because of the infrequent use of the right-sided DLT. A common problem with the left-sided DLT is the lack of objective guidelines to choose properly the correct or approximate size of DLT.

A left-sided DLT that is too small requires a large endobronchial cuff volume, which might increase the incidence of malposition. In addition, a small DLT does not readily allow fiberoptic bronchoscope placement and can make suction difficult. A properly sized DLT is one in which the main body of the tube passes without resistance through the glottis and advances easily within the trachea and in which the bronchial component passes into the intended bronchus without difficulty. In a study performed in adult cadavers, it was shown that the cricoid ring diameter never exceeds the diameter of the glottis. If a DLT encounters resistance when passing the glottis, it is likely that the DLT would encounter resistance while passing the cricoid ring [7].

There are increasing reports of complications related to the use of an undersized DLT. Sivalingam and Tio [8] described a complication (tension pneumothorax and pneumomediastinum) that occurred after the endobronchial tip of a smaller-than-predicted DLT had migrated too far into the left lower bronchus, and the whole tidal volume was delivered

---
Support was provided by the Department of Anesthesia, University of Iowa Health Care.

E-mail address: javier-campos@uiowa.edu

into a single lobe. Also a small-sized DLT might present with more resistance to gas flow and more intrinsic auto–positive end-expiratory pressure compared with the wider lumen of a larger DLT tube [9].

Airway-related complications have been reported with undersized left-sided DLTs. Sakuragi et al [10] reported a rupture of the left main stem bronchus by the tracheal portion of a DLT. A longitudinal laceration of the left main stem bronchus occurred, originating below the tracheal carina and extending to the left upper lobe bronchial orifice. The cause of this complication was believed to be an undersized DLT, which allowed the endotracheal portion of the DLT to enter the left main stem bronchus. An oversized DLT also can be associated with bronchial rupture in a small adult patient [11].

In the 1990s, a number of methods were proposed for determining proper left-sided DLT size. Brodsky et al [12] reported that measurement of tracheal diameter at the level of the clavicles on the preoperative posteroanterior chest radiograph can be used to determine proper left-sided DLT size. This method led to a 90% increase in the use of larger left-sided DLTs (ie, 41F DLT in men and 39F and 41F DLT in women). Chow et al [13], using the methodology of Brodsky et al [12], found this approach less reliable in Asian patients. In this study [13], the overall positive predictive value for proper size of left-sided DLT was 77% for men and 45% for women. This method seems to have limited use in patients with small stature, such as Asians and women, and an alternative method should be sought.

Another method for selecting a left-sided DLT uses measurements of left main stem bronchial diameter from a CT scan [14,15]. Seymour [16] showed that the mean diameter of the cricoid ring is the same as that of the left main stem bronchus. In this cadaver study [16], the left main stem bronchus-to-cricoid ratio almost invariably exceeded 83% in both sexes. A CT scan can identify the bronchial wall or cricoid ring, facilitating measurement of bronchial diameter. For this method to be reliable, the distal outside diameter of the bronchial portion of the DLT must be known. Currently this information is not included in the manufacturer's package insert. A properly sized, left-sided DLT should have a bronchial tip 1 to 2 mm smaller than the patient's left bronchus diameter to allow for the space occupied by the deflated bronchial cuff.

In another study, Eberle et al [17] used a three-dimensional image reconstruction of tracheobronchial anatomy from the spinal CT scans combined with superimposed transparencies of DLTs to predict proper size for a right-sided or left-sided DLT. Taken together, these studies suggest that chest radiographs and CT scans are valuable tools for selection of proper DLT size, in addition to their proven value in assessment of any abnormal tracheobronchial anatomy, and they should be reviewed before the placement of a DLT.

Methods of insertion

Two techniques are used most commonly by anesthesiologists when inserting and placing a DLT. The first is the blind technique, that is, when the DLT is passed with direct laryngoscopy, then turned 90° counterclockwise, either left for a left-sided DLT or right for a right-sided DLT, after the endobronchial cuff has passed beyond the vocal cords. The DLT is advanced until moderate resistance is felt, which usually indicates that the endobronchial lumen of the DLT has entered the bronchus, or, alternatively, the tube is advanced until the depth of insertion at the teeth is approximately 29 cm for either men or women if their height is at least 170 cm [18].

The second technique employs fiberoptic bronchoscopy guidance, in which the tip of the endobronchial lumen is guided after the DLT passes the vocal cords; direction is sought with the aid of a flexible fiberoptic bronchoscope. In a study by Boucek et al [19], comparing the blind technique versus the fiberoptic bronchoscopy–guided technique, it was shown that of the 32 patients who underwent the blind technique approach, primary success occurred in 27 patients and complete success occurred in 30 patients. In contrast, in the 27 patients using the bronchoscopy-guided technique, primary success was achieved only in 21 patients and eventual success in 25 patients. This study also showed that the average time spent placing a DLT was an average of 88 seconds for the blind technique and 181 seconds for the directed bronchoscopic approach [19]. Although both methods resulted in successful left main stem bronchus placement in most patients, slightly more time was required when the fiberoptic bronchoscopy guidance technique was used. In addition, two patients in each group required an alternative method for tube placement. Either method may fail when used alone.

Right-sided double-lumen endotracheal tubes

Indications

Although a left-sided DLT is used more commonly for most elective thoracic procedures [4], there

Box 1. Indications for right-sided double-lumen endotracheal tubes

Distorted anatomy of the entrance of left main stem bronchus due to:

External or intraluminal tumor compression
Descending thoracic aortic aneurysm

Site of surgery involving the left main stem bronchus

Left lung transplantation
Left-sided tracheobronchial disruption
Left-sided pneumonectomy
Left-sided sleeve resection

are specific clinical situations in which the use of a right-sided DLT is indicated (Box 1) [6]. The anatomic differences between the right and left main stem bronchus are reflected in the fundamentally different designs of the right-sided and left-sided DLTs. Because the right main stem bronchus is shorter than the left bronchus and because the right upper lobe bronchus originates at a distance of 1.5 to 2 cm from the carina, techniques using right endobronchial intubation must take into account the location and potential for obstruction of the orifice of the right upper lobe bronchus. The right-sided DLT incorporates a modified cuff, or slot, on the endobronchial side that allows ventilation for the right upper lobe.

Safety of right-sided double-lumen endotracheal tubes

In theory, the left-sided DLT and right-sided DLT should be equally safe and efficacious for collapse of either the right or the left lung. In practice, however, use of the right-sided DLT has become controversial. An early study showed that because of bronchial anatomy, the left-sided DLT is simpler to use and has a greater margin of safety than the right-sided DLT [20]. Another study [21] has shown failure to ventilate the right upper lobe in 11% of patients and obstruction of the right upper bronchus in 89% of patients after right-sided DLT placement; studies relying on fiberoptic bronchoscopy guidance techniques have shown no increased risk of obstruction of the right upper lobe bronchus orifice [5,6]. The only absolute contraindication for right-sided DLT use, besides the usual contraindications to use any DLT, is the presence of an anomalous right upper lobe

takeoff from the trachea, which has been estimated to be present in 1 of 250 otherwise normal subjects [22].

In a study by Campos et al [5], right-sided DLTs compared favorably with left-sided DLTs in patients requiring OLV for left-sided surgery thoracic surgery. In this study, the incidence of right upper lobe collapse was assessed intraoperatively by a chest radiograph, which showed good expansion of the right upper lobe in all patients who received right-sided DLTs.

Technique

The preferred technique for placement of a right-sided DLT is with the use of a bronchoscope, with the patient first in the supine position, then in the lateral decubitus position for tube placement confirmation. After the right-sided DLT is passed beyond the vocal cords, the fiberoptic bronchoscope is advanced through the endobronchial lumen. Before advancing the DLT, the tracheal carina, the entrance of the right main stem bronchus, and the takeoff of the right upper lobe bronchus are identified. Then the DLT is rotated 90° to the right and advanced with the aid of the fiberoptic bronchoscope. The proper position of a right-sided DLT is one that provides a good alignment between the opening slot of the endobronchial lumen in relationship to the takeoff of the right upper lobe bronchus and, distally (endobronchial lumen), a free view of the bronchus intermedius and the right lower lobe bronchus. From the tracheal view, the optimal position for a right-sided DLT provides a view of the edge of the blue cuff (the endobronchial balloon) when inflated just below tracheal carina and a view into the entrance of the right main stem bronchus. Fig. 1 shows the optimal position of a right-sided DLT seen from the endobronchial or endotracheal view with a fiberoptic bronchoscope.

Placement and positioning of a left-sided DLT can be accomplished with either technique discussed earlier: the blind technique, in which the left-sided DLT is passed beyond the vocal cords (endobronchial cuff) and the tube is rotated 90° counterclockwise and advanced until the tip of the tube enters the left main stem bronchus, or the bronchoscopy-guided technique, in which the endobronchial tip is passed beyond the vocal cords and guided through the endobronchial tube with the aid of the fiberoptic bronchoscope until the entrance of the left main stem bronchus is identified and the tube is introduced into the left bronchus. The optimal position for a left-sided DLT as seen with the fiberoptic bronchoscope is the one that allows, from the endotracheal view, observation of a fully inflated endobronchial cuff (no more

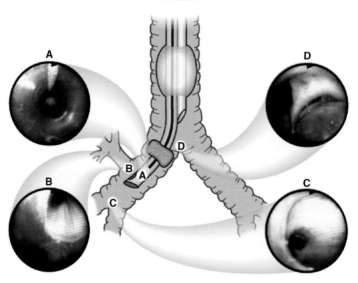

Fig. 1. Fiberoptic bronchoscopic examination for a right-sided double-lumen tube. (*A*) Shows the white line marker when the bronchoscope is passed through the endobronchial lumen. (*B*) Slot of the endobronchial lumen properly aligned within the entrance of the right upper bronchus. (*C*) Part of the bronchus intermedius when the bronchoscope is advanced through the distal portion of the endobronchial lumen. (*D*) Edge of the endobronchial cuff around the entrance of the right main stem bronchus when the bronchoscope is passed through the tracheal lumen. (*From* Campos JH. Current techniques for perioperative lung isolation in adults. Anesthesiology 2002;97:1295–301; with permission.)

then 3 mL of air) located 5 to 10 mm below the tracheal carina inside the left main stem bronchus. The second and important view is the endobronchial bronchoscopy view. Two observations are relevant: First, the fiberoptic bronchoscope is advanced inside the endobronchial lumen, and the patency of the lumen is observed before advancing through to the blue portion of the tube; the second view is at the distal end of the endobronchial tip of the tube, where a clear and unobstructed view of the left upper and lower lobe bronchus entrance orifices are visualized. Fig. 2 shows the optimal position of a left-sided DLT when seen with a fiberoptic bronchoscope.

Confirmation of double-lumen endotracheal tube placement

Evidence strongly suggests that auscultation alone is unreliable for confirmation of proper DLT placement. One study had shown that when fiberoptic bronchoscopy was used in DLTs believed to be well positioned by auscultation, more than 78% of left-sided DLTs and 83% of right-sided DLTs had to be repositioned [23]. A second study involving 200 patients who were intubated by the blind technique followed by confirmation with a fiberoptic bronchoscope found that more than one third of the DLTs required repositioning by at least 0.5 cm [24].

A study by Brodsky and Lemmens [4] reported clinical experience with the use of left-sided DLTs in 1170 patients. Using auscultation and clinical signs, there were 71 patients (6.2%) in whom the DLT was found not to be in satisfactory position and required

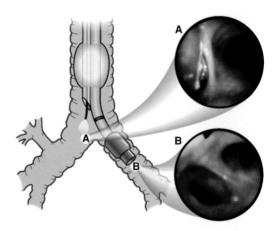

Fig. 2. Fiberoptic bronchoscopic examination for a left-sided double-lumen tube. (*A*) Edge of the endobronchial cuff around the entrance of the left main stem bronchus when the bronchoscope is passed through the tracheal lumen. (*B*) Clear view of the bronchial bifurcation (left upper and lower bronchi) when the left-sided double-lumen tube is in the optimal position, and the fiberoptic bronchoscope is being advanced through the endobronchial lumen.

readjustment after initial placement. What is important from the Brodsky study [4] is the fact that in 56 patients the DLT was too deep into the left bronchus, and, indirectly, this was a cause of hypoxemia in 21 of 56 patients who had a malpositioned tube. Anesthesiologists should be able to avoid this complication with the use of a fiberoptic bronchoscope.

In a report related to the national confidential inquiry into perioperative deaths in Great Britain [25] detailing the management of patients undergoing esophagogastrectomy, it was shown that 30% of deaths reported were associated with malposition of DLTs. The problems ranged from use of multiple DLTs to prolonged periods of hypoxia and hypoventilation. The anesthesiologist did not use a fiberoptic bronchoscope to confirm DLT position before surgery, during surgery, or when the DLT tube was incorrectly placed. Part of this report is highlighted in an editorial forum [26].

In another controversial editorial, Slinger [27] pointed out the importance of use of fiberoptic bronchoscopy to confirm placement of DLTs. It is the author's opinion that fiberoptic bronchoscopy is essential to achieve 100% success in placement and positioning of DLTs. Auscultation and clinical signs have to be followed by fiberoptic bronchoscopy assessment in a supine position first, then in a lateral decubitus position. Because left-sided DLTs have been shown typically to be displaced proximally when changing from supine into a lateral decubitus position, the edge of the bronchial cuff should be initially at least 5 to 10 mm deeper into the bronchus to prevent herniation or displacement [28]. The fiberoptic bronchoscope should be available throughout the procedure in case a malposition needs to be corrected.

Current problems associated with double-lumen endotracheal tubes

The most common problems and complications from the use of DLTs are malposition and airway trauma. A malpositioned DLT fails to allow collapse of the lung, causing gas trapping during positive-pressure ventilation, or it may partially collapse the ventilated or dependent lung, producing hypoxemia. A common cause of malposition is dislodgment of the endobronchial cuff because of overinflation, surgical manipulation of the bronchus, or extension of the head and neck during or after patient positioning [29]. Although right-sided DLTs seem to be more likely to dislodge intraoperatively than left-sided DLTs, studies [5] have shown that the incidence of

malposition is not different when comparing left-sided or right-sided DLT placement.

Airway trauma and rupture of the membranous part of the trachea or the bronchus continue to be an isolated problem with the use of DLTs [10–31]. This problem can occur during insertion and placement, while the case is in progress, or during extubation [32]. Another problem that has been reported is the development of bilateral pneumothoraces or a tension pneumothorax in the dependent and ventilated lung during OLV [33,34]. A 25-year review of the literature by Fitzmaurice and Brodsky [35] found that most airway injuries were associated with undersized DLTs, particularly in women who received a 35F or 37F disposable DLT. It is likely that airway damage occurs when an undersized DLT migrates distally into the bronchus, and the main (ie, tracheal) body of the DLT comes into contact with the bronchus, producing lacerations or rupture of the airway. Airway damage during the use of DLTs can present as unexpected air leaks, subcutaneous emphysema, massive airway bleeding into the lumen of the DLT, or protrusion of the endotracheal or endobronchial cuff into the surgical field, with visualization of this by the surgeon. If any of the above-mentioned problems occur, a bronchoscopic examination should be performed and perhaps surgical repair performed.

Bronchial blockers for lung separation

An alternative method to achieve lung separation involves blockade of a main stem bronchus to allow lung collapse distal to the occlusion [3]. Bronchial blockers also can be used selectively to achieve lobar collapse if necessary [36–38]. Currently, there are different bronchial blockers available to facilitate lung separation collapse; these devices either are attached to a single-lumen endotracheal tube with an enclosed bronchial blocker (Torque Control Blocker Univent [TCBU]; Vitaid, Lewinston, NY) [39] or are used independently over a conventional single-lumen endotracheal tube, as with the wire-guided endobronchial blocker (Arndt blocker; Cook Critical Care, Bloomington, IN) [40] or the Cohen tip deflecting endobronchial blocker (Cook Critical Care, Bloomington, IN).

Although DLTs are still the most common device used during lung separation techniques [4–41], bronchial blockade technology is on the rise, and in some specific clinical situations it can offer more advantages over DLTs. Only the newest generation of bronchial blockers is discussed in this section.

Single-lumen endotracheal tube with an enclosed bronchial blocker (Torque Control Blocker Univent)

The TCBU, which is a variant of the former Univent, was introduced in 2001. This unit has a shape similar to that of a standard endotracheal tube (Fig. 3). Within the Univent, there is a channel enclosing a movable bronchial blocker that can be used to block the left or right main stem or any specific secondary bronchus. The enclosed bronchial blocker is made of flexible nonlatex material, and it includes a flexible shaft that is easier to guide into a bronchus than the previous model. The bronchial balloon has a high-pressure, low-volume cuff that requires approximately 2 mL of air to produce an airtight seal if selective lobar blockade is used or 4 to 8 mL of air if total blockade of the bronchus is desired. The bronchial blocker has a 2-mm diameter lumen that can be used for suctioning or for oxygen administration, and it should be closed before insertion. An advantage of the TCBU is its utility in patients in whom the airway is considered difficult for

direct laryngoscopy and during unanticipated difficult endotracheal intubation [42–48].

The translaryngeal placement of the silicone TCBU is straightforward. Before use, the bronchial blocker is lubricated to facilitate passage. The enclosed bronchial blocker is fully retracted into the standard lumen of the tube. Conventional endotracheal tube placement is performed, then a fiberoptic bronchoscope is passed through the Portex swivel adaptor. Under direct vision, the enclosed bronchial blocker is advanced into the targeted bronchus. When the TCBU tube is used, the enclosed bronchial blocker must be directed into the bronchus of the surgical side, where the lung collapse is to occur.

The Univent has been used in tracheostomy patients who require OLV [49,50]. Another feature of the Univent or the newest version TCBU is its efficacy as a selective lobar blocker to improve oxygenation [36,37]. Because of its relative ease of placement, the Univent has been effective with different modalities of ventilation, including jet ventilation during sleeve pneumonectomy [51,52]. The TCBU can be converted to a conventional single-lumen endotracheal tube by deflating and withdrawing the bronchial blocker; this alleviates the need for endotracheal tube exchange, particularly if a large-size tube is been used (ie, Univent or TCBU no. 8.0 and larger sizes), if postoperative mechanical ventilation is required.

Complications related to the Torque Control Blocker Univent

A structural complication in the TCBU has been reported in which a fracture of the blocker cap connector occurred in 2 of the first 50 tubes used [53]. Failure to achieve lung separation because of abnormal anatomy (early takeoff of the entrance of the right upper lobe bronchus above tracheal carina) or lack of seal within the bronchus also has been reported [54,55]. Inclusion of the enclosed bronchial blocker into the stapling line has been reported during a right upper lobectomy [56]. Communication with the surgical team regarding the presence of a bronchial blocker in the surgical side is crucial. Another potential and dangerous complication with the bronchial blocker cuff of the Univent has been reported: The cuff of the bronchial blocker was inflated mistakenly near the tracheal lumen, precluding all airflow and producing a respiratory arrest [57].

Another common problem with the TCBU is malposition and dislodgment of the bronchial blocker while turning the patient from the supine to the lateral decubitus position. The author recommends cuff

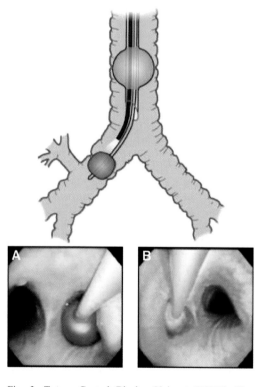

Fig. 3. Torque Control Blocker Univent (TCBU). The optimal position of the TCBU in the right (*A*) and the left (*B*) main stem bronchus. (*From* Campos JH. An update on bronchial blockers during lung separation techniques in adults. Anesth Analg 2003;97:1269; with permission.)

deflation of the blocker after the original placement and before turning the patient into a lateral decubitus position, then reinflation of the bronchial blocker. Although malpositions are of concern, one study had reported that when comparing a right-sided DLT versus Univent tubes for right-sided surgeries, it was found that the rate of malpositions was neither statistically different nor clinically significant. It was concluded that Univents can be used easily in the right main stem bronchus if indicated [58].

Independent bronchial blockers during lung separation

Another alternative to achieve lung separation is by using an independent blocker passed through an in situ single-lumen endotracheal tube. Two available devices considered to be independent blockers include the wire-guided endobronchial blocker (Arndt blocker) and the Cohen tip-deflecting endobronchial set; both devices are made by Cook Critical Care (Bloomington, IN).

Arndt blocker
Description of device. The Arndt blocker [40] is attached to a 5F, 7F, or 9F catheter that is available in 65-cm and 78-cm lengths with an inner lumen that measures 1.4 mm in diameter. Near the distal end of the catheter, there are side holes (Murphy eyes) incorporated to facilitate lung deflation. These side holes are present only in the 9F Arndt blocker. The

Arndt blocker has a high-volume, low-pressure cuff with either an elliptical (more commonly used for the left main stem bronchus) or spherical (used for the right main stem bronchus) shape. A unique feature of the Arndt blocker compared with other blockers is that the inner lumen contains a flexible nylon wire passing through the proximal end of the catheter and extending to the distal end, which exits as a small flexible wire-loop. Fig. 4 shows the Arndt blocker and its multiport connector. The wire-loop of the Arndt blocker is coupled with the fiberoptic bronchoscope and serves as a guidewire to introduce the blocker into a bronchus. For the Arndt blocker to function properly and allow manipulation with the adult fiberoptic bronchoscope, the proper size endotracheal tube must be used: For a 7F blocker, a 7.0-mm ID single-lumen endotracheal tube is used, and for the larger 9F Arndt blocker, at least an 8.0-mm ID single-lumen endotracheal tube is used.

The advantages of the Arndt blocker include its use in patients who are already tracheally intubated [59], who present a difficult airway [60], or who require OLV during acute trauma to the chest [61]. Another advantage is that it can be passed through an existing nasotracheal tube in patients who require nasal intubation and OLV, in patients with airway abnormalities, or in patients with previous tracheostomy requiring OLV [62–64]. In addition, it can be used as a selective lobar blocker in patients with previous pneumonectomy who require selective one-lobe ventilation [62–65] or as a selective blocker dur-

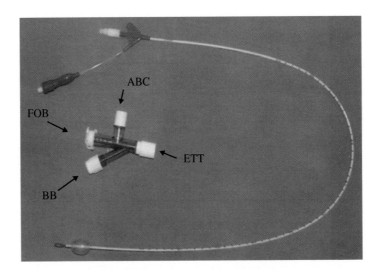

Fig. 4. The wire-guided endobronchial blocker (Arndt blocker) and the multiport connector. ABC, anesthesia breathing circuit; BB, bronchial blocker port; ETT, connection to the endotracheal tube; FOB, fiberoptic bronchoscopy port.

ing severe pulmonary bleeding [66]. Because the
Arndt blocker requires a single-lumen endotracheal
tube, it maximizes the cross-sectional diameter and
eliminates the need for tube exchange if mechanical ventilation is contemplated in the postoperative period.

Limitations of the Arndt blocker include the fact
that it is difficult to use when a 9F blocker is passed
through a 7.0-mm ID or smaller single-lumen endotracheal tube. Another limitation is with the nylon
wire-guided loop; once it is removed, it cannot be re-
inserted, and intraoperative reposition of the blocker
can be difficult, especially during left main stem
bronchus intubation.

*Placement and optimal position of the Arndt
blocker.* The Arndt blocker is an independent
endobronchial blocker that is passed through an
existing single-lumen endotracheal tube. To facilitate
insertion through the endotracheal tube, the blocker
and the fiberoptic bronchoscope are lubricated. For
a right-sided main stem bronchus intubation, the
spherically shaped blocker is recommended; for left
main stem bronchus intubation, the elliptical or the
spherical blocker is used.

The placement of the Arndt blocker involves
placing the endobronchial blocker through the endotracheal tube and using the fiberoptic bronchoscope
and wire-guided loop to direct the blocker into a main
stem bronchus. The fiberoptic bronchoscope has to be
advanced distally enough so that the Arndt blocker
enters the bronchus while it is being advanced. When
the deflated cuff is beyond the entrance of the
bronchus, the fiberoptic bronchoscope is withdrawn,
and the cuff is fully inflated with fiberoptic visualization with 5 to 8 mL of air to obtain total bronchial
blockade. For a right main stem bronchus blockade,
the Arndt blocker can be advanced independently of
the wire-loop by observing its entrance into the right
main stem bronchus under fiberoptic visualization.
Before turning the patient into a lateral decubitus
position, the cuff of the blocker should be deflated,
then advanced 1 cm deeper to avoid proximal dislodgment while changing the patient's position, then
placement again is confirmed in the lateral decubitus
position. The wire loop can be withdrawn to convert
the 1.4-mm channel into a suction port to expedite
lung collapse. It is important to remove the wire loop
to avoid inclusion in the stapling line of the bronchus
[67,68]. The optimal position of the Arndt blocker
in the left or in the right bronchus is achieved when
the blocker balloon's outer surface is seen with the
fiberoptic bronchoscope at least 5 mm below

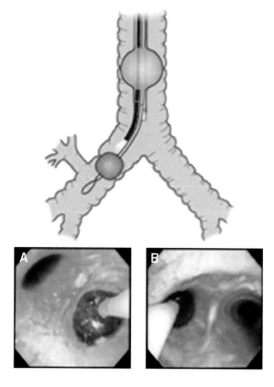

Fig. 5. Wire-guided endobronchial blocker (Arndt blocker).
The optimal position of the Arndt blocker in the right
(*A*) and the left (*B*) main stem bronchus.

the tracheal carina on the target bronchus and the
proper seal is obtained. Fig. 5 shows the proper position of the Arndt blocker in the right or left main
stem bronchus.

Cohen endobronchial blocker

Description of device. In principle, the Cohen
blocker is similar to the Arndt blocker. The Cohen
blocker is an independent endobronchial blocker that
is available only in size 9F and 65-cm length with an
inner lumen also measuring 1.4 mm in diameter. This
device comes with a spherically shaped balloon. Near
the distal end of the catheter, there are side holes
(Murphy eyes) incorporated to facilitate lung deflation. This bronchial blocker also has a high-volume,
low-pressure cuff. The Cohen blocker relies on a
wheel-twisting device located in the most proximal
part of the unit that allows deflecting of the tip of the
distal part of the blocker into the desired bronchus.
This device has been purposely preangled at the distal
tip to facilitate insertion into a target bronchus. Also
there is a torque grip located at the 55-cm mark to

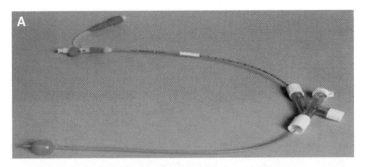

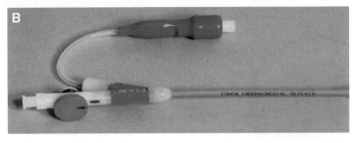

Fig. 6. (*A*) The Cohen endobronchial blocker and the (*B*) Arndt multiport connector.

allow rotation of the blocker. In the distal tip above the balloon, there is an arrow that when seen with the fiberoptic bronchoscope indicates in which direction the tip deflects. This Cohen blocker also comes with a multiport adaptor to facilitate an airtight seal when in place.

The advantages of the Cohen blocker are similar to the advantages of the Arndt blocker. Fig. 6 shows the Cohen endobronchial blocker.

Placement and optimal position of the Cohen endobronchial blocker. The Cohen endobronchial blocker is a single unit that is passed through an 8.0-mm ID single-lumen endotracheal tube. Before insertion, the blocker balloon is tested, then fully deflated. This blocker needs to be lubricated to facilitate insertion and passage through the single-lumen endotracheal tube.

The placement of the Cohen blocker involves placing the endobronchial blocker through the endotracheal tube and using the fiberoptic bronchoscope to observe the direction of the blocker into a mainstem bronchus. One of the limitations of the Cohen blocker is the lack of a precise guidance system; this blocker tends to migrate to the right main stem bronchus. For blocking the right main stem bronchus, the optimal position is the one that provides a view of the outer surface of the fully inflated balloon (4–8 mL of air) with the fiberoptic bronchoscope at least

5 mm below the tracheal carina on the right main stem bronchus.

Intubation of the left main stem bronchus can be facilitated by allowing the tip of the single-lumen endotracheal tube to be near the entrance of the left bronchus, then twisting the Cohen blocker to the left side (arrow pointed to the left when seen with the fiberoptic bronchoscope). After the blocker is seen inside the left bronchus, the single-lumen endotracheal tube is withdrawn a few centimeters. The optimal position in the left main stem bronchus is achieved when the blocker balloon's outer surface is seen with the fiberoptic bronchoscope at least 5 mm below the trachea carina inside the left main stem bronchus. Fig. 7 shows the optimal position of the Cohen bronchial blocker in the right main stem bronchus. Table 1 shows the differences between the Arndt and the Cohen endobronchial blockers.

Complications with the Arndt and Cohen endobronchial blockers

There are not many reports of complications, although these blockers were introduced only more recently (Arndt in 1999 and Cohen in 2003). There is a report of a sheared balloon of the Arndt blocker that occurred when the blocker was removed through the multiport blocker side [69]. It is advised that when the Arndt or Cohen blocker is not in use it needs to be

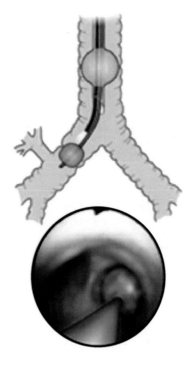

Fig. 7. The Cohen endobronchial blocker. The optimal position seen in the right main stem bronchus.

removed with the multiport connector in place rather than through the connector.

Comparison of lung separation techniques

Lung isolation is used mainly to facilitate surgical exposure, to facilitate gas exchange to the other bronchus as with a bronchopleural fistula, or to prevent contamination to the contralateral lung (eg, abscess, or hemorrhage). All this can be accomplished with either a DLT or a bronchial blocker. A left-sided DLT is used in most cases that require OLV [4]. One of the advantages of a DLT over a bronchial blocker is that the large lumen of the DLT facilitates the suctioning of blood or secretions from the bronchus, and usually the conversion from two-lung ventilation to OLV is easy and reliable. In the case of absolute lung separation (eg, bronchopulmonary lavage or presence of contamination to the other lung with massive bleeding or pus where a large suction lumen is needed), use of a DLT should be the first-line intervention for lung separation.

In many cases, a DLT placement can be difficult, including difficulties in selecting the proper tube size (specifically in patients of short stature, Asians, and women). Also the potential exists for tearing the tracheal cuff during intubation requiring multiple DLTs. A bronchial blocker could be an alternative. Perhaps when difficulties are encountered predicting a DLT size, a bronchial blocker might be preferred over DLT.

To consider the advantage that a bronchial blocker or a DLT can offer, some facts need to be discussed. A study [39] showed that when a cardiothoracic anesthesiologist placed a left-sided DLT, it took less time to place (an average of 2:08 minutes when compared with the TCBU, 2:38 minutes, or the Arndt blocker, 3:34 minutes). The same study showed that lung collapse is faster with the DLT compared with the TCBU or the Arndt blocker. Also, most patients who received bronchial blockers required assisted suction to expedite lung collapse. In another study [70], comparing a bronchial blocker (Wiruthan bronchial blocker) with the left-sided DLT during thoracoscopic surgery, it was found that the frequency of malpositions occurred more often with the bronchial blocker; also, placement of the blocker in the left main stem bronchus was more difficult.

An important issue is the effectiveness of the surgical exposure. In the Campos and Kernstine study [39], after OLV was achieved either with a DLT or bronchial blocker (TCBU or Arndt blocker), surgical exposure was clinically equivalent among the three

Table 1
Characteristics of the Arndt and Cohen endobronchial blockers

	Arndt blocker	Cohen blocker
Size	5F, 7F, and 9F	9F
Balloon shape	Spherical or elliptical	Spherical
Guidance mechanism	Nylon wire-loop that is coupled with the fiberoptic bronchoscope	Wheel device to deflect the tip
Smallest recommended ETT for coaxial use	5F (4.5 ETT), 7F (7.0 ETT), 9F (8.0 ETT)	9F (8.0 ETT)
Murphy eye	Present in 9F	Present

Abbreviation: ETT, endotracheal tube.

groups studied during elective thoracic surgery. During lung re-expansion to check for any air leaks, no contamination with secretions to the contralateral lung occurred. No difficulties recollapsing the lung were encountered in the bronchial blocker group.

In the author's opinion, bronchial blockers can be used in many cases that require OLV, taking into consideration that (1) bronchial blockers might require longer time for placement, (2) assisted suction to expedite lung collapse might be required, and (3) a fiberoptic bronchoscope may need to be used in the event that dislodgment of the blocker occurs. Anesthesiologists should become familiar with this technology and be skilled enough to use it when appropriate. Thoracic surgeons also should be aware of the different alternatives for lung isolation depending on the individual case so that the right device is suggested.

Summary

The progress in lung separation technology has allowed anesthesiologists to become skillful in fiberoptic bronchoscopy techniques and to provide excellent lung exposure in thoracic surgery patients. Given the availability of two technologies—DLTs (right-sided and left-sided) and bronchial blocker technology (TCBU, Arndt, and Cohen)—every case that requires lung collapse and OLV should receive the benefit of these devices.

Because of its greater margin of safety, a left-sided DLT is the more common device used in lung separation. If any contraindication to placing a left-sided DLT exists, a right-sided DLT is an option for any specific situation (eg, left lung transplantation). For a patient who requires lung separation and presents with the dilemma of a difficult or abnormal airway, bronchial blockers offer more advantages. Regardless of the device used, the optimal position of these devices (DLTs and bronchial blockers) is achieved best with the use of fiberoptic bronchoscopy techniques first in supine and then in lateral decubitus position or whenever repositioning of the device is needed.

References

[1] Björk VO, Carlens E. The prevention of spread during pulmonary resection by the use of a double lumen catheter. J Thorac Surg 1950;20:151–7.

[2] Campos JH. Current techniques for perioperative lung isolation in adults. Anesthesiology 2002;97:1295–301.

[3] Campos JH. An update on bronchial blockers during lung separation techniques in adults. Anesth Analg 2003;97:1266–74.

[4] Brodsky JB, Lemmens JMH. Left double-lumen tubes: clinical experience with 1,170 patients. J Cardiothorac Vasc Anesth 2003;17:289–98.

[5] Campos JH, Massa CF, Kernstine KH. The incidence of right upper-lobe collapse when comparing a right-sided double-lumen tube versus a modified left double-lumen tube for left-sided thoracic surgery. Anesth Analg 2000;90:535–40.

[6] Campos JH, Gomez MN. Pro: right-sided double-lumen endotracheal tubes should be routinely used in thoracic surgery. J Cardiothorac Vasc Anesth 2002;16: 246–8.

[7] Seymour AH, Prakash N. A cadaver study to measure the adult glottis and subglottis: defining a problem associated with the use of double-lumen tubes. J Cardiothorac Vasc Anesth 2002;16:196–8.

[8] Sivalingam P, Tio R. Tension pneumothorax, pneumomediastinum, pneumoperitoneum, and subcutaneous emphysema in a 15-year old Chinese girl after a double-lumen tube intubation and one-lung ventilation. J Cardiothorac Vasc Anesth 1999;13:312–5.

[9] Bardoczky G, d'Hollander A, Yernault JC, Van Meuylem A, Moures JM, Rocmans P. On-line expiratory flow-volume curves during thoracic surgery: occurrence of auto-PEEP. Br J Anaesth 1994;72:25–8.

[10] Sakuragi T, Kumano K, Yasumoto M, Dan K. Rupture of the left mainstem bronchus by the tracheal portion of a double-lumen endobronchial tube. Acta Anaesthesiol Scand 1997;41:1218–20.

[11] Hannallah M, Gomes M. Bronchial rupture associated with the use of a double-lumen tube in a small adult. Anesthesiology 1989;71:457–9.

[12] Brodsky JD, Macario A, Mark JBD. Tracheal diameter predicts double-lumen tube size: a method for selecting left double-lumen tubes. Anesth Analg 1996;82: 861–4.

[13] Chow MYH, Liam BL, Lew TWK, Chelliah RY, Ong BC. Predicting the size of a double-lumen endobronchial tube based on tracheal diameter. Anesth Analg 1998;87:158–60.

[14] Hannallah M, Benumof JL, Silverman PM, Kelly LC, Lea D. Evaluation of an approach to choosing a left double-lumen tube size base on chest computed tomographic scan measurement of the left mainstem bronchial diameter. J Cardiothorac Vasc Anesth 1997; 11:168–71.

[15] Chow MYH, Liam BL, Thng CH, Chong BK. Predicting the size of a double-lumen endobronchial tube using computed tomographic scan measurements of the left main bronchus diameter. Anesth Analg 1999;88:302–5.

[16] Seymour AH. The relationship between the diameters of the adult cricoid ring and main tracheobronchial tree: a cadaver study to investigate the basis for double-lumen tube selection. J Cardiothorac Vasc Anesth 2003;17:299–301.

[17] Eberle B, Weiler N, Vogel N, Kauczor HU, Heinrichs

W. Computed tomography-based tracheobronchial image reconstruction allows selection of the individually appropriate double-lumen tube size. J Cardiothorac Vasc Anesth 1999;13:532–7.

[18] Brodsky JB, Benumof JL, Ehrenwerth J. Depth of placement of left double-lumen endobronchial tubes. Anesth Analg 1991;73:570–2.

[19] Boucek CD, Landreneau R, Freeman JA, Strollo D, Bircher NG. A comparison of techniques for placement of double-lumen endobronchial tubes. J Clin Anesth 1998;10:557–60.

[20] Benumof JL, Partridge BL, Salvatierra C, Keating J. Margin of safety in positioning modern double-lumen endotracheal tubes. Anesthesiology 1987;67:729–38.

[21] McKenna MJ, Wilson RS, Botelho RJ. Right upper lobe obstruction with right-sided double-lumen endobronchial tubes: a comparison of two tube types. J Cardiothorac Anesth 1988;2:734–40.

[22] Stene R, Rose M, Weigner MB, Benumof JL, Harrell J. Bronchial trifurcation at the carina complicating use of a double-lumen tracheal tube. Anesthesiology 1994;80:1162–4.

[23] Alliaume BA, Coddens J, Deloaf T. Reliability of auscultation in positioning of double-lumen endobronchial tubes. Can J Anaesth 1992;39:687–90.

[24] Klein U, Karzai W, Bloos F, Wohlfarth M, Gottschall R, Fritz H, et al. Role of fiberoptic bronchoscopy in conjunction with the use of double-lumen tubes for thoracic anesthesia. Anesthesiology 1998;88:346–50.

[25] Sherry K. Management of patients undergoing esophagectomy. In: Gray AJG, Hoile RW, Ingram JS, Sherry KM, editors. The report of the National Confidential Enquiry into Perioperative Deaths 1996/1997. London: National Confidential Enquiry into Perioperative Deaths; 1998. p. 57–61.

[26] Pennefather SH, Russell GN. Placement of double lumen tubes—time to shed light on an old problem [editorial III]. Br J Anaesth 2000;84:308–10.

[27] Slinger P. A view of and through double-lumen tubes. J Cardiothorac Vasc Anesth 2003;17:287–8.

[28] Desiderio DP, Burt M, Kolker AC, Fischer ME, Reinsel R, Wilson RS. The effects of endobronchial cuff inflation on double-lumen endobronchial tube movement after lateral decubitus positioning. J Cardiothorac Vasc Anesth 1997;11:595–8.

[29] Saito S, Dohi S, Naito H. Alteration of double lumen endobronchial tube position by flexion and extension of the neck. Anesthesiology 1985;52:696–7.

[30] Ayorinde BT, Hanning CD, Wemyss-Holden S, Veitch PS. Tracheal rupture with a double-lumen tracheal tube. Anaesthesia 2000;55:820.

[31] Yüceyar L, Kaynak K, Canturk E, Aykac B. Bronchial rupture with a left-sided polyvinylchloride double-lumen tube. Acta Anaesthesiol Scand 2003;47:622–5.

[32] Benumof JL, Dickson W. Tracheal tear caused by extubation of a double-lumen tube. Anesthesiology 2002;97:1007–8.

[33] Sucato DJ, Girgis M. Bilateral pneumothoraces, pneumomediastinum, pneumoperitoneum, pneumoret-roperitoneum, and subcutaneous emphysema following intubation with a double-lumen endotracheal tube for thoracoscopic anterior spinal release and fusion in a patient with idiopathic scoliosis. J Spinal Disord Tech 2002;15:133–8.

[34] Weng W, DeCrosta DJ, Zhang H. Tension pneumothorax during one-lung ventilation: a case report. J Clin Anesth 2002;14:529–31.

[35] Fitzmaurice BG, Brodsky JB. Airway rupture from double-lumen tubes. J Cardiothorac Vasc Anesth 1999;13:322–9.

[36] Campos JH. Effects on oxygenation during selective lobar versus total lung collapse with or without continuous positive airway pressure. Anesth Analg 1997;85:583–6.

[37] Campos JH, Ledet C, Moyers JR. Improvement of arterial oxygen saturation with selective lobar bronchial block during hemorrhage in a patient with previous contralateral lobectomy. Anesth Analg 1995;81:1095–6.

[38] Amar D, Desiderio DP, Bains MS, Wilson RS. A novel method of one-lung isolation using a double endobronchial blocker technique. Anesthesiology 2001;95:1528–30.

[39] Campos JH, Kernstine KH. A comparison of a left-sided Broncho-Cath, with the torque control blocker Univent and the wire-guided blocker. Anesth Analg 2003;96:283–9.

[40] Arndt GA, Kranner PW, Rusy DA, Love R. Single-lung ventilation in a critically ill patient using fiber-optically directed wire-guided endobronchial blocker. Anesthesiology 1999;90:1484–6.

[41] Lewis JW, Serwin JP, Gabriel FS, Bastanfar M, Jacobsen G. The utility of a double-lumen tube for one-lung ventilation in a variety of noncardiac thoracic surgical procedures. J Cardiothorac Vasc Anesth 1992;6:705–10.

[42] Hagihira S, Takashina M, Mori T, Yoshiya I. One-lung ventilation in patients with difficult airways. J Cardiothorac Vasc Anesth 1998;12:186–8.

[43] Baraka A. The Univent tube can facilitate difficult intubation in a patient undergoing thoracoscopy. J Cardiothorac Vasc Anesth 1996;10:693–4.

[44] Ransom ES, Carter LS, Mund GD. Univent tube: a useful device in patients with difficult airways. J Cardiothorac Vasc Anesth 1995;9:725–7.

[45] Campos JH. Difficult airway and one-lung ventilation. Curr Rev Clin Anesth 2002;22:197–208.

[46] Garcia-Aguado R, Mateo EM, Tommasi-Rosso M, Grau F, Galbis J, Canto A, et al. Thoracic surgery and difficult intubation: another application of the Univent tube for one-lung ventilation. J Cardiothorac Vasc Anesth 1997;7:925–6.

[47] Garcia-Aguado R, Mateo EM, Onrubia VJ, Bolinches R. Use of the Univent system for difficult intubation and for achieving one-lung anesthesia. Acta Anaesthesiol Scand 1996;40:765–7.

[48] Takenaka I, Aoyama K, Kadoya T. Use of the Univent bronchial-blocker tube for unanticipated difficult

endotracheal intubation. Anesthesiology 2000;93:590–1.

[49] Bellver J, Garcia-Aguado R, DeAndres J, Valia JC, Bolinches R. Selective bronchial intubation with the Univent system in patients with a tracheostomy. Anesthesiology 1993;79:1453–4.

[50] Dhamee MS. One-lung ventilation in a patient with a fresh tracheostomy using the tracheostomy tube and a Univent endobronchial blocker. J Cardiothorac Vasc Anesth 1997;11:124–5.

[51] Ransom E, Detterbeck F, Klein JI, Norfleet EA. Univent tube provides a new technique for jet ventilation. Anesthesiology 1996;84:724–6.

[52] Williams H, Gothard J. Jet ventilation in a Univent tube for sleeve pneumonectomy. Eur J Anaesthesiol 2000;18:407–9.

[53] Campos JH, Kernstine KH. A structural complication in the torque control blocker Univent fracture of the blocker cap connector. Anesth Analg 2003;96:630–1.

[54] Peragallo RA, Swenson JD. Congenital tracheal bronchus: the inability to isolate the right lung with a Univent bronchial blocker tube. Anesth Analg 2000; 91:300–1.

[55] Asai T. Failure of the Univent bronchial blocker in sealing the bronchus [letter]. Anaesthesia 1999;54:97.

[56] Thelimeier KA, Anwar M. Complication of the Univent tube. Anesthesiology 1996;84:491.

[57] Dougherty P, Hannallah M. A potentially serious complication that resulted from improper use of the Univent tube. Anesthesiology 1992;77:835–6.

[58] Campos JH, Massa CF. Is there a better right-sided tube for one-lung ventilation? A comparison of the right-sided double lumen tube with the single-lumen tube with right-sided enclosed bronchial blocker. Anesth Analg 1998;86:696–700.

[59] Arndt GA, DeLessio ST, Kranner PW, Ceranski B, Valtysson B. One-lung ventilation when intubation is difficult: presentation of a new endobronchial blocker. Acta Anaesthesiol Scand 1999;43:356–8.

[60] Arndt GA, Buchika S, Kranner PW, DeLessio ST. Wire-guided endobronchial blockade in a patient with a limited mouth opening. Can J Anaesth 1999; 46:87–9.

[61] Grocott HP, Scales G, Schinderle D, King A. A new technique for lung isolation in acute thoracic trauma. J Trauma 2000;49:940–2.

[62] Campos JH, Kernstine KH. Use of the wire-guided endobronchial blocker for one-lung anesthesia in patients with airway abnormalities. J Cardiothorac Vasc Anesth 2003;17:352–4.

[63] Tobias JD. Variations on one-lung ventilation. J Clin Anesth 2001;13:35–9.

[64] Matthews AJ, Sanders DJ. Single-lung ventilation via a tracheostomy using a fiberoptically-directed 'steerable' endobronchial blocker [letter]. Anaesthesia 2001; 56:492.

[65] Ng JM, Hartigan PM. Selective lobar bronchial blockade following contralateral pneumonectomy. Anesthesiology 2003;98:268–70.

[66] Kabon B, Waltl B, Leitgeb J, Kapral S, Zimpfer M. First experience with fiberoptically directed wire-guided endobronchial blockade in severe pulmonary bleeding in an emergency setting. Chest 2001;120: 1399–402.

[67] Karzai W. Alternative method to deflate the operated lung when using wire-guided endobronchial blockade [letter]. Anesthesiology 2003;99:240.

[68] Campos JH. In response: alternative method to deflate the operated lung when using wire-guided endobronchial blockade [letter]. Anesthesiology 2003;99:241.

[69] Prabhu MR, Smith JH. Use of the Arndt wire-guided endobronchial blocker [letter]. Anesthesiology 2002; 97:1325.

[70] Bauer C, Winter C, Hentz JG, Ducrocq X, Steib A, Dupeyron JP. Bronchial blocker compared to double-lumen tube for one-lung ventilation during thoracoscopy. Acta Anaesthesiol Scand 2001;45:250–4.

ELSEVIER
SAUNDERS

Thorac Surg Clin 15 (2005) 85 – 103

THORACIC
SURGERY
CLINICS

Pathophysiology and Management of One-Lung Ventilation

Katherine P. Grichnik, MD[a],*, Jeffrey A. Clark, MD[b]

[a]*Department of Anesthesiology, Duke University Medical Center, Box 3094, Duke University Health Care Systems,
Durham, NC 27710, USA*
[b]*Department of Anesthesiology, Dartmouth Hitchcock Medical Center, One Medical Center Drive, Lebanon, NH 03756, USA*

Thoracic surgical volume is continually expanding with increased potential to care for patients with advanced surgical and respiratory disease. To care for these patients optimally, the clinician must understand the pathophysiology of the maneuvers necessary for thoracic surgery, including lateral positioning, one-lung ventilation (OLV), and the intraoperative variables that affect outcome. It is crucial to recognize and manage the consequences of OLV during surgery.

Physiology of positioning, anesthesia, ventilation, and chest opening

Ventilation

Lateral, awake, spontaneous respiration, chest closed

Benumof [1] eloquently depicted ventilation pressure to volume patterns with lateral positioning and chest incision (Fig. 1). With the assumption of a lateral position in an awake patient, the nondependent lung behaves as the superior portion of the upright lung, and the dependent lung behaves as the inferior portion of the upright lung. The dependent lung is on a steep portion of the pulmonary compliance curve, and the nondependent lung is on a less compliant portion on the curve. The shape of the dependent hemidiaphragm is altered and is subjected to increased loading from the abdominal contents; these effects serve to improve diaphragmatic effi-

ciency with subsequent increased ventilation. With relatively more perfusion directed to the dependent lung, these factors keep ventilation-perfusion (V/Q) relatively matched.

Lateral, anesthetized, spontaneous respiration, chest closed

With the induction of anesthesia, overall functional residual capacity (FRC) decreases [2], but with the lateral position, the nondependent lung moves to a more compliant portion, and the dependent lung moves to a less compliant portion of the pulmonary compliance curve. FRC increases for the nondependent lung and declines for the dependent lung [1,3] with 55% of the tidal volume directed to the nondependent lung in the lateral, anesthetized position [4]. A significant V/Q mismatch is introduced because perfusion changes little.

Lateral, anesthetized, controlled respiration, chest closed

With the onset of muscle relaxation and application of controlled ventilation, tidal volume continues to be redistributed away from the dependent lung. Without spontaneous diaphragmatic contraction, there is increased tension on the dependent hemidiaphragm from the abdominal compartment, which impairs rather than augments ventilation. The mediastinum may push downward, and improper positioning may limit the lung movement—all of which decrease the proportion of the tidal volume ventilation distributed to the dependent lung. Further V/Q mismatch results.

---

* Corresponding author.
E-mail address: grich002@mc.duke.edu (K.P. Grichnik).

thoracic.theclinics.com

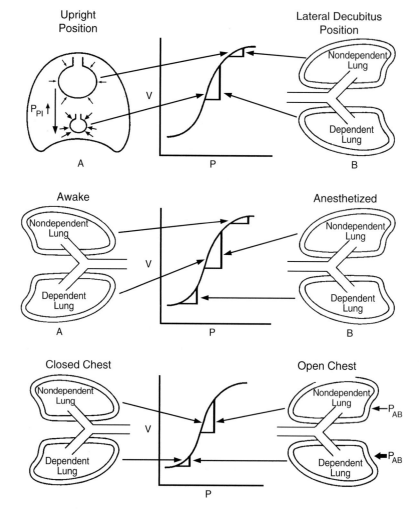

Fig. 1. Positional distribution of ventilation. The distribution of ventilation in various positions as related to a pressure-volume curve. P, pressure; P_{AB}, pressure of abdomen; V, volume. (*Adapted from* Benumof JL, editor. Anesthesia for thoracic surgery. 2nd edition. Philadelphia: WB Saunders, 1995; with permission.)

Lateral, anesthetized, controlled respiration, chest open

Opening the nondependent hemithorax of a lateral, anesthetized, paralyzed patient leads to further redirection of ventilation to the nondependent lung. The dependent lung experiences the full weight of the mediastinum because it is no longer held in place by the negative intrapleural pressure of the nondependent hemithorax at the same time that the nondependent lung is no longer constrained by the chest wall. Decreased dependent lung FRC with less compliance results. Because perfusion is altered little by chest opening, increased V/Q mismatch occurs.

Perfusion

Gravity has been proposed as the primary force for the distribution of perfusion with proportionally more blood flow in the dependent areas of a lung (Fig. 2) [5]. As with ventilation, in the lateral position, the nondependent lung behaves as the superior portions of the upright lung, and the dependent lung behaves as the inferior portions of the upright lung. The importance of gravity and position is illustrated by the finding that oxygenation with OLV is best preserved in the lateral versus the supine or semilateral position (Fig. 3) [6,7]. Other investigators have reported that blood flow distribution

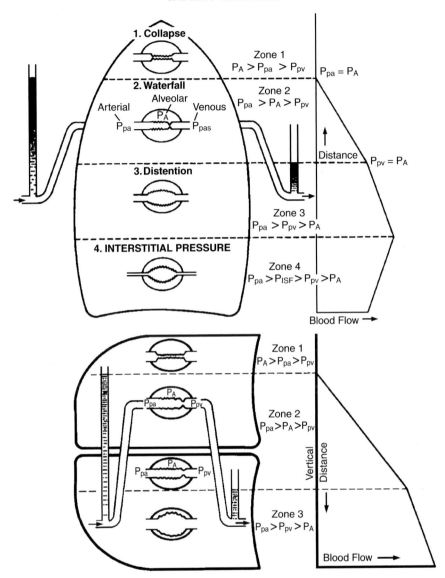

Fig. 2. The zones of West: The classic zones of West depicting the flow of blood in the lung as related to the alveolar pressure, the arterial pressure, and the venous pressure at various gravitational levels. Note the similarity of the zones in the upright and lateral positions such that in the lateral position, the nondependent lung behaves as the superior portions of the upright lung, and the dependent lung behaves as the inferior portion of the upright lung. P_A, alveolar pressure; P_{pa}, pulmonary artery pressure; P_{pv}, pulmonary vein pressure. (*Adapted from* West JB: Respiratory physiology: the essentials. 5th edition. Chapter 4. Baltimore: Williams and Wilkins; 1995; *and from* Benumof JL, editor. Anesthesia for thoracic surgery. 2nd edition. Chapter 4. Philadelphia: WB Saunders, 1995; with permission.)

changes little, however, from supine to lateral positioning [8].

Nongravitational forces also are important. In spontaneously breathing volunteers, Hakim et al [9] found central to peripheral blood flow distribution along isogravitational planes using single-photon emission computed tomography (Fig. 4). Other in-

vestigators have noted that (1) lung regions with high blood flow remained high-flow areas, and low-flow areas remained low-flow areas despite extreme changes in pulmonary artery pressure and cardiac output with exercise; (2) blood flow distribution heterogeneity was stable over time; and (3) gravity influenced blood flow distribution only mildly in

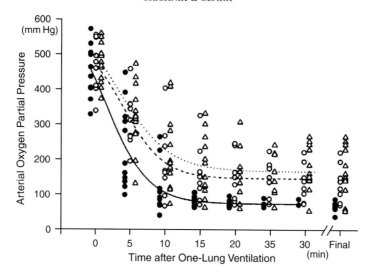

Fig. 3. Arterial oxygen pressure as a function of position. Arterial oxygenation during one-lung ventilation in the supine, semilateral, and lateral positions. △, lateral; ○, semilateral; ●, supine. (*From* Wantabe S, Noguchi E, Yamada S, et al. Sequential changes of arterial oxygen tension in the supine position during one-lung ventilation. Anesth Analg 2000;90:28–34; with permission.)

upright versus inverted lungs [10]. Geometric differences in chest cavity dimensions, preexisting pulmonary hypertension, and preexisting structural lung abnormalities also influence the primary effects of gravity on perfusion.

Mediastinal shift, paradoxical respiration

Spontaneous ventilation leads to mediastinal shift and paradoxical respiration under lateral, open chest conditions. With a closed chest, the descent of the diaphragm leads to decreased intrathoracic pressure, which is equalized by entrance of atmospheric pressure via the trachea. With an open chest, descent of the diaphragm leads to decreased intrathoracic pressure only in the closed, dependent hemithorax. The continuous application of atmospheric pressure from the open hemithorax to the mediastinum leads to mediastinal movement toward the dependent hemithorax during inspiration and movement away during expiration. Tidal volume to the dependent lung is reduced. Paradoxical respiration also may occur— nondependent lung collapse during inspiration and expansion during exhalation. As the pressure decreases in the dependent hemithorax during inspiration, volume to the dependent lung is partially entrained from the nondependent lung. The process is reversed during expiration, and part of the dependent lung tidal volume is exhaled into the nondependent lung, causing paradoxical expansion.

Mediastinal shift and paradoxical respiration decrease the efficiency of spontaneous ventilation with rebreathing of exhaled gases. Controlled ventilation with neuromuscular blockade during open chest conditions eliminates these problems.

Physiology of one-lung ventilation

Overview

With current lung separation techniques, the entire tidal volume can be delivered to the dependent lung with relative ease. The introduction of OLV results in changes in airway resistance and mean airway pressure in addition to the aforementioned physiologic changes. The individual lumens of double-lumen endotracheal tubes vary in diameter from 5 to 6.5 mm. Slinger and Leiuk [11] noted increased airflow resistance with OLV through a double-lumen tube compared with a single-lumen tube or a Univent tube. Other factors that decrease airway caliber and increase resistance include external compression from the mediastinum and diaphragm, suboptimal positioning, surgical packing, and endobronchial secretions [12]. Mean airway pressure cannot be allowed to increase unchecked because eventually it leads to increased pulmonary artery pressure and further shunting through the nondependent lung.

With collapse of the nondependent lung during OLV, perfusion to the nondependent lung continues,

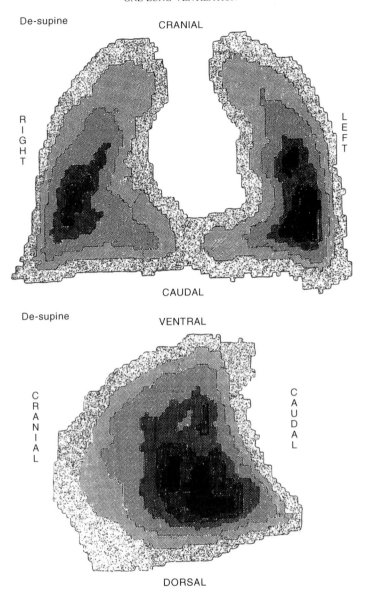

Fig. 4. Isogravitational pulmonary blood flow. The assessment of pulmonary blood flow using single-photon emission computed tomography. Note the central-to-peripheral distribution of blood flow along isogravitational planes. Darker areas represent higher blood flow, and lighter areas represent lower blood flow. (*From* Hakim TS, Lisbona R, Dean GW. Gravity-independent inequality in pulmonary blood flow in humans. J Appl Physiol 1987;63:1114–21; with permission.)

although it may be decreased initially by physical kinking of pulmonary vessels with lung deflation. Continued perfusion of an unventilated lung leads to a large increase in V/Q mismatch or shunt fraction in addition to positional effects. The main change in perfusion is from hypoxic pulmonary vasoconstriction (HPV), stimulated after the onset of OLV; it serves to decrease the V/Q mismatch and is described subsequently. Pulmonary artery pressure also may

increase from elevated airway pressure, hypoxia, hypercarbia, heart failure, or preexisting pulmonary disease, all of which may overcome HPV and lead to increased shunting through the nonventilated lung.

OLV often leads to greater changes in oxygenation than ventilation because of the physical character-istics of the red blood cell. During oxygen loading, hemoglobin is at a relatively flat portion of the dis-sociation curve and is unable to increase the amount loaded, even if excess is available. In contrast, the carbon dioxide (CO_2) elimination curve is relatively linear at physiologic values so that excessively ventilated alveoli are able to remove more CO_2 and serve to balance underventilated alveoli. There are greater increases in partial pressure of oxygen alveolar-to-arterial gradients compared with CO_2 gradients with OLV, although the partial pressure for carbon dioxide ($PaCO_2$) may increase in excess of that estimated by the end-tidal CO_2 ($ETCO_2$) [13]. Ultimately the degree of deoxygenation depends on the degree of shunt flow, a condition that is limited by the degree of the HPV response.

Hypoxic pulmonary vasoconstriction

Description

The principal mechanism to achieve more effective V/Q matching is to decrease blood flow to under-oxygenated alveoli; this is accomplished primarily by HPV, an acute or chronic reflex response of the pulmonary circulation to alveolar hypoxia [14]. This local phenomenon occurs within 1 minute, is maximal at 15 minutes, and is reversible; the magnitude is proportional to the amount of lung rendered hypoxic [1,15]. HPV diverts pulmonary blood flow from low oxygen tension regions to better aerated lung. It is unique to the pulmonary vascular system because vasodilation occurs with hypoxia in systemic vasculature [16]. HPV may be provoked by primary hypoxia or by atelectasis resulting in hypoxia. Small segments of hypoxic lung also favor the partial pressure for oxygen (PaO_2) as the primary stimulus, whereas large hypoxic segments with atelectasis favor the partial pressure of venous oxygen as the main stimulus [17]. HPV can limit what theoretically would be a 40% shunt to a 22% shunt (Fig. 5) [18,19].

The mechanisms mediating HPV locally seem to alter the balance of vasodilatory and vasoconstrictive compounds. Proposed etiologies include (1) mediators that inhibit prostaglandin synthesis, enhance leukotriene synthesis, or alter calcium channel pathways or (2) changes in nitric oxide (NO) production [20–22]. Potential humoral agents include endothelin, angiotensin II, NO, and adrenomedullin. A biologic systems unit to explain HPV mechanisms has been proposed (Fig. 6) [23]. Each unit has a sensor, a mediator, and effectors to preserve the critical variable of pulmonary PaO_2. In this model, the sensor resides in the pulmonary artery smooth muscle cells and uses the vascular redox system of the electron transport chain of mitochondria, the mediators are activated oxygen species, the signal is transmitted by

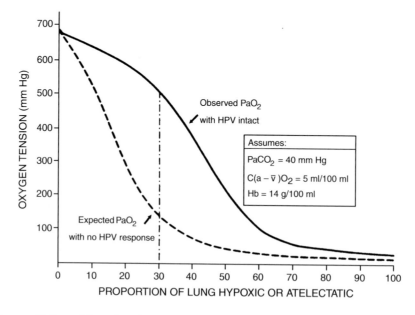

Fig. 5. One-lung ventilation and hypoxic pulmonary vasoconstriction (HPV). The dashed line of the graph illustrates the expected partial pressure of oxygen (PaO_2) in dogs in response to increasing proportion of lung hypoxia or atelectasis under normocapnia. The solid line illustrates the actual observed PaO_2. The higher than predicted PaO_2 can be attributed to a hypoxic pulmonary ventilatory response in the hypoxic or atelectatic lung, which limits perfusion to that lung segment. (*From* Cohen E, editor. The practice of thoracic anesthesia. Chapter 4, Figs. 4–14. Philadelphia: JB Lippincott; 1995; with permission.)

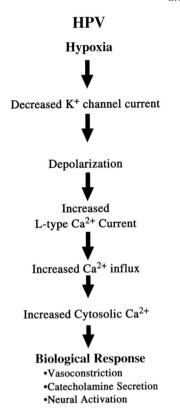

HPV

Hypoxia

↓

Decreased K⁺ channel current

↓

Depolarization

↓

**Increased
L-type Ca²⁺ Current**

↓

Increased Ca²⁺ influx

↓

Increased Cytosolic Ca²⁺

↓

Biological Response
- •Vasoconstriction
- •Catecholamine Secretion
- •Neural Activation

Fig. 6. A flow chart of the biological response to hypoxia. HPV, hypoxic pulmonary vasoconstriction. (*From* Archer S, Michelakis E. The mechanism(s) of hypoxic pulmonary vasoconstriction: potassium channels, redox O2 sensors, and controversies. News Physiol Sci 2002;17:131–7; with permission.)

voltage-sensitive potassium channels, and the effector is the membrane potential to control calcium entry and tone. Vasoconstriction results in response to hypoxia. Supporting evidence is the known phenomenon that HPV is inhibited by antagonists of voltage-dependent calcium channels [24,25].

Physiologic factors also affect HPV. Increases in cardiac output increase pulmonary perfusion, which can inhibit HPV [26]. Intermittent hypoxia variably affects the HPV response [27,28], but hyperoxia has no effect [29]. Surgical manipulation may limit or augment the HPV response.

Effects of inhalational and intravenous anesthetics

In general, it is believed that intravenous anesthetics (IVA) have little effect on HPV, whereas inhalational anesthetics (IHA) directly inhibit HPV. Conflicting results have been obtained, however, when comparing IHA with each other and with IVA

clinically during OLV [30–34]. Benumof et al [30] showed that PaO_2 was less during IHA compared with IVA in patients undergoing thoracic surgery in a crossover study. Abe et al [35] also found that propofol decreased shunt and improved oxygenation in contrast to IHA. Propofol compared with IHA for thoracotomy caused less impairment of postoperative lung function [36]. It also is controversial whether various IHAs have differential effects; for example, desflurane has been reported to preserve arterial oxygenation to a greater extent than isoflurane with OLV [37]. In contrast, Beck et al [38] found that propofol and sevoflurane were not significantly different with respect to shunt fraction under OLV (Fig. 7). Similarly, Yondov et al [39] found no difference in intraoperative PaO_2 with IVA compared with IHA.

IHA may not cause V/Q mismatch owing to specific inhibition of HPV—a more global vasodilator response may contribute. Loeckinger et al [40] examined IVA versus IHA during two-lung ventilation (TLV) *without* the influence of OLV. IHA vasodilated basal, poorly aerated lung without a change in pulmonary vascular resistance.

Interpretation of these studies is confounded by the effects of surgically induced lung trauma; unpredictable individual HPV responses; and other effects of IHA and IVA, such as depression of cardiac output with subsequent decreases in mixed venous oxygen tension. IHA may inhibit HPV, but the effect seems to be clinically insignificant.

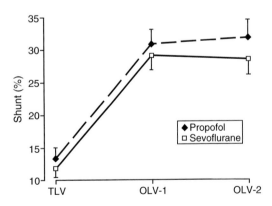

Fig. 7. Sevoflurane versus propofol and shunt fraction during one-lung ventilation. There was no significant difference between sevoflurane and propofol during thoracic surgery with respect to shunt fraction. OLV-1, one-lung ventilation supine; OLV-2, one-lung ventilation lateral; TLV, two-lung ventilation. (*From* Beck DH, Doepfmer UR, Sinemus C, et al. Effects of sevoflurane and propofol on pulmonary shunt fraction during one-lung ventilation for thoracic surgery. Br J Anaesth 2001;86:38–43; with permission.)

Vasoactive agents and hypoxic pulmonary vasoconstriction

The teaching that vasodilators, such as sodium nitroprusside and nitroglycerin, blunt the HPV response [41] has been challenged [42] because no change in shunt fraction or oxygenation with sodium nitroprusside during thoracotomy has been shown [43]. Prostaglandin $F_{2\alpha}$, a pulmonary vasodilator, inhibits HPV only when injected into the atelectatic lung pulmonary artery [44]. Dopamine and dobutamine may inhibit HPV indirectly by increasing cardiac output [45].

Novel ideas for hypoxic pulmonary vasoconstriction augmentation

Sepsis and endotoxemia inhibit HPV [46], which could be due to the generation of reactive oxygen species (ROS) [47,48]. Scavengers of ROS may prevent or reverse HPV inhibition. OLV of a rat caused increased contralateral lung pulmonary vascular resistance, a surrogate for HPV [49]. This pulmonary vascular resistance was decreased by the administration of lipopolysaccharide to simulate endotoxemia, but ROS scavengers attenuated this impairment of HPV [49].

Management of one-lung ventilation

Lung protective strategy

Description

Traditional guidelines for OLV recommend a tidal volume of 8 to 10 mL/kg to avoid dependent lung atelectasis and maintenance of a minute ventilation to defend a $PaCO_2$ of 40 mm Hg. This management strategy may be harmful, however.

The lung injury literature suggests that acute lung injury (ALI) may be directly related to volutrauma—delivery of a large tidal volume with high inspiratory pressures [50,51]. This suggestion is directly applicable to patients undergoing OLV, in which a dependent lung is ventilated with a relatively high tidal volume, often requiring a high inspiratory driving pressure. Initiation of OLV immediately increases peak and plateau airway pressures by 49% and 51% [12].

Sustained high intraoperative airway pressure has been identified as a risk factor for ALI. Licker [52] defined a "ventilatory hyperpressure index" as the product of inspiratory plateau pressure greater than 10 cm H_2O and the duration of OLV. Patients who developed ALI after OLV and thoracic surgery were managed intraoperatively with almost twice the ventilatory hyperpressure index than patients who did not develop ALI. This was the strongest risk factor for ALI identified in their study. van der Werff et al [53] found that 42% of patients with consistent intraoperative peak inspiratory pressures of greater than 40 cm H_2O pressure developed signs of ALI. Pulmonary damage also may occur with difficult intraoperative ventilation or as a result of multiple cycles of deflation and reinflation of a dependent lung [54].

The theory of lung protection is that allowing a lung to experience lower inspiratory and peak pressures while preventing cyclic alveolar collapse should avoid mechanical and inflammatory lung injury [55]. Amato et al [56] described lung protective strategies for use in medical patients with ARDS (Table 1). They found improved survival and a higher rate of

Table 1

Lung-protective strategy for reduction of volutrauma and barotrauma in patients with acute lung injury

Maneuver	Recommended value
Limit inspiratory driving pressure (P_{PLAT} − $PEEP_{TOTAL}$)	<20 cm H_2O pressure
Limit peak airway pressure	<40 cm H_2O pressure
Pressure limited or pressure support ventilation	Pressure controlled inverse ratio ventilation if FIO_2 >0.5
Relatively high PEEP (if $PEEP_{AUTO}$ occurs, then $PEEP_{TOTAL}$ = $PEEP_{EXT}$ + $PEEP_{AUTO}$)	$PEEP_{TOTAL}$ 2 cm H_2O pressure >P_{FLEX}
Frequent lung recruitment measures	Hold continuous positive airway pressure at 30–40 cm H_2O pressure for 40 sec
Respiratory rate	<30

Abbreviations: FIO_2, fraction of inspired oxygen; P_{PLAT}, plateau pressure after inspiratory pause; P_{FLEX}, the inflection point corresponding to the upward shift in the slope of the pressure-volume curve; $PEEP_{AUTO}$, the difference between alveolar pressure at end expiration and airway pressure; $PEEP_{EXT}$, PEEP applied externally to the respiratory circuit; $PEEP_{TOTAL}$, $PEEP_{EXT}$ + $PEEP_{AUTO}$.

Data from Amato MBP, Barbas CSV, Medeiros DM, et al. Effect of a protective-ventilation strategy on mortality in the acute respiratory distress syndrome. N Engl J Med 1998;338:347–54.

weaning from mechanical ventilation. The use of low tidal volume (5–6 mL/kg) based on ideal body weight also has been validated in a large multicenter randomized trial of ALI [57]. One can extrapolate this tidal volume recommendation for use with OLV.

Experimental studies

A rabbit model was used to investigate TLV, OLV protective ventilation, and OLV nonprotective ventilation [58]. Protective ventilation resulted in less alveolar collapse and overdistention, whereas the nonprotected group had greater lung water gain, more inflammation, and higher inspiratory pressures.

Adverse ventilatory settings in patients with concurrent pulmonary disease may cause release of pulmonary-derived cytokines and permit bacterial and endotoxin translocation from the lung to the systemic circulation [59]. In rabbits, the response to tracheally instilled endotoxin was investigated under protective lung ventilation versus nonprotective lung ventilation conditions. Plasma endotoxin levels and tumor necrosis factor-α increased in the nonprotected ventilation group concurrent with a decrease in PaO_2 and mean arterial pressure, resulting in requirement for pressor and bicarbonate support. These results suggest a pathophysiologic link between ventilatory strategy and outcome. Other investigators have not found differences, however, in cytokine release between lung protective and lung nonprotective ventilation strategies during thoracic surgery [60].

Positive end-expiratory pressure

Anesthesiologists traditionally use positive end-expiratory pressure (PEEP) in the dependent lung as a therapeutic maneuver only after hypoxia has occurred, but PEEP instituted at the beginning of OLV may prevent lung injury. In a sheep model of lung injury, the use of PEEP at the initiation of OLV at two different levels was associated with a greater PaO_2-to-fraction of inspired oxygen (FIO_2)ratio and less shunt, but more importantly less inflammation and histologic- injury [61].

To be comparable to OLV in humans, who often develop intrinsic PEEP, investigators must ensure that the addition of external PEEP would not be injurious. Slinger and Hickey [62] showed that external PEEP does not increase total PEEP or aggravate auto-PEEP if the expiratory time is appropriately long. Slinger et al [63] also showed that adding external PEEP may improve dependent lung compliance, FRC, and oxygenation in selected patients. Kinglstedt et al [64] showed improved V/Q distribution by adding PEEP to the dependent lung. The use of PEEP from the start

of surgery may necessitate the use of concurrent continuous positive airway pressure to the nonventilated lung to oxygenate blood shunted from dependent lung.

Lung recruitment

Tusman et al [13,65] reported on the benefits of an alveolar recruitment strategy for improving oxygenation and dead space during OLV. They found that dependent lung application of tidal volumes with peak inspiratory pressures of 40 cm H_2O and PEEP of 20 cm H_2O for 5 breaths augmented intraoperative PaO_2 (Fig. 8). They also noted that dead space ventilation decreased, and there were no adverse consequences of this limited ventilatory maneuver.

Inspired oxygen concentration

Traditionally the use of 100% oxygen has been advocated to prevent and treat oxygen desaturation during OLV. The FIO_2 used during surgery may contribute to morbidity, however. High levels of

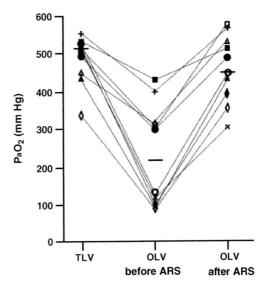

Fig. 8. Partial pressure of oxygen (PaO_2) (mm Hg) in all patients during two-lung ventilation (TLV) and during one-lung ventilation (OLV) before and after the alveolar-recruitment strategy (ARS). Each symbol represents one patient in every point of the study. Horizontal bars represent mean values at each point. (*From* Tusman G, Bohm SH, Melkun F, et al. Alveolar recruitment strategy increases arterial oxygenation during one-lung ventilation. Ann Thorac Surg 2002;73:1204–9; with permission.)

inspired oxygen cause physiologic and pathologic changes similar to other forms of ALI [66–68].

Fracica et al [69] examined three groups of primates exposed to 100% oxygen for 40, 60, and 80 hours. Histopathologic changes were noted in all lungs at 60 hours, and significant increases in pulmonary leukocyte accumulation, extravascular lung water, and permeability were noted by 80 hours, with decrements in cardiac output and stroke volume. Histopathology included early endothelial injury, later endothelial cell destruction, interstitial edema, alveolar basement membrane exposure, and capillary congestion [69]. Hyperoxia also may promote the release ROS to perpetuate an inflammatory response [70,71]; ROS also are generated during pulmonary surgery with OLV [72]. Proposed markers are protein thiol loss and protein carbonyl formation. Protein thiol levels declined and protein carbonyl levels increased after pulmonary resection with OLV. Protein thiol recovery after surgery was greater after minor resections than after extensive resections, suggesting a spectrum of injury.

Diseased lungs may be more susceptible to injury from moderate hyperoxia [73], but the role of hyperoxia in lung injury acquired during thoracic surgery is unknown. Although this relationship is not defined, a FIO_2 less than or equal to 0.6 is usually considered to be safe [74].

Ventilator strategies

Pressure-controlled ventilator

A pressure-controlled ventilator (PCV) may augment a lung protection strategy during OLV. Limiting peak and plateau transalveolar airway pressures may limit mechanical lung trauma; combined with a decelerating flow pattern, the distribution of gas flow may improve [75]. With PCV, tidal volume varies but can be kept low by setting the maximal peak pressures allowed.

Turul et al [76] found that peak airway pressure, plateau pressure, and shunt fraction increased during volume-controlled ventilation compared with PCV with OLV. PaO_2 was higher with PCV, and this correlated inversely with preoperative pulmonary function tests; patients with the poorest preoperative pulmonary function derived the greatest benefit from PCV.

Flow-volume loops

Intraoperative flow-volume loops also may be used to assess individual patient responses to lateral positioning and OLV. In-line flow-volume loops allow monitoring for the development of incomplete expiration from interrupted expiratory flow (Fig. 9) [77]. Flow-volume loops also can detect endotracheal tube movement into an incorrect position [78].

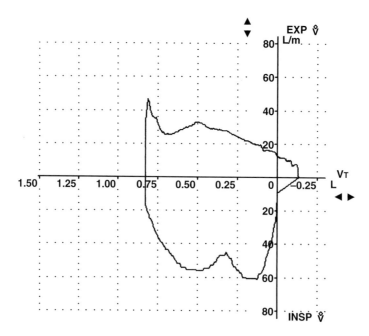

Fig. 9. An example of a flow-volume loop showing interrupted expiratory flow at the arrow. Flow is in liters/min (L/m), and pulmonary volume is in liters (L).

Adequacy of ventilation

Traditionally, $PaCO_2$ is estimated by $ETCO_2$ intraoperatively. Multiple authors have challenged the accuracy of $ETCO_2$ monitoring during abnormal patient positioning and in the presence of shunts [79,80]. Yam et al [81] described a large discrepancy between $PaCO_2$ and $ETCO_2$ during OLV as a result of changes in shunt and dead space. Transcutaneous CO_2 monitoring may be more accurate during OLV to estimate $PaCO_2$ [82].

Intraoperative fluids

Controversy

The operative volume of fluid administered to a patient during thoracic surgery has been implicated as a contributor to lung injury. Several studies support the finding that perioperative fluid administration greater than 2 L is associated with postpneumonectomy pulmonary edema or ALI [52,83,84]. This condition also occurs in patients without high perioperative fluid load [85,86], however, leading to the speculation that fluid therapy may be one contributory but not necessarily causative factor [87,88].

Given the unclear role of fluid administration in ALI during OLV for thoracic surgery, it would seem prudent to manage fluids perioperatively conservatively. The amount and type of fluids used for thoracic procedures are contentious, however.

Colloids versus crystalloids

Proposed benefits of colloid fluids include the longer duration of time for translocation to the extravascular space and perhaps less total volume of fluid translocated to the extravascular space compared with crystalloid fluid movement [89,90]. Improved tissue microperfusion, less endothelial swelling, and improved tissue oxygen tension also are reported [91]. Some investigators have found, however, increased long-term mortality with colloid use in sepsis patients [92,93]. Colloids have been found to increase the volume of the extravascular space in excess of the volume administered in septic patients [92]. Others found that colloids promote lung water retention in burn patients [94]. A meta-analysis of isotonic crystalloid versus colloid in all types of patients found no difference in pulmonary edema or mortality [95].

Fluid amount

The second issue is the amount of fluid to administer. In a review of the literature, the total *volume* of fluid seems to be a crucial factor for ALI

syndromes [52,83,96]. A combination of crystalloid and colloid is one strategy to attempt to avoid contributing to ALI during OLV. A minimal amount of crystalloid can be administered initially, after which colloids can be given to replace intravascular volume because less total fluid volume is needed. Practical, but not scientifically proven, suggestions include total positive fluid balance in the first 24 hours not greater than 20 mL/kg, less than 3 L of crystalloid use in the first 24 hours (as there is no "third space" in the chest), and use of invasive monitoring or inotropes for hemodynamic support if the urine output is at least 0.5 mL/kg/h [97].

Transfusion

A patient at risk of hypoxemia during OLV because of severe pulmonary disease may need to maintain a higher hemoglobin than a patient with normal lungs. The hemoglobin level considered safe is unknown. Arguments against liberal transfusion include the known infectious risks [98], the immunosuppressive effects of transfusion [99], and the association of transfusion with poorer outcomes [100,101].

Intraoperative problems with one-lung ventilation

Hypoxemia

Onset and prediction

PaO_2 falls sharply initially, then declines less precipitously after 15 to 20 minutes of OLV (Fig. 10) [102,103]. The ability to predict which patient would become hypoxic with OLV would be ideal. A list of postulated factors follows, which then are considered individually.

Preoperative percentage of predicted forced expiratory volume in 1 second (FEV_1)—inverse correlation
Thoracotomy for nonpulmonary surgery
Amount of perfusion to operative half of thorax
Poor preoperative PaO_2
Cardiac output and pulmonary artery pressure
Hemoglobin
Elderly
Side of surgical procedure
Supine versus lateral position

Some investigators have found a correlation between a poor predicted postoperative FEV_1 and less hypoxemia intraoperatively (Fig. 11) [103]. Explanations include (1) slow nondependent lung

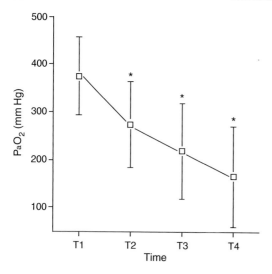

Fig. 10. The decline in partial pressure of oxygen (PaO₂) with one-lung ventilation (OLV) over time. T1 = 10 minutes of two-lung ventilation; T2 = 5 minutes of OLV in the lateral decubitus position; T3 = 15 minutes of OLV in the lateral decubitus position; T4 = 5 minutes after thoracotomy. (*From* Guenoun T, Journois D, Silleran-Chassany J, et al. Prediction of arterial oxygen tension during one-lung ventilation: analysis of preoperative and intraoperative variables. J Cardiothorac Vasc Anesth 2002;16:199–203; with permission.)

collapse after OLV institution with a prolonged period of residual oxygenation; (2) preexisting reduced perfusion in the nondependent lung secondary to intrinsic pathology or chronic HPV; (3) kinked pulmonary vessels in the deflated, nondependent lung that inhibit perfusion; and (4) development of intrinsic PEEP in dependent lung, augmenting FRC and decreasing atelectasis. Patients with relatively high perfusion of the operative, nondependent lung have a high incidence of an unacceptable PaO₂ compared with patients with relatively less perfusion of an operative lung (Fig. 12) [104]. When the blood flow to the operative lung is greater than 45%, the likelihood of hypoxemia is increased [105].

Slinger et al [106] found three factors important to the prediction of oxygen desaturation with OLV: (1) the side of surgery, (2) the PaO₂ on TLV, and (3) the percentage of predicted FEV₁ (also an inverse correlation). The right lung receives 10% more blood flow than the left and may be more subject to hypoxemia under OLV. The PaO₂ after induction of anesthesia during TLV reflects the reserve of the patient's respiratory system to maintain oxygenation with general anesthesia, positive-pressure ventilation, and lateral position. Guenoun et al [102] examined 49 variables possibly related to intraoperative hypoxemia. Only PaO₂ with TLV was an independent predictor.

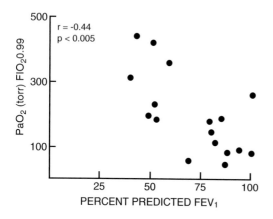

Fig. 11. Partial pressure of oxygen (PaO₂) during one-lung ventilation as a function of predicted postoperative forced expiratory volume in 1 second (FEV₁). Note the relationship of a higher predicted postoperative FEV₁ with a lower intraoperative PaO₂ during one-lung ventilation. FIO₂, fraction of inspired oxygen. (*From* Katz JA, Laverne RG, Fairley HB, et al. Pulmonary oxygen exchange during endobronchial anesthesia: effect of tidal volume and PEEP. Anesthesiology 1982;56:164–72; with permission.)

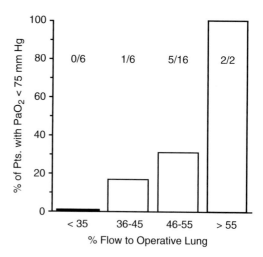

Fig. 12. The proportion of patients with hypoxemia during one-lung ventilation grouped according to the relative preoperative perfusion to the operative lung. PaO₂, partial pressure for oxygen. (*From* Hurford WE, Kolker AC, Strauss HW. The use of ventilation/perfusion lung scans to predict oxygenation during one-lung anesthesia. Anesthesiology 1987;67:841–4; with permission.)

Acceptable level

Oxygen desaturation to 88% to 90% is common; many have used this level as a threshold for intervention [106–108]. No adequate studies exist, however, to define acceptable arterial oxygen saturation with OLV. Treatment should be considered with mild desaturation to avoid significant declines in oxygenation while the intervention is being initiated. The anticipated ability of the patient to tolerate a significant decrease in oxygen delivery depends on patient pathology, comorbid diseases, operative blood losses, and duration of desaturation.

Conventional treatment

Conventional treatment for hypoxemia always should be initiated—hand ventilation to assess dynamic compliance of the pulmonary system, optimization of ventilator settings, suction of blood and secretions, and confirmation of the correct endotracheal tube position. Nonocclusive insufflation of oxygen through the open endobronchial double-lumen tube, continuous positive airway pressure to the nonventilated lung, and PEEP to the ventilated lung are other therapies. Occlusion of the artery to the tissue to be resected is most useful for large lung resections, especially pneumonectomy. Intermittent TLV occasionally may be necessary. Usually, continuous positive airway pressure is initiated before PEEP to avoid PEEP-induced compression of pulmonary blood vessels, which promote diversion of blood flow to the nonventilated lung [1]. The subset of patients who do not develop auto-PEEP (good FEV_1) may benefit more, however, from PEEP to the dependent lung first [62,63]. Ishikawa et al [109] noted that some OLV patients responded to physical compression of the nonventilated lung after hypoxemia occurred, possibly as a result of redirection of blood flow toward the ventilated lung.

Use of inhaled vasodilators and vasoconstrictors

Many groups have investigated the use of inhaled NO to the dependent ventilated lung, with variable results [110,111]. Rocca et al [112] found improved oxygenation and decreased pulmonary vascular resistance in patients with profound hypoxemia during OLV. Other patients, such as patients with a prior shunt or pulmonary hypertension, did not benefit from NO. The dose of NO used in published studies has been labeled inconsistent and excessive [113]. In a porcine study, hypoxia with OLV was improved most effectively by 4 ppm of NO compared with higher doses (Fig. 13) [113]. This finding may be due to changes in V/Q matching, some of which may be aggravated by larger NO doses. NO also is proposed to be a mediator for inhibition of HPV in sepsis and endotoxemia, when released within the nondependent, nonventilated lung [114]. It remains to be

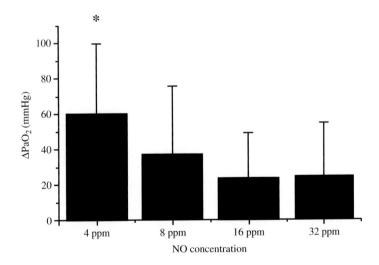

Fig. 13. Improvement in oxygenation with nitric oxide (NO). Small doses of NO improve oxygenation to a greater degree than larger doses in a porcine model of one-lung ventilation. NO was administered after hypoxia had occurred. ΔPaO_2, improvement in partial pressure for oxygen as the result of the NO administration. (*From* Sticher J, Scholz S, Böning O, et al. Small-dose nitric oxide improves oxygenation during one-lung ventilation: an experimental study. Anesth Analg 2002;95: 1557–62; with permission.)

proven that exogenous inhaled NO is clinically useful in humans under OLV conditions.

Inhaled prostacyclin may be an alternative to NO [115]. Haché et al [116] found that inhaled prostacyclin decreases pulmonary artery pressures and variably improves PaO_2-to FIO_2 ratios in thoracotomy patients. Low cost and ease of use may propel further use in thoracic surgery [117].

Almitrine is a systemic vasoconstrictor used in patients to potentiate HPV and improve oxygenation [118]. An approach to treat hypoxia with OLV is to combine an inhaled vasodilator to the dependent, ventilated lung with a vasoconstrictor for the nondependent, nonventilated lung for better V/Q matching (Fig. 14) [119]. Almitrine also is used independently to slow deceases in PaO_2 with OLV without significant hemodynamic changes [120]. Phenylephrine may be considered because almitrine may have undesirable side effects and is pending consideration by the US Food and Drug Administration [121,122].

Hypercapnia

The use of a lung protective strategy may conflict with the goal of maintaining normocapnia. Permissive hypercapnia has been advocated [123,124]. Sticher et al [125] investigated OLV patients randomized to low tidal volume ventilation versus normal tidal volume ventilation; the $PaCO_2$ was allowed to increase (to 60–70 mm Hg) without intervention. Cardiac index and pulmonary vascular resistance increased in the hypercapnia group, but oxygenation remained unchanged.

Dynamic pulmonary hyperinflation

A traditional ventilatory strategy may result in dynamic pulmonary hyperinflation or auto-PEEP. Most patients develop auto-PEEP with OLV [126, 127], and the use of high tidal volume may exacerbate further the inability of patients with diseased lungs to empty the dependent lung with each expiration. Other causes include inappropriate inspiration to expiration settings, small diameter, high-resistance endotracheal tubes, application of excessive external PEEP, or use of a volume-controlled ventilator without alarms for increasing baseline pressure levels [11]. Hemodynamic consequences include impaired venous return, right ventricular and left ventricular dysfunction, and decreased cardiac output [128].

Standard anesthesia machines and most ICU ventilatory monitors do not readily detect retained pulmonary volume [129]. Dynamic pulmonary hyperinflation may be an underappreciated cause of cardiac arrest resulting from electromechanical dissociation [130,131]. Ideally an expiratory flowmeter can monitor for dynamic pulmonary hyperinflation [132]. When this is suspected clinically, the patient should be disconnected from the ventilator immediately and allowed to exhale completely, which may take seconds to minutes. Hemodynamic parameters should improve, but resuscitation measures may be necessary.

Ducros et al [133] investigated auto-PEEP and air-trapping under supine TLV, lateral TLV, and lateral OLV conditions. Patients with mild lung disease had minimal air-trapping and developed auto-PEEP only with OLV, whereas patients with restrictive lung disease had little air-trapping or auto-PEEP overall.

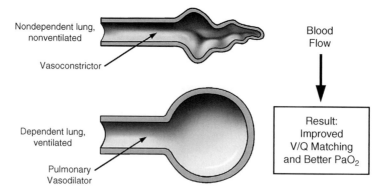

Fig. 14. A model for optimization of hypoxic pulmonary vasoconstriction. The use of a pulmonary vasoconstrictor directed toward the nondependent lung and a pulmonary vasodilator directed toward the dependent lung is proposed to improve ventilation-perfusion (V/Q) matching during one lung-ventilation. PaO_2, partial pressure for oxygen. (*Conceived from the text of* Moutafis M, Liu N, Dalibon N, et al. The effects of inhaled nitric oxide and its combination with intravenous almitrine on PaO_2 during one-lung ventilation in patients undergoing thoracoscopic procedures. Anesth Analg 1997;85:1130–5; with permission.)

Patients with severe obstructive lung disease showed high levels of auto-PEEP and trapped air with TLV, however, which increased with OLV.

Barotrauma

Barotrauma occurs from sustained increased alveolar overdistention. Because alveolar volume does not correlate with alveolar pressure, it is not easily measurable. The risk of barotrauma increases with increased expiratory resistance resulting from endotracheal tubes, increased resistance with coughing or "bucking" against the ventilator, and inappropriate levels of extrinsic PEEP. The hemodynamic effects of barotrauma in the dependent, ventilated lung are similar to dynamic pulmonary hyperinflation, but also include mediastinal shift toward the nondependent lung and increased inflation pressures.

Avoidance of barotrauma is aided by the use of muscle relaxants, intermittent disconnection from the ventilator, long expiratory relative to inspiratory times, limitation of inflation pressures, and vigilance. A "lung protective strategy" has led to decreased barotrauma in ICU patients [56].

Barotrauma-induced pneumothorax in the contralateral dependent lung during OLV can become a tension pneumothorax quickly with positive-pressure ventilation [134]. Emergent treatment includes resuscitative medications and relief of intrapleural pressure. Barotrauma also can manifest as pneumomediastinum, pneumoperitoneum, and subcutaneous emphysema.

Summary

The ability to manage OLV effectively in patients with significant pulmonary disease is increasing. Knowledge of pulmonary ventilation and perfusion physiology, improvements in the ability to prevent and treat hypoxia, and a thorough grasp of traditional and novel ventilatory techniques may promote improved perioperative outcomes.

References

[1] Benumof JL. Chapter 2: distribution of ventilation and perfusion. In: Benumof JL, editor. Anesthesia for thoracic surgery. 2nd edition. Philadelphia: WB Saunders; 1995. p. 35–52.

[2] Wahba RWM. Perioperative functional residual capacity. Can J Anaesth 1991;38:384–400.

[3] Lumb AB, Nunn JF. Respiratory function and ribcage contribution to ventilation in body positions commonly used during anesthesia. Anesth Analg 1991; 73:422–6.

[4] Larsson A, Malmkivist G, Werner O. Variations in lung volume and compliance during pulmonary surgery. Br J Anaesth 1987;59:585–91.

[5] West JB. Respiratory physiology: the essentials. 5th edition. Baltimore: Williams & Wilkins; 1995.

[6] Wantabe S, Noguchi E, Yamada S, et al. Sequential changes of arterial oxygen tension in the supine position during one-lung ventilation. Anesth Analg 2000;90:28–34.

[7] Bardoczky GI, Szegedi LL, d'Hollander AA, et al. Two-lung and one-lung ventilation in patients with chronic obstructive pulmonary disease: the effects of position and FIO2. Anesth Analg 2000;90:35–41.

[8] Mure M, Domino KB, Robertson T, et al. Pulmonary blood flow does not redistribute in dogs with reposition from supine to left lateral position. Anesthesiology 1998;89:483–92.

[9] Hakim TS, Lisbona R, Dean GW. Gravity-independent inequality in pulmonary blood flow in humans. J Appl Physiol 1987;63:1114–21.

[10] Glenny RW. Blood flow distribution in the lung. Chest 1998;114:8S–16S.

[11] Slinger PD, Leiuk L. Flow resistances of disposable double lumen, single lumen and univent tubes. J Cardiothorac Vasc Anesth 1998;12:142–4.

[12] Szegedi LL, Bardoczky GI, Engleman EE, d'Hollander AA. Airway pressure changes during one lung ventilation. Anesth Analg 1997;84:1034–7.

[13] Tusman G, Bohm SH, Sipmann FS, Maisch S. Lung recruitment improves efficiency of ventilation and gas exchange during one lung ventilation anesthesia. Anesth Analg 2004;98:1604–9.

[14] Dumas JP, Bardou M, Goirand F, Dumas M. Hypoxic pulmonary vasoconstriction. Gen Pharmacol 1999; 33:289–97.

[15] Leach RM, Treacher DF. Clinical aspects of hypoxic pulmonary vasoconstriction. Exp Physiol 1995;80: 865–75.

[16] Farhi LE, Sheehan DW. Pulmonary circulation and systemic circulation: similar problems, different solutions. Adv Exp Med Biol 1990;277:579–86.

[17] Domino KB, Wetstein L, Glasser SA. Influence of mixed venous oxygen tension (PvO2) on blood flow to atelectatic lung. Anesthesiology 1983;59:428.

[18] Benumof JL. One-lung ventilation and hypoxic pulmonary vasoconstriction: implications for anesthetic management. Anesth Analg 1985;64:821–33.

[19] Grichnik KP, McIvor W, Slinger PD. Intraoperative management for thoracotomy. In: Kaplan JA, Slinger PD, editors. Thoracic anesthesia. 3rd edition. Philadelphia: Churchill Livingstone; 2003. p. 138.

[20] Dumas JP, Bardou M, Goirand F. Hypoxic pulmonary vasoconstriction. Gen Pharmacol 1999;33:289–97.

[21] Wilkins MR, Zhao L, Al-Tubuly R. The regulation of pulmonary vascular tone. Br J Clin Pharmacol 1996; 42:127–31.

[22] Naeije R, Brimioulle S. Physiology in medicine: importance of hypoxic pulmonary vasoconstriction in maintaining arterial oxygenation during acute respiratory failure. Crit Care 2001;5:67–71.

[23] Archer S, Michelakis E. The mechanism(s) of hypoxic pulmonary vasoconstriction: potassium channels, redox O2 sensors, and controversies. News Physiol Sci 2002;17:131–7.

[24] Robertson TP, Hague D, Aaronson PI, Ward JP. Voltage-independent calcium entry in hypoxic pulmonary vasoconstriction of intrapulmonary arteries of the rat. J Physiol 2000;525(Pt 3):669–80.

[25] Minami T, Inoue H, Ogawa J, Shohtsu A. Effect of Ca-antagonists on pulmonary blood flow during single-lung ventilation in the dog. Jap J Thorac Dis 1993;31:1207–14.

[26] Domino KB, Eisenstein BL, Tran T. Increased pulmonary perfusion worsens ventilation-perfusion matching. Anesthesiology 1993;79:817–26.

[27] Benumof JL. Intermittent hypoxia increases lobar hypoxic pulmonary vasoconstriction. Anesthesiology 1983;58:399–404.

[28] Chen L, Miller FL, Williams JJ, et al. Hypoxic pulmonary vasoconstriction is not potentiated by repeated intermittent hypoxia in closed chest dogs. Anesthesiology 1985;63:608–10.

[29] Hambraeus-Jonzon K, Bindslev L, Millgard AJ, et al. Hypoxic pulmonary vasoconstriction in human lungs. Anesthesiology 1997;8:308–15.

[30] Benumof JL, Augustine SD, Gibbons JA. Halothane and isoflurane only slightly impair arterial oxygenation during one-lung ventilation in patients undergoing thoracotomy. Anesthesiology 1987;67:910–5.

[31] Slinger P, Scott WA. Arterial oxygenation during one-lung ventilation: a comparison of enflurane and isoflurane. Anesthesiology 1995;82:940–6.

[32] Karzai W, Haberstroh J, Preibe HJ. Effects of desflurane and propofol on arterial oxygenation during one-lung ventilation in the pig. Acta Anaesthesiol Scand 1998;42:648–52.

[33] Kellow NH, Scott AD, White SA, et al. Comparison of the effects of propofol and isoflurane anesthesia on right ventricular function and shunt fraction during thoracic surgery. Br J Anaesth 1995;75:578–82.

[34] Shimizu T, Abe K, Kinouchi K, et al. Arterial oxygenation during one-lung ventilation. Can J Anaesth 1997;44:1162–6.

[35] Abe K, Shimizu T, Tacashina M, Shiozaki H, Yoshiya I. The effects of propofol, isoflurane, sevoflurane on oxygenation and shunt fraction during one lung ventilation. Anesth Analg 1998;87:1164–9.

[36] Speicher A, Jessberger J, Braun R, et al. Postoperative pulmonary function after lung surgery: total intravenous anesthesia with propofol in comparison to balanced anesthesia with isoflurane. Anaesthetist 1995;44:265–73.

[37] Pagel PS, Fu JJL, Damask MC, et al. Desflurane and isoflurane produce similar alterations in systemic and pulmonary hemodynamics and arterial oxygenation in patients undergoing one-lung ventilation during thoracotomy. Anesth Analg 1998;87:800–7.

[38] Beck DH, Doepfmer UR, Sinemus C, et al. Effects of sevoflurane and propofol on pulmonary shunt fraction during one-lung ventilation for thoracic surgery. Br J Anaesth 2001;86:38–43.

[39] Yondov D, Kounev V, Ivanov O, et al. A comparative study of the effect of halothane, isoflurane and propofol on partial arterial oxygen pressure during one-lung ventilation in thoracic surgery. Folia Med 1999;41:45–51.

[40] Loeckinger A, Keller C, Lindner KH, et al. Pulmonary gas exchange in coronary artery surgery patients during sevoflurane and isoflurane anesthesia. Anesth Analg 2002;94:1107–12.

[41] D'Oliveira M, Sykes MK, Chakrabarti MK, et al. Depression of hypoxic pulmonary vasoconstriction by sodium nitroprusside and nitroglycerine. Br J Anaesth 1981;53:11–8.

[42] Miller JR, Benumof JL, Trousdale FR. Combined effects of sodium nitroprusside and propranolol on hypoxic pulmonary vasoconstriction. Anesthesiology 1982;57:267–71.

[43] D'Oliveira M, Sykes MK, Chakrabarti MK, Ochard J, Keslin J. Depression of hypoxic pulmonary vasoconstriction by sodium nitroprusside and nitroglycerine. Br J Anaesth 1981;53:11.

[44] Scherer RW, Vigfusson G, Hultsch E, et al. Prostaglandin F2 alpha improves oxygen tension and reduces venous admixture during one-lung ventilation in anesthetized paralyzed dogs. Anesthesiology 1985;62:23–8.

[45] Gardaz JP, McFarlane PA, Sykes M. Mechanisms by which dopamine alters blood flow distribution during lobar collapse in dogs. J Appl Physiol 1986;60:959–64.

[46] Ichinose F, Zapol WM, Sapirstein A, et al. Attenuation of hypoxic pulmonary vasoconstriction by endotoxemia requires 5-lipoxygenase in mice. Circ Res 2001;88:832–8.

[47] Van DV, Eiserich JP, Shigenaga MK, Cross CE. Reactive nitrogen species and tyrosine nitration in the respiratory tract: epiphenomena or a pathobiologic mechanism of disease? Am J Respir Crit Care Med 1999;160:1–9.

[48] Chabot F, Mitchell JA, Gutteridge JM, Evans TW. Reactive oxygen species in acute lung injury. Eur Respir J 1998;11:745–57.

[49] Baboolal HA, Ichinose F, Ullrich R, et al. Reactive oxygen species scavengers attenuate endotoxin-induced impairment of hypoxic pulmonary vasoconstriction in mice. Anesthesiology 2002;97:1227–33.

[50] Tsuno K, Miura K, Takeya M, Kolobow T, Morioka T. Histopathologic pulmonary changes from mechanical ventilation at high peak airway pressures. Am Rev Respir Dis 1991;143:1115–20.

[51] Parker JC, Hernandez LA, Peevy KJ. Mechanisms of ventilator-induced lung injury. Crit Care Med 1993; 21:131–43.

[52] Licker M, De Perrot M, Spiliopoulos A, et al. Risk

factors for acute lung injury after thoracic surgery for lung cancer. Anesth Analg 2003;97:1558–65.

[53] Van der Werff YD, van der Houwen HK, Heilmans PJM, et al. Postpneumonectomy pulmonary edema: a retrospective analysis of incidence and possible risk factors. Chest 1997;111:1278–84.

[54] Dos Santos CC, Slutsky AS. Mechanisms of ventilator-induced lung injury: a perspective. J Appl Physiol 2000;89:1645–55.

[55] Hickling KG, Walsh I, Henderson S, Jackson R. Low mortality rate in adult respiratory distress syndrome using low-volume, pressure limited ventilation with permissive hypercapnea: a prospective study. Crit Care Med 1994;22:1568–78.

[56] Amato MBP, Barbas CSV, Medeiros DM, et al. Effect of a protective-ventilation strategy on mortality in the acute respiratory distress syndrome. N Engl J Med 1998;338:347–54.

[57] The Acute Respiratory Distress Syndrome Network. Ventilation with lower tidal volumes as compared with traditional tidal volumes for acute lung injury and the acute respiratory distress syndrome. N Engl J Med 2000;342:1301–8.

[58] de Abreu MG, Heintz M, Heller A, et al. One-lung ventilation with high tidal volume and zero positive end-expiratory pressure is injurious in the isolated rabbit lung model. Anesth Analg 2003;96:220–8.

[59] Murphy DB, Cregg N, Tremblay L, et al. Adverse ventilatory strategy causes pulmonary to systemic translocation of endotoxin. Am J Respir Crit Care Med 2000;162:27–33.

[60] Wrigge H, Uhlig U, Zinserling J, et al. The effects of different ventilatory settings on pulmonary and systemic inflammatory responses during major surgery. Anesth Analg 2004;98:775–81.

[61] Takeuchi M, Goddon S, Dolhnikoff M, et al. Set positive end-expiratory pressure during protective ventilation affects lung injury. Anesthesiology 2002; 97:682–92.

[62] Slinger PD, Hickey DR. The interaction between applied PEEP and auto-PEEP during one-lung ventilation. J Cardiothorac Vasc Anesth 1998;12:133–6.

[63] Slinger PD, Kruger M, McRae K, et al. Relation of the static compliance curve and positive end-expiratory pressure to oxygenation during one-lung ventilation. Anesthesiology 2001;95:1096–102.

[64] Kinglstedt C, Hedenstierna G, Baehrendtz S, et al. Ventilation-perfusion relationships and atelectasis formation in the supine and lateral positions during conventional mechanical and differential ventilation. Acta Anaesthesiol Scand 1990;34:421–99.

[65] Tusman G, Bohm SH, Melkun F, et al. Alveolar recruitment strategy increases arterial oxygenation during one-lung ventilation. Ann Thorac Surg 2002; 73:1204–9.

[66] Fox RB, Hoidal JR, Brown DM, et al. Pulmonary inflammation due to oxygen toxicity: involvement of chemotactic factors and polymorphonuclear leukocytes. Am Rev Respir Dis 1981;123:521–3.

[67] Royer F, Martin DJ, Benchetrit G, et al. Increase in pulmonary capillary permeability in dogs exposed to 100% O2. J Appl Physiol 1988;65:1140–6.

[68] Royston BD, Webster NR, Nunn JF. Time course of changes in lung permeability and edema in the rat exposed to 100% oxygen. J Appl Physiol 1990;69: 1532–7.

[69] Fracica PJ, Knapp MJ, Piantadosi CA, et al. Responses of baboons to prolonged hyperoxia: physiology and qualitative pathology. J Appl Physiol 1991; 71:2352–62.

[70] Carvalho CR, Schettino GPP, Maranhao B, Bethlem EP. Hyperoxia and lung disease. Curr Opin Pulm Med 1998;4:300.

[71] Szarek JL, Ramsay HL, Andringa A, Miller ML. Time course of airway hyperresponsiveness and remodeling induced by hyperoxia in rats. Am J Physiol 1995;269:L227.

[72] Williams E, Quinlan GJ, Goldstraw P, Gothard JW, Evans TW. Postoperative lung injury and oxidative damage in patients undergoing pulmonary resection. Eur Respir J 1998;11:1028–34.

[73] Witschi HR, Haschek WM, Klein-Szanto AJ, et al. Potentiation of diffuse lung damage by oxygen: determining variables. Am Rev Respir Dis 1981;123:98–103.

[74] Brower RG, Ware L, Berthiaume Y, Matthay MA. Treatment of ARDS. Chest 2001;120:1347–67.

[75] Campbell RS, Davis BR. Pressure-controlled versus volume-controlled ventilation: does it matter? Respir Care 2002;47:416–24.

[76] Turul M, Camci E, Karadeniz H, et al. Comparison of volume controlled with pressure controlled ventilation during one-lung anaesthesia. Br J Anaesth 1997; 79:306–10.

[77] Bardoczky GI, d'Hollander A. Continuous monitoring of the flow-volume loops and compliance during anaesthesia. J Clin Monit 1992;8:251–2.

[78] Bardoczky GI, Levarlet M, Engelman E, et al. Continuous spirometry for detection of double-lumen endobronchial tube displacement. Br J Anaesth 1993; 70:499–502.

[79] Grenier B, Verchere E, Mesli A, et al. Capnography monitoring during neurosurgery: reliability in relation to various intraoperative positions. Anesth Analg 1999;88:43–8.

[80] Short JA, Paris ST, Booker PD, et al. Arterial to end-tidal carbon dioxide tension difference in children with congenital heart disease. Br J Anaesth 2001;86: 349–53.

[81] Yam PC, Innes PA, Jackson M, et al. Variation in the arterial to end-tidal PCO2 difference during one-lung thoracic anaesthesia. Br J Anaesth 1994;72:21–4.

[82] Tobias JD. Noninvasive carbon dioxide monitoring during one-lung ventilation: end-tidal versus transcutaneous techniques. J Cardiothorac Vasc Anesth 2003;17:306–8.

[83] Zeldin RA, Normandin D, Landtwing D, Peters RM. Postpneumonectomy pulmonary edema. J Thorac Cardiovasc Surg 1984;87:359.

[84] Verheijen-Breemharr L, Bogaard JM, van den Berg B. Noncardiogenic pulmonary edema complicating lung resection. Ann Thorac Surg 1988;43:323–6.

[85] Alvarez JM, Bairstow BM, Tang C, Newman MA. Post-lung resection pulmonary edema: a case for aggressive management. J Cardiothorac Vasc Anesth 1998;12:199–205.

[86] Turnage WS, Lunn JJ. Postpneumonectomy pulmonary edema: a retrospective analysis of associated variables. Chest 1993;103:1646–50.

[87] Slinger PD. Perioperative fluid management for thoracic surgery: the puzzle of postpneumonectomy pulmonary edema. J Cardiothorac Vasc Anesth 1999; 9:442.

[88] Slinger PD. Acute lung injury after pulmonary resection: more pieces of the puzzle. Anesth Analg 2003;97:155–7.

[89] Vaupshasl HJ, Levy M. Distribution of saline following acute volume loading: postural effects. Clin Invest Med 1990;13:165–77.

[90] Ernest D, Belzberg AS, Dodeck PM. Distribution of normal saline and 5% albumin infusions in septic patients. Crit Care Med 1999;27:46–50.

[91] Lang K, Boldt J, Suttner S, Haisch G. Colloids versus crystalloids and tissue oxygen tension in patients undergoing major abdominal surgery. Anesth Analg 2001;93:405–9.

[92] Boldt J. The good, the bad, and the ugly: should we completely banish human albumin from our intensive care units? Anesth Analg 2000;91:887–95.

[93] Schierhout G, Roberts I. Fluid resuscitation with colloid or crystalloid solutions in critically ill patients: a systematic review of randomized trials. BMJ 1998; 316:961–4.

[94] Goodwin CW, Dorethy J, Lam V, Pruitt BA. Randomized trial of efficacy of crystalloid and colloid resuscitation on hemodynamic response and lung water following thermal injury. Ann Surg 1983; 197:520–31.

[95] Choi PT-L, Yip G, Quinonez LG, Cook DJ. Crystalloids vs. colloids in fluid resuscitation: a systematic review. Crit Care Med 1999;27:200–10.

[96] Parquin F, Marchal M, Meehiri S, et al. Postpneumonectomy pulmonary edema: analysis and risk factors. Eur J Cardiothorac Surg 1996;10: 929–33.

[97] Slinger P. Post-pneumonectomy pulmonary edema. Curr Opin Anesthesiol 1999;12:49–54.

[98] Klein HG. Will blood transfusion ever be safe enough? Transfus Med 2001;11:122.

[99] Claas FH, Roelen DL, van Rood JJ, Brand A. Modulation of the alloimmune response by blood transfusions. Transfus Clin Biol 2001;8:315.

[100] Leal-Noval SR, Rincon-Ferrari MD, Garcia-Curiel A, et al. Transfusion of blood components and postoperative infection in patients undergoing cardiac surgery. Chest 2001;119:1461.

[101] Langley SM, Alexiou C, Bailey DH, Weeden DF. The influence of perioperative blood transfusion on survival after esophageal resection for carcinoma. Ann Thorac Surg 2002;73:1704–9.

[102] Guenoun T, Journois D, Silleran-Chassany J, et al. Prediction of arterial oxygen tension during one-lung ventilation: analysis of preoperative and intraoperative variables. J Cardiothorac Vasc Anesth 2002;16: 199–203.

[103] Katz JA, Laverne RG, Fairley HB, et al. Pulmonary oxygen exchange during endobronchial anesthesia: effect of tidal volume and PEEP. Anesthesiology 1982;56:164–72.

[104] Hurford WE, Kolker AC, Strauss HW. The use of ventilation/perfusion lung scans to predict oxygenation during one-lung anesthesia. Anesthesiology 1987;67:841–4.

[105] Dunn PF. Physiology of the lateral decubitus position and one-lung ventilation. Int Anesthesiol Clin 2000; 38:25–53.

[106] Slinger P, Suissa S, Triolet W. Predicting arterial oxygenation during one-lung anaesthesia. Can J Anaesth 1992;39:1030–5.

[107] Kerr JH, Crampton Smith A, Prys-Roberts C, et al. Observations during endobronchial anaesthesia: II. oxygenation. Br J Anaesth 1974;46:84–92.

[108] Severinghaus JW, Naifeh KH. Accuracy of response of six pulse oximeters to profound hypoxemia. Anesthesiology 1987;67:551–8.

[109] Ishikawa S, Nakazawa K, Makita R. Progressive changes in arterial oxygenation during one-lung anaesthesia are related to the response to compression of the non-dependent lung. Br J Anaesth 2003;90:21–6.

[110] del Barrio E, Varela G, Sastre JA, et al. Inhalation administration of nitric oxide during selective pulmonary ventilation decreased the intrapulmonary shunt. Rev Esp Anestesiol Reanim 1999;46:247–51.

[111] Fradj K, Samain E, Delefosse D, et al. Placebo-controlled study of inhaled nitric oxide to treat hypoxaemia during one-lung ventilation. Br J Anaesth 1999;82:208–12.

[112] Rocca GD, Passariello M, Coccia C, et al. Inhaled nitric oxide administration during one-lung ventilation in patients undergoing thoracic surgery. J Cardiothorac Vasc Anesth 2001;15:218–23.

[113] Sticher J, Scholz S, Böning O, et al. Small-dose nitric oxide improves oxygenation during one-lung ventilation: an experimental study. Anesth Analg 2002; 95:1557–62.

[114] Ullrich R, Bloch KD, Ichinose F, Steudel W, Zapol WM. Hypoxic pulmonary blood flow redistribution and arterial oxygenation in endotoxin-challenged NOS2-deficient mice. J Clin Invest 1999;104: 1421–9.

[115] Lowson SM. Inhaled alternatives to nitric oxide. Anesthesiology 2002;96:1504–13.

[116] Haché M, Denault AN, Bélisle S, et al. Inhaled prostacyclin (PDI2) is an effective addition to the treatment of pulmonary hypertension and hypoxia in the operating room and intensive care unit. Can J Anaesth 2001;48:924–9.

[117] Sutcliffe N, McCluskey A. Simple apparatus for continuous nebulisation of prostacyclin. Anaesthesia 2000;55:405.

[118] Jolliet P, Bulpa P, Ritz M, et al. Additive beneficial effects of the prone position, nitric oxide, and almitrine bismesylate on gas exchange and oxygen transport in acute respiratory distress syndrome. Crit Care Med 1997;25:786–94.

[119] Moutafis M, Liu N, Dalibon N, et al. The effects of inhaled nitric oxide and its combination with intravenous almitrine on PaO2 during one-lung ventilation in patients undergoing thoracoscopic procedures. Anesth Analg 1997;85:1130–5.

[120] Moutafis M, Dalibon N, Liu N, et al. The effects of intravenous almitrine on oxygenation and hemodynamics during one-lung ventilation. Anesth Analg 2002;94:830–4.

[121] B'chir A, Mebazaa A, Losser MR, Romieu M, Payen D. Intravenous almitrine bismesylate reversibly induces lactic acidosis and hepatic dysfunction in patients with acute lung injury. Anesthesiology 1998; 89:823–30.

[122] Bouche P, Lacomblez L, Leger JM, et al. Peripheral neuropathies during treatment with almitrine: report of 46 cases. J Neurol 1989;236:29–33.

[123] Tuxen D, Williams T, Scheinkestel C, et al. Limiting dynamic hyperinflation in mechanically ventilated patients with severe asthma reduces complications. Anaesth Intensive Care 1993;21:718.

[124] Zollinger A, Zaugg M, Wedeer W, et al. Video-assisted thoracoscopic volume reduction surgery inpatients with diffuse pulmonary emphysema: gas exchange and anesthesiological management. Anesth Analg 1997;84:845–51.

[125] Sticher J, Müller M, Scholz S, et al. Controlled hypercapnea during one-lung ventilation in patients undergoing pulmonary resection. Acta Anaesthesiol Scand 2001;45:842–7.

[126] Bardoczy GI, Yernault JC, Engleman E, et al. Intrinsic positive end-expiratory pressure during one-lung ventilation using double lumen endobronchial tube. Chest 1996;110:180–4.

[127] Yokota K, Toriumi T, Sari A, et al. Auto-positive end-expiratory pressure during one-lung ventilation for thoracic surgery. Anesth Analg 1996;82:1007–10.

[128] Myles PS, Ryder IG, Weeks AM, et al. Diagnosis and management of dynamic hyperinflation during lung transplantation. J Cardiothorac Vasc Anesth 1997; 11:100.

[129] Rogers PL, Schlichtig R, Miro A, Pinsky M. Auto-PEEP during CPR: an "occult" cause of electromechanical dissociation? Chest 1991;99:492–3.

[130] Lapinsky SE, Leung RS. Auto-PEEP and electromechanical dissociation. N Engl J Med 1996;335:674.

[131] Connery LE, Deignan MJ, Gujer MW, Richardson MG. Cardiovascular collapse associated with extreme iatrogenic PEEPi in patients with obstructive airways disease. Br J Anaesth 1999;83:493–5.

[132] Bardoczky G, d'Hollander A, Cappello M, Yernault J. Interrupted expiratory flow on automatically constructed flow-volume curves may determine the presence of intrinsic positive end-expiratory pressure during one lung ventilation. Anesth Analg 1998; 86:880.

[133] Ducros L, Moutafis M, Castelain M-H, et al. Pulmonary air trapping and one-lung ventilation. J Cardiothorac Vasc Anesth 1999;13:35.

[134] Keller CA, Naunheim KS. Perioperative management of lung reduction patients. Clin Chest Med 1997; 18:285.

THORACIC
SURGERY
CLINICS

ELSEVIER
SAUNDERS

Thorac Surg Clin 15 (2005) 105 – 121

Impact of Acute Pain and its Management for Thoracic Surgical Patients

E. Andrew Ochroch, MD[a],*, Allan Gottschalk, MD, PhD[b]

[a]Department of Anesthesia, University of Pennsylvania Health System, 3400 Spruce Street, 680 Dulles Building,
Philadelphia, PA 19104, USA
[b]Department of Anesthesiology and Critical Care Medicine, The Johns Hopkins Hospital, 720 Rutland Avenue,
Baltimore, MD 21205, USA

Despite efforts to recognize the undertreatment of perioperative pain and promulgate guidelines to improve this situation [1], perioperative pain remains prevalent and is one of the aspects of the perioperative experience that generates the greatest concern for patients about to undergo surgery [2]. Thoracic surgery can produce some of the most intense perioperative pain that patients can experience [3–5]. Beyond the discomfort, pain and the body's response to pain contribute significantly to perioperative morbidity. There is also a growing recognition of the extent to which acute painful experiences can lead to longer term painful consequences, even when tissue healing appears to be complete [6].

The neurobiologic basis of acute painful experiences and the processes whereby these lead to longer term pain and its consequences have been elucidated partially [7]. The key observations are that (1) multiple sites and multiple receptors collectively contribute and that (2) a painful experience initiates a cascade of events that sensitize the nervous system so that subsequent noxious stimuli are perceived with greater intensity (*hyperalgesia*), and even previously nonpainful stimuli can be painful (*allodynia*) (Box 1). Incorporating these observations into effective perioperative regimens designed to limit acute pain and its consequences leads to a multimodal preemptive approach to acute pain management. Multimodal analgesia recognizes the multitude of sites and receptors that contribute to painful experience and the process whereby the nervous system becomes sensitized. In practice, multimodal analgesia employs an array of drugs and techniques with the expectation that the effects of each will be at least additive if not synergistic. Preemptive analgesia recognizes the importance of initiating an analgesic regimen capable of preventing sensitization of the nervous system *before* the onset of noxious stimuli and maintaining such an intervention for the duration of time (length unknown) when untreated pain could otherwise sensitize the nervous system.

Thoracic surgical pain is an ideal setting for the use of preemptive analgesic techniques because the timing of noxious stimuli is known in advance, and sensitization of the nervous system is ongoing during surgery despite adequate levels of general anesthesia with volatile anesthetics [8]. This article reviews the physiologic impact of thoracic surgery and research on current treatment regimens, which are the basis for advocating an aggressive, multimodal, preemptive approach to acute pain therapy throughout the entire perioperative period.

This article was supported in part by National Institutes of Health grants 1-R01-NH-40545 and 1-K23-HD/NS-40914.

* Corresponding author.
E-mail address: OchrochA@uphs.upenn (E.A. Ochroch).

Physiologic and pharmacologic basis of acute pain

Pain begins with mechanical, thermal, or chemical stimulation of peripheral nociceptors. These nociceptors fall into two basic classes: faster conducting

> **Box 1. Glossary of pain terms**
>
> *Allodynia:* when a typically nonpainful stimulus produces pain.
> *Hyperalgesia:* an increase in the perceived pain for the same level of noxious stimulation.
> *Multimodal analgesia:* combinations of analgesics, routes of analgesia, and analgesic techniques designed to prevent sensitization (see below) and maximize analgesia, while minimizing side effects.
> *Preemptive analgesia:* the analgesic strategy of initiating an analgesic regimen before the onset of noxious stimulation with the goal of preventing the cascade of neurophysiologic events that can lead to hyperalgesia and allodynia.
> *Sensitization:* a physiologic state in which it is more likely that a peripheral stimulus will be interpreted as being painful and that pain information will be transmitted to the brain.

Many pathways and factors are present to decrease the likelihood of nociceptor activation. Activation of opioid receptors reduces nociceptor output and decreases the release of excitatory proinflammatory neuropeptides, such as substance P and CGRP [13]. Peripheral opioid receptors appear on peripheral nerve endings in response to peripheral inflammation and are the natural targets of endogenous opioids released locally by cells of the immune system [13]. Muscarinic agonists [14–16], α_2-agonists [17], and N-methyl-D-aspartate (NMDA) antagonists [18,19] also may play a role in modulating peripheral nociception.

Pain information travels proximally along the peripheral nerve, which divides into sensory and motor roots, and passes through the cell bodies that comprise the dorsal root ganglia. Within the sensory root, the large-diameter (Aα and Aβ) and small-diameter (Aδ and C) fibers further segregate, with the small-diameter fibers entering the spinal cord through Lissauer's tract, terminating primarily in laminae I, II (substantia gelatinosa), and V of the dorsal horn of the spinal cord [9]. Activity in descending pathways [20] and Aα and Aβ fibers [9] can inhibit the firing of dorsal horn neurons that typically occurs in response to noxious stimuli. This activity is the neurobiologic basis for the gate control theory of pain [21], which has been examined and updated continually since its initial description in the 1960s [22].

Painful experience can lead to an enhanced sensitivity to subsequent noxious stimuli (hyperalgesia) and sensitize the pain pathway so that previously nonpainful stimuli produce pain (allodynia). Teleologically, this sensitization plays a vital role by limiting use of injured body parts so that they are permitted to heal. Through the above-described mechanisms, the peripheral nervous system contributes to hyperalgesia, and this process generally is referred to as *peripheral sensitization*. Phenomena involving just the peripheral nociceptive system are not sufficient, however, to explain the sensitization induced by noxious input.

Peripheral nociceptor activity also can enhance the response of spinal neurons; this became clear with the observation that noxious stimuli can enhance the response of spinal neurons, even when the subsequent stimulus is applied at the same dermatome on the *contralateral* side [23]. Although this process has been described as "windup," the term *central sensitization* may be more appropriate [24,25]. Even relatively brief applications of noxious stimuli are capable of inducing central sensitization [26,27]. Substance P, CGRP, and excitatory amino acid transmitters acting at NMDA receptors seem to play

myelinated Aδ and slower conducting unmyelinated C nerve fibers The Aδ fibers give rise to an early, sharp, and generally short-lived sensation, often referred to as *first pain,* whereas the C fibers give rise to a delayed dull sensation, which is more sustained and often referred to as *second pain* (Fig. 1) [9].

Several clinical situations can enhance the output of the peripheral nociceptors. Repeated application of a noxious stimulus can enhance the intensity and duration of the nociceptor response to subsequent applications of the same stimulus, sometimes inducing previously unresponsive receptors to fire [10–12]. Tissue injury leads to the release of mediators, which can activate directly or enhance nociceptor activity. Agents that are known to initiate firing of nociceptors in the absence of other stimuli include potassium, kinins (bradykinin and kallidin), and histamine. Substance P, calcitonin gene–related peptide (CGRP), and various prostanoids (prostaglandins, leukotrienes, and hydroxy acids) increase the likelihood of the nociceptor reaching activation threshold. These factors are intimately involved with the inflammatory response and interact via multiple feedback pathways [7]. Overall the effect is one of increased sensitivity of the nerves to an increased range of inputs over a wider receptive field.

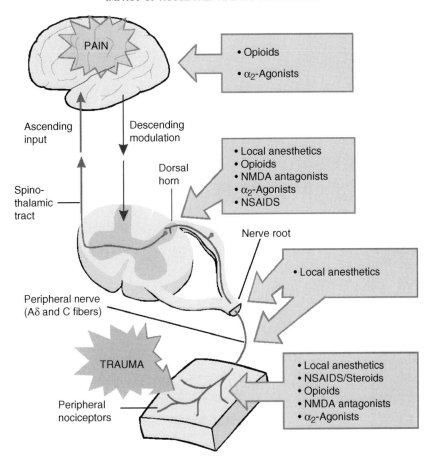

Fig. 1. The pain pathway from the peripheral nerve to the brain. The medications are listed in relationship to the areas where they are effective. In particular, local anesthetics are effective when used subcutaneously, for regional anesthesia on the peripheral nerve fibers, for epidural analgesia on the nerve roots, and for spinal anesthesia. No attempt was made to rank the effectiveness of the medications at each site. (*Adapted from* Kehlet H. The value of "multimodal" or "balanced analgesia" in postoperative pain treatment. Anesth Analg 1993;77:1048–56, artwork by David Klemm, Inc; with permission.)

important interactive roles in the process of central sensitization [28–33].

Postthoracotomy pain and its physiologic impact

Thoracotomy can be one of the most painful types of incision that patients can experience [3–5]. Noxious input from the skin incision, cut or retracted muscle, fractured or excised ribs, and damaged parietal pleura are transmitted along the intercostal nerves to the dorsal horn. Input from damaged visceral pleura is relayed through autonomic nerves; noxious stimuli originating in the lung also may be carried by the vagus nerve, and noxious stimuli from the mediastinum, diaphragm, and pericardial pleura may be relayed by the phrenic nerve [34].

No matter what its anatomic origin, the pain from thoracotomy is profound and protracted. Ochroch et al [35] studied 120 subjects undergoing thoracotomy; 38 underwent classic posterolateral thoracotomy, and 82 underwent axillary vertical muscle-sparing thoracotomy. They all were treated with aggressive patient-controlled thoracic epidural analgesia and nonsteroidal anti-inflammatory drugs (NSAIDs). As seen in Fig. 2, their "worst pain over the past 24 hours" (eg, coughing, chest physiotherapy) was 5.5 out of 10, and their "average pain over the past 24 hours" was 3.2 out of 10. These scores did not decrease for the duration of the hospitalization and remained nearly as severe 4 weeks after the operation, probably owing to the extensive tissue trauma. Their "current pain" was less than 2 out of 10 at all times during hospitalization. This phenomenon of patients

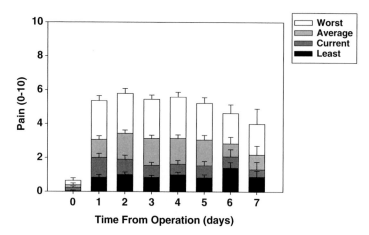

Fig. 2. Pain scores are for preoperative levels (day 0) and postoperative days 1–7. The scores were collected using the Brief Pain Inventory [191]. This survey asks for worst, average, current, and least pain over the previous 24 hours to be ranked from 0 (no pain) to 10 (worst pain imaginable).

rating pain at the time of interview as less than "average pain" highlights the need to assess multiple aspects of pain to develop a detailed image of its scope because physicians possibly would be led to undertreat pain if they relied solely on the one pain measure.

The impact of postthoracotomy pain is profound, and it may be the most important factor for the decrease in respiratory function after thoracotomy [36], but it is difficult to separate out from the effects of the surgery and anesthesia. Decrements in pulmonary function after thoracic surgery also result from loss of functional lung units, atelectasis from anesthesia and surgery, loss of function of incised or retracted intercostal muscles, rib dislocation, exacerbation of preexisting lung disease, and diaphragmatic dysfunction [36,37]. General anesthesia causes a reduction in functional residual capacity of approximately 20% [38,39], and this is exacerbated by the lateral decubitus position [40], but the effect from the anesthesia typically is reversed with pulmonary toilet by 2 to 3 days after surgery [41,42]. The amount of functional tissue removed can be calculated preoperatively, but the measured postoperative pulmonary function tests are typically far worse than the predicted function [36]. This situation is echoed in the statistically significant decrease in forced vital capacity of 19%, in forced expiratory volume in 1 second of 15%, and total lung capacity of 11% that did not return to preoperative baseline until 2 years after thoracotomy without lung resection in patients undergoing anterior spinal fusion [43]. This occurred despite an average correction of the thoracic coronal scoliosis from 53 to 24 degrees.

Beyond the impact on pulmonary function, thoracotomy can affect catecholamine levels, glucose homeostasis, nitrogen balance, coagulation, sodium balance, and a myriad of other systems secondary to the activation of the stress response [44,45]. The stress response has been implicated in perioperative myocardial infarction, deep venous thrombosis, pulmonary embolus, fluid overload, and other complications [44,45]. Although not well studied in thoracic surgery, most studies that randomize between standard analgesia and a more aggressive analgesic regimen indicate that the more aggressive the regimen, the less that hormone levels and other measures change from preoperative levels [46–49]. The increase in exercise tolerance several weeks after surgery in patients who receive aggressive analgesia [50] may be related to decreased catabolism [51] or long-term reductions in pain [49]. In one of the largest trials, Rigg et al [52] randomized 915 patients undergoing major intra-abdominal surgery to receive epidural or intravenous patient-controlled analgesia (IV PCA) morphine. The rate of postoperative respiratory failure was reduced by 7% for the patients receiving epidural analgesia. Another study suggests a favorable association between neuraxial anesthesia/analgesia and reduced morbidity and mortality [53].

Current treatment options

Analgesic options are as diverse as thoracic surgical techniques. Choice of medication or combinations of medications and their route and frequency of administration can be considered only in light of the patient's medical history and surgical intervention. The primary modes of analgesia—systemic opioids, regional local anesthetic, epidural local anesthetics, and epidural opioids—are reviewed with respect to measures of pain and physiologic outcome where available.

Intravenous patient-controlled analgesia

Systemic opioids have long been a mainstay of postoperative analgesia. Since the 1980s, dosing regimens have evolved from as-needed intramuscular doses to IV PCA because it has been shown that as-needed or set-dose opioids fail greater than 60% of the time to achieve adequate analgesia [54]. Typical medications and programming for the PCA pump are morphine, 0.5 to 2.5 mg; fentanyl, 10 to 30 μg; or hydromorphone, 0.1 to 0.3 mg, demand bolus with a 5- to 10-minute lockout period (Table 1). Background (basal) infusions are used less frequently because of reports of increased frequency of respiratory depression, although respiratory depression typically is seen in older patients or patients receiving sedatives in combination with the opioids [55,56].

A meta-analysis that included 30 trials involving thoracic surgery [57] showed that for recovery after thoracotomy, IV PCA opioids were inferior to epidural opioids or local anesthetics (lumbar or thoracic) in terms of higher pain scores and longer times to mobilization and discharge. The visual analog pain scores were significantly lower in the epidural group ($P < .002$). Incidences of nausea and vomiting were lower in the lumbar epidural patients than in the PCA patients. More importantly, epidural use has been associated with decreased postoperative

atelectasis [58]. Epidural analgesia in video-assisted thoracic surgery (VATS) is largely unevaluated because it has been broadly assumed that VATS is not painful enough to require epidural analgesia. It has been shown that pain and pulmonary function of VATS patients having PCA analgesia are similar to pain and pulmonary function of thoracotomy patients having epidural analgesia [59].

Intercostal and paravertebral nerve block

Intercostal nerve blockade has been shown to be a valued, albeit short-duration, analgesic [60,61]. Intercostal catheters have been faulted for the unreliable spread of local anesthetic and the potential for rapid systemic absorption and high blood levels of local anesthetic [62,63]. When they have been compared directly, epidural analgesia is at least as effective and usually superior to continuous intercostal nerve blockade [64–66]. Most of these studies are too small for even nontrivial differences to be detected.

A more effective version of the intercostal catheter is the paravertebral catheter. The paravertebral space is continuous along the entire length of the vertebral column; it extends laterally from the vertebral column and merges into the intercostal space. It is continuous medially with the epidural space via the intervertebral foramen [67]. This space includes the sympathetic chain, the rami communicans, the dorsal ramus, and the intercostal nerves [68]. In the paravertebral space, the intercostal nerves are devoid of a fascial sheath and easily blocked by local anesthetic [69]. A reported advantage of continuous paravertebral blockade is the lower likelihood of hypotension [70], but because the paravertebral space is contin-

Table 1
Drugs and dosages for intravenous patient-controlled analgesia (IV PCA)

	Equipotent doses	Half-life	IV PCA ranges*	Receptor	Comments
Morphine	1 mg	2.5–3.5 h	1–3 mg q 10 min	μ agonist	Histamine release
Hydromorphone (Dilaudid)	0.125 mg	2–3 h	0.1–0.3 mg q 10 min	μ agonist	
Meperidine (Demerol)	8 mg	1.5–2.5 h	10–25 mg q 10 min	μ and κ agonist	Rarely used due to risk of seizures in patients with renal insufficiency
Fentanyl	20 μg	3 h in steady state, but extreme lipophilicity makes first doses have shorter effect	15–35 μg q 10 min	μ agonist	Preferred in patients with renal insufficiency

* Doses are approximate and need to be adjusted for many factors, including, but not limited to, patient weight, age, central nervous system disease, concomitant medications, opioid tolerance, renal function, and hepatic function.

uous with the epidural space, there may be no profound differences between these techniques. When compared in randomized trials, analgesia from paravertebral blockade was either equivalent or superior to epidural analgesia [70,71]. In a meta-analysis, paravertebral blockade was shown to preserve spirometric lung function better than epidural blockade [72]. A potential advantage is that the paravertebral catheter can be placed under direct vision at the time of surgery [73], although this does not improve success compared with a posterior approach. These catheters also tend to become dislodged or to malfunction prematurely [61,63,66, 74,75].

Blocking the intercostal nerves by cryotherapy during surgery would seem to be an appealing option because it avoids the side effects associated with systemic opioid or epidural analgesia. Because of the many other routes for noxious input previously described, the pain relief from cryoanalgesia is considerably less than the pain relief from epidural analgesia [76–79]. Far more important is that cryoanalgesia does not preserve lung function as effectively as epidural analgesia [72,78]. When comparing cryoanalgesia with systemic morphine alone, the quantity of systemic morphine was reduced after cryoanalgesia; however, the differences were small, and the rates of side effects were not always different [78,79]. There have been reports of neuroma formation and chronic pain after cryotherapy during thoracotomy [79], although this has not been a consistent finding [80]. Consequently, cryotherapy should be reserved for situations when epidural analgesia and paravertebral blockade are not feasible.

Epidural analgesia

Epidural analgesia is the *de facto* standard for postthoracotomy analgesia [81]. It is reliable and effective. Compared with opioid analgesia, patients receiving epidural analgesia have less pain (particularly with activity) [57,82], are extubated sooner [83,84], and have fewer pulmonary complications [81,85]. Debate focuses on the optimal location for the placement of the catheter (lumbar versus thoracic), medications administered (opioid, local anesthetic, α_2-agoinsts, NMDA antagonists, or combinations), timing of the initiation of blockade (preemptive analgesia, which is discussed in the following section), use of patient control, and use of adjuvant analgesics (multimodal analgesia, which is discussed later).

The selection of the dermatomal level for the entrance of the epidural catheter weighs the potential advantages of having the catheter tip at the mid dermatome of the incision versus the theoretical safety benefit of a lumbar placement. The concept is that needle insertion at the level of the thoracic vertebrae has the potential to damage the spinal cord. There are no systematically collected data to support this finding; it is merely an observation based on anatomy of the spinal cord. To permit feedback in the case of a needle contacting a nerve root or the spinal cord, patients generally should not have thoracic catheters placed while they are heavily sedated or under general anesthesia.

Potential benefits associated with placement of the epidural catheter at a thoracic dermatome near the site of surgery include improved analgesia [86], reduced drug use [87], and improved pulmonary function [88]. It was shown in a review that the benefits of epidural analgesia are greatest when thoracic catheters are used in high-risk patients, and these benefits include reduction in ICU care, faster recovery, and decreased cost [89]. The authors believe that proper drug selection is crucial in maximizing benefit and minimizing risk from thoracic epidural placement. Dilute local anesthetics (bupivacaine, 0.5–1 mg/mL) should be combined with lipophilic opioids (fentanyl, 2–5 μg/mL; meperidine, 0.5–2 mg/mL) because these combinations provide better segmental analgesia, while minimizing the risk of respiratory depression, motor block, and hypotension.

Patient-controlled epidural analgesia combines a continuous infusion of epidural medications with a supplemental bolus that is controlled by the patient. Similar to IV PCA, the pump is programmed to limit the boluses to allow one every few minutes. Although no studies show a significant advantage over a simple continuous infusion, it is reasonable to assume that the added psychological benefit the patient gains is worth the slightly increased technical demand.

Approximately one third of patients who are receiving epidural analgesia commonly report shoulder pain on the side ipsilateral to the incision [90]. The origin of this pain is unclear. Suprascapular nerve block does not reduce this pain in the recovery room, indicating that this pain is not primarily of shoulder origin [91]. Infiltration of 10 mL of 1% lidocaine into the periphrenic fat pad at the conclusion of surgery provided a 2-hour window during which patients did not complain of shoulder pain [92]; this suggests that the origin of this pain may be phrenic irritation, although pleural injury also may play a role. Phrenic nerve blockade can cause significant decrements in respiratory function, and it is not a reasonable technique to maintain analgesia into the postoperative period. Given the presumed inflammatory origin of perioperative shoulder pain associated with thoracotomy, NSAIDs commonly are used to treat this pain, but there are no published efficacy data.

Long-term postthoracotomy pain

With the exception of the pain syndromes associated with limb amputation [93], long-term postthoracotomy pain syndrome may be the most recognized pain syndrome associated with a particular type of surgery. Several studies indicated that more than half the patients who undergo open thoracotomy continue to experience pain, sometimes severe, 1 year after surgery [94,95]. Despite the minimally invasive aspects of VATS, the rate of long-term pain is similar to open thoracotomy [89]. Risk factors for developing long-term postthoracotomy pain are thought to include female gender [35,96–100] and chest wall resection. Patients who experience the most severe pain during the first few postoperative days are most likely to have persistent long-term pain [35,95], but it is unknown whether this relationship is causal or simply represents a greater susceptibility to noxious input. Aggressive perioperative epidural analgesia seems to have reduced the rate of pain 1 year after surgery to 21% [35] (compared with >50% [94,95]).

Preemptive analgesia in thoracic surgery

Because the intense perioperative pain associated with thoracic surgery may represent a nociceptor barrage capable of sensitizing the peripheral and central nervous systems, leading to long-term pain, efforts to modulate this process have been explored. Preemptive analgesia is the practice of initiating an analgesic regimen before the onset of noxious stimuli, with the expectation that this will lead to decreased pain and analgesic consumption [101–103]. The ability to realize these benefits is controversial [104–109]. Much of this controversy stems from ambiguity with respect to terminology and clinical studies with small numbers of subjects and interventions lacking profound impact [108,110,111]. Pain experienced at any point during the perioperative period can sensitize the pain pathways. Consequently, regimens must be designed to prevent sensitization throughout the entire perioperative period, not just at the time of incision or during the invasive procedure. Researchers also must recognize that analgesic regimens used in a preemptive fashion show efficacy only if they are capable of preventing sensitization, not simply because they were initiated before the onset of surgery. Failure to prevent sensitization throughout the perioperative period may overwhelm benefits obtained during one portion of the perioperative period, and analgesic therapy in the control group itself may decrease sensitization and bias studies in favor of the null hypothesis. A meta-analysis of preemptive analgesia [106] using a restrictive definition of preemptive analgesia was generally not supportive of this strategy for acute pain control, but it did highlight the many methodologic challenges that remain for realizing the clinical potential of preemptive analgesia.

Similar to the findings of the meta-analysis [106], trials of preemptive analgesia in thoracic surgery have produced equivocal results [35,112–118]. Most of these rely on the timing of an epidural intervention [35,114,116–118], in which the potentially beneficial effect may have been lost because of small numbers of patients, inappropriate dosages, or inappropriate concentrations of epidural medications or simply overwhelmed by the long duration of postoperative pain. The definition of preemptive analgesia is paramount. The intervention must be profound and continue over the entire period when nociceptor output is sufficiently intense that sensitization of the nervous system could occur. The duration and level of pain that initiates sensitization are unknown, so the duration of analgesia that is needed to prevent it remains unknown. Although epidurals provide profound analgesia, it seems unlikely that they can prevent sensitization originating from the various pain pathways from the lung, pleura, or diaphragm that were previously described. Consequently, future trials should focus on combining dense epidural blockade with NSAIDs, NMDA receptor antagonists, α_2-blockers, and other novel analgesics.

Adjuvant medications

Nonsteroidal anti-inflammatory drugs

Prostaglandins are important mediators of the pain pathway. They increase the sensitivity and receptive field of peripheral and central nociceptors, making it far more likely that noxious information will be transmitted to the central nervous system [119,120]. The analgesic properties of NSAIDs can be attributed to their inhibition of cyclooxygenases and the subsequent decrease in prostaglandins in the peripheral and central nervous systems [121]. Cyclooxygenase catalyzes the transformation of arachidonic acid to form prostaglandins [122]. Clinically applicable medications that inhibit the cyclooxygenase type 1 (COX-1) and cyclooxygenase type 2 (COX-2) isoforms are widely available. The properties of a third, more recently identified cyclooxygenase isoform are now being elucidated [123]. COX-1 is constitutively expressed in the peripheral and central nervous systems, and its expression can be induced by many factors, including many of the mediators of pain and inflammation. COX-2 is present and ubiquitous in the central nervous system, but is not present in the periphery except for the kidney and vas deferens. It becomes a major source for prostaglandins in the periphery only after induction, which requires several hours after tissue injury. The COX-2 isoform is up-regulated by bacterial lipopolysaccharide, cytokines, growth factors, tumor promoters, and multiple factors released during cell damage and death, including the mediators of pain and inflammation previously described [121,124]. These observations prompted speculation as to the role of peripheral COX-2 in prostaglandin formation during inflammation and in response to noxious stimuli [119,120].

NSAIDs have been shown repeatedly to provide analgesia and decrease opioid consumption after thoracotomy [125–130]. Typically studied doses of NSAIDs are ibuprofen, 400 to 600 mg orally three or four times daily; ketorolac (Toradol), 15 mg intra-venously or intramuscularly every 6 to 8 hours; indo-methacin, 100 mg per rectum every 8 to 12 hours; rofecoxib (Vioxx), 50 mg orally daily; valdecoxib (Bextra), 20 to 40 mg orally daily; and parecoxib (Dynastat, Rayzon, Zapit), 40 mg intravenously daily (Table 2). The magnitude of opioid sparing and improved analgesia is seen in the low number-needed-to-treat (number of patients needed to see a significant effect), which is typically 2 to 3 [131], which is similar to that of opioids.

Beyond augmenting analgesia and limiting opioid dosing, NSAIDs have potential benefits that may be more important in thoracic surgical patients than in general surgical patients. In one study, NSAIDs had no significant impact on hemodynamic indices. There were minimal changes in cardiac output, stroke volume, mean arterial pressure, and systemic vascular resistance after intravenous ketorolac injections, whereas cardiac output and mean arterial pressure decreased after administration of morphine [132]. Most important is that the pulmonary circulation was unaffected by ketorolac administration, whereas mor-phine administration induced an increase in pulmo-nary vascular resistance [132]. Morphine caused a decrease in minute ventilation, which allowed an increase in arterial concentration of carbon dioxide, which causes pulmonary vasoconstriction [132]. This effect may be particularly important in chronic smokers and chronic obstructive pulmonary disease patients, who commonly have pulmonary hyper-tension [133,134].

Regardless of the potential benefits of NSAIDs, many clinicians are appropriately concerned about using NSAIDs in the postoperative setting because of fears of renal failure, operative site bleeding, and gastrointestinal bleeding. Fear of renal failure from NSAID use in patients with normal preoperative renal function seems to be unfounded. In a Cochrane Database systematic review of 14 studies, Lee et al [135] found that NSAIDs caused a minimal and clinically unimportant reduction in creatinine clear-ance postoperatively compared with placebo. Urine production remained unchanged during recovery, and no cases of acute renal failure were reported with NSAID use. The investigators concluded that, "NSAIDs should not be withheld from adults with normal preoperative renal function because of con-cerns about postoperative renal impairment "[135]. COX-2 inhibitors hold no advantage over nonselec-tive NSAIDs in reducing the risk of renal failure [136]. Thoracic surgical patients may be at increased risk of NSAID-induced renal dysfunction compared with other surgical populations because of advanced age and fluid restriction. Trials of NSAIDs in thoracic

Table 2
Dosages of nonsteroidal anti-inflammatory drugs (NSAIDs)

NSAID	Dose	Comments[a]
COX-2-specific inhibitors		
Parecoxib (Dynastat,Rayzon,Zapit)	20–40 mg IV qd	Less risk of gastrointestinal ulceration
Valdecoxib (Bextra)	20–40 mg PO qd	No increased blood loss
Celecoxib (Celebrex)	100–200 mg PO qd	Same renal effects as nonspecific COX inhibitors
Rofecoxib (Vioxx)	25–50 mg PO qd	Doubtful increased risk of myocardial infarction
Nonspecific COX inhibitors		
Ibuprofen	600–800 mg PO q 6–8 h	
Ketorolac (Toradol)	15–30 mg IV or IM q 6–8 h	
Indomethacin	25–100 mg PO or PR q 8–12 h	

Abbreviation: COX, cyclooxygenase.
  [a] All comments listed above apply to all of the COX-2 inhibitors.

surgery have not reported increased rates of renal failure, however [112,113,125,137–140].

Operative site bleeding from NSAID inhibition of platelet function is worrisome but does not seem to be a significant issue. A meta-analysis of more than 1800 patients undergoing tonsillectomy showed no clear effect on perioperative bleeding [141]. The trials of NSAIDs in thoracic surgery all have been too small to determine an effect, and a meta-analysis including these studies would be helpful. Some data suggest that COX-2 inhibitors may be safer. Valdecoxib did not inhibit platelet function (bleeding time and platelet aggregation) in healthy adults or in the elderly [142], and this drug is similar to other COX-2 inhibitors [136]. Small perioperative trials of COX-2 inhibitors have not shown increased bleeding [143,144].

Risk of gastrointestinal erosion and ulceration may be the one area where COX-2-specific inhibitors may be better than nonselective NSAIDs. Lower rates of endoscopic gastroduodenal ulcer formation were found with valdecoxib compared with ibuprofen, naproxen, and diclofenac ($P < .001$ to $P < .05$) [142]. Gastrointestinal ulceration has not been a significant concern, however, in large reviews of perioperative NSAID use [136,145,146]. Overall, the risk-benefit balance of causing renal failure or bleeding versus preventing pain, hypoventilation, and pneumonia strongly favors NSAID use and improved analgesia.

A potential for an increased rate of cardiovascular thromboembolic events with COX-2-selective inhibitors is particularly worrisome in thoracic surgical patients. Prostacyclin, a product of COX-2 in vascular endothelium, has important physiologic roles, such as increasing blood flow to injured tissues, reducing leukocyte adherence, and inhibiting platelet aggregation [147]. Although controversial, it has been hypothesized that COX-2-specific inhibitors may increase the risk of cardiovascular thromboembolic events because of their inhibition of vascular prostacyclin synthesis and lack of an effect on platelet thromboxane A_2 production and aggregation [148,149]. Large-scale, population-based studies mostly have found no differences in rate of stroke or myocardial infarction in patients receiving COX-2 inhibitors, nonselective NSAIDs, or no therapy when examining Medicaid/Medicare databases of patients older than 45 years of age [149–152]. In higher doses (>25 mg/d), rofecoxib has been associated with higher rates of cardiovascular thromboembolism [151], and celecoxib has been shown to produce higher rates of cardiovascular thromboembolism [153]. Consequently, there may be a class effect for COX-2 inhibitors that is just being recognized that

increases the risk of cardiovascular thromboembolism, and this potentially could magnify the risk of perioperative thromboembolism in the elderly population of smokers who present for thoracic surgery. More data need to be collected before widespread perioperative use is adopted, unless the patient has significant risk factors for gastrointestinal ulceration, which would tip the balance of safety toward using a COX-2 inhibitor instead of a nonselective NSAID.

N-methyl-D-aspartate antagonists

As discussed previously, central sensitization can be augmented by the action of excitatory amino acids acting at NMDA receptors. Ketamine is a phencyclidine derivative that can be used as an intravenous general anesthetic that is an NMDA antagonist. Systemic ketamine decreases wound hyperalgesia after abdominal surgery, but it is not associated with decreased pain [18,154]. Other studies involving abdominal surgery indicate that low-dose ketamine does not reduce postoperative pain consistently [155–158]. When systemic ketamine is combined with epidural analgesics, however, its use can result in persistent reductions in postoperative pain [159,160]. Preoperative oral dextromethorphan, another NMDA antagonist, can decrease pain and analgesic consumption in a dose-dependent manner [161–164] and can augment the benefits of performing the surgical procedure under epidural anesthesia with a combination of a short-acting local anesthetic and morphine [165].

There are few studies of NMDA antagonists in thoracic surgery. Overall, low-dose ketamine (0.1 mg/kg/h) seems to improve analgesia in combination with either epidural analgesia or IV PCA, to reduce morphine consumption by 40%, and not to increase the risk of respiratory depression [166,167]. It is unclear whether it has a preemptive effect in reducing pain. Apart from their more direct analgesic benefits, NMDA antagonists also may contribute to perioperative pain control by decreasing acute opioid tolerance [168,169]. Consequently an infusion of ketamine is a good candidate to supplement epidural and NSAID analgesia in thoracic surgical patients whose pain is not sufficiently controlled for them to participate in pulmonary toilet and other activities that are essential for rapid recovery.

α₂-Agonists

α_2-Adrenergic receptors are present in the central and peripheral nervous systems at autonomic ganglia and presynaptic and postsynaptic sites. Central nervous system activation of postsynaptic receptors by α_2-agonists leads to inhibition of sympathetic activity, which decreases blood pressure and heart rate, causes sedation, and inhibits respiration minimally [170]. In the spinal cord, activation of α_2-receptors causes analgesia. Although there are many studies of α_2-agonists in analgesia, epidural clonidine for cancer and neuropathic pain is the only approved analgesic application of this class of drugs. Consequently, all uses of these drugs for analgesia are off-label or for research purposes [171], and practitioners should be aware that oral, intramuscular, intravenous, and epidural delivery of these drugs can produce dose-dependent decreases in heart rate and blood pressure.

Epinephrine has been used widely in epidural analgesia. It produces analgesia via activation of α_2-receptors and prolonging the duration of other drugs in the epidural space secondary to α_1-mediated vasoconstriction [172]. The addition of 1.5 μg/mL of epinephrine to 1 mg/mL of bupivacaine with 2 μg/mL of fentanyl has been shown to reduce significantly pain at rest and pain with coughing when infused in a thoracic epidural catheter during recovery from thoracic surgery [173,174]. The addition of epinephrine to 1 mg/mL of ropivacaine with 2 μg/mL of fentanyl reduced side effects and decreased time to mobilization compared with 1 mg/mL of ropivacaine alone [172,173]. Although there is concern that the vasoconstriction could threaten the segmental blood supply in the spinal cord, particularly in the elderly, there is not clear documentation of dilute epinephrine causing this potentially catastrophic side effect.

Clonidine has been shown to be an effective analgesic when delivered epidurally alone [175–179] and in combination with opioids or local anesthetics [180]. The analgesia produced is improved and significantly different from that of local anesthetics or opioids alone [170,179,180]. Epidural clonidine can cause more frequent and profound hypotension than local anesthetics alone [170,180]. Dexmedetomidine is a newer α_2-agonist that was approved for ICU sedation in intubated patients for 24 hours. Its main advantage over clonidine is a shorter half-life and greater specificity for the α_2-receptor [181]. It significantly decreases opioid requirements after major surgery when used intraoperatively and postoperatively [182]. Further research on clonidine and dexmedetomidine is needed before their adoption into standard postthoracotomy analgesia care.

Multimodal analgesia

The best analgesic plan prevents sensitization throughout the entire perioperative period to reduce the total pain experience [108]. This may be possible only by directing therapy at multiple anatomic and pharmacologic sites of action, an approach called *multimodal analgesia* (see Fig. 1) [183]. Components of multimodal analgesia include (1) neuronal blockade by local anesthetics, which may take the form of epidural anesthesia, spinal anesthesia, nerve blocks, skin infiltration before incision, or wound infiltration before closure; (2) infusion of opioids by the intravenous, intrathecal, or epidural routes before incision and throughout the perioperative period; (3) use of NSAIDs before incision, throughout surgery, and postoperatively [8,101,183,184]; and (4) other analgesic agents the use of which have not yet gained wide acceptance, such as α_2-agonists (clonidine and dexmedetomidine) [106,185,186] and NMDA antagonists (ketamine and dextromethorphan) [18,106, 185–187]. Current practice of postthoracotomy analgesia is multimodal because NSAIDs frequently are employed along with epidural or intravenous opioid analgesics. Future inclusion of NMDA antagonists and α_2-agonists and other drugs and modalities will help to reduce pain and improve recovery after thoracic surgery.

Anticoagulation and regional anesthesia

Spinal or epidural hematoma after epidural placement is rare, occurring in less than 1 in 150,000 epidural anesthetics [188]. This condition is a medical emergency that requires immediate treatment. The key to making the diagnosis is an awareness that epidural local anesthetics infused for postoperative analgesia, typically dilute bupivacaine 0.1% to 0.05% (1–0.5 mg/mL), *rarely* cause profound motor weakness. Neurologic compromise from hematoma commonly presents as progressing motor or sensory blockade, less commonly as bowel or bladder dysfunction, and rarely as severe radicular back pain [189]. Symptoms of motor block out of proportion to the local anesthetics should trigger immediate spine CT or MRI and an emergency consultation with either a neurologist or a neurosurgeon. Neurologic consequences from spinal cord ischemia were minimized when patients had decompressive laminectomies within 8 hours of the onset of symptoms [190].

Anticoagulation that is initiated before, during, or after thoracic surgery can increase the risk of hematoma in the epidural or spinal space. Owing to the rarity of such occurrences, no study ever could be used definitively to determine which anticoagulants are safe for surgery and regional anesthesia. Clear practice guidelines were set forth in a consensus panel from the American Society for Regional Anesthesia, and the rest of this section and Table 3

Table 3
Low-molecular-weight heparins and their impact on the timing of regional analgesia

Low-molecular-weight heparins	Systemic anticoagulation*	Thromboprophylaxis[†]
Enoxaparin (Lovenox)	1 mg/kg q 12 h	30 mg q 12 h
	1.5 mg/kg qd	
Dalteparin (Fragmin)	120 U/kg q 12 h	5000 U qd
	200 U qd	
Tinzaparin (Innohep)	175 U/kg	3500 U qd

* 24 hours delay for placement or removal from last dose.
[†] 12 hours delay for placement or removal from last dose.

are a summary of their conclusions [189]. The most important message is that an indwelling catheter should not be placed or removed while the patient is significantly anticoagulated, which is defined by the class of the anticoagulant. Anticoagulation should not be initiated or resumed for 2 hours after catheter placement or removal, particularly if blood is noted in the epidural space or catheter placement was technically difficult.

Unfractionated heparin should not be given intravenously for at least 1 hour after epidural placement, and the partial thromboplastin time should be within normal range at the time of catheter removal with heparinization being held for 2 hours after removal. There are no contraindications for subcutaneous doses of 5000 U of unfractionated heparin. Recommendations for low-molecular-weight heparin are presented in Table 3. For warfarin therapy, the international normalized ratio should be less than 1.5, with no dose taken within the last 24 hours for catheter placement or removal. Aspirin and NSAIDs alone are not contraindications, but epidural hematomas have been reported when these drugs are combined with other anticoagulants. Platelet glycoprotein IIb/IIIa inhibitor abciximab (ReoPro) should be held for 24 hours, and eptifibatide (Integrilin) and tirofiban (Aggrastat) should be held for 4 to 8 hours before catheter placement or removal. Ticlopidine (Ticlid) should be stopped 14 days before surgery, and clopidogrel (Plavix) should be stopped 7 days before surgery.

Summary

Perioperative analgesia for thoracotomy has evolved in concert with increasing knowledge of the impact of pain on recovery, the origin of this pain, and new methods for treating it. Thoracic surgery is one of the few areas where there is more general agreement between surgeons and anesthesiologists as to the importance of aggressive pain management,

often with an indwelling epidural catheter left in place until after thoracostomy tube removal. The reasons for this agreement is that it has become increasingly clear to both specialties that pain puts patients with decreased pulmonary reserve who undergo thoracotomy at greater risk for morbidity. Future studies need to examine drugs or drug combinations that can lead to further reductions in the often intense pain that patients receiving aggressive epidural analgesia still experience. Studies directed at finding interventions capable of reducing the rate of long-term postthoracotomy pain still need to be performed.

References

[1] Carr DB, Jacox AK, Chapman CR. Clinical practice guidelines for acute pain management: operative or medical procedures and trauma. Washington, DC: Agency for Health Care Policy and Research, US Departement of Health and Human Services; 1992.

[2] Warfield CA, Kahn CH. Acute pain management: programs in US hospitals and experiences and attitudes among US adults. Anesthesiology 1995;83: 1090–4.

[3] Kruger M, McRae K. Pain management in cardiothoracic practice. Surg Clin North Am 1999;79:387–400.

[4] Jain S, Datta S. Postoperative pain management. Chest Surg Clin N Am 1997;7:773–99.

[5] Jain S, Datta S, Tundis D. Management of chronic postthoracotomy pain. Semin Cardiothorac Vasc Anesth 1999;3:191–203.

[6] Perkins FM, Kehlet H. Chronic pain as an outcome of surgery: a review of predictive factors. Anesthesiology 2000;93:1123–33.

[7] Kelly DJ, Ahmad M, Brull SJ. Preemptive analgesia: I. physiological pathways and pharmacological modalities. Can J Anaesth 2001;48:1000–10.

[8] Abram SE, Yaksh TL. Morphine, but not inhalation anesthesia, blocks post-injury facilitation: the role of preemptive suppression of afferent transmission. Anesthesiology 1993;78:713–21.

[9] Fields HL. Pain. New York: McGraw-Hill; 1987.

[10] Fitzgerald M, Lynn B. The sensitization of high

threshold mechanoreceptors with myelinated axons by repeated heating. J Physiol 1977;265:549–63.

[11] Campbell JN, Meyer RA, LaMotte RH. Sensitization of myelinated nociceptive afferents that innervate monkey hand. J Neurophysiol 1979;42:1669–79.

[12] Meyer RA, Campbell JN. Myelinated nociceptive afferents account for the hyperalgesia that follows a burn to the hand. Science 1981;213:1527–9.

[13] Stein C. The control of pain in peripheral tissue by opioids. N Engl J Med 1995;332:1685–90.

[14] Yang LC, Chen LM, Wang CJ, Buerkle H. Postoperative analgesia by intra-articular neostigmine in patients undergoing knee arthroscopy. Anesthesiology 1998;88:334–9.

[15] Bernardini N, Reeh PW, Sauer SK. Muscarinic M2 receptors inhibit heat-induced CGRP release from isolated rat skin. Neuroreport 2001;12:2457–60.

[16] Bernardini N, Roza C, Sauer SK, Gomeza J, Wess J, Reeh PW. Muscarinic M2 receptors on peripheral nerve endings: a molecular target of antinociception. J Neurosci 2002;22:RC229.

[17] Gentili M, Juhel A, Bonnet F. Peripheral analgesic effect of intra-articular clonidine. Pain 1996;64:593–6.

[18] Tverskoy M, Oren M, Vaskovich M, Dashkovsky I, Kissin I. Ketamine enhances local anesthetic and analgesic effects of bupivacaine by peripheral mechanism: a study in postoperative patients. Neurosci Lett 1996;215:5–8.

[19] Carlton SM. Peripheral excitatory amino acids. Curr Opin Pharmacol 2001;1:52–6.

[20] Watkins LR, Mayer DJ. Multiple endogenous opiate and non-opiate analgesia systems: evidence of their existence and clinical implications. Ann N Y Acad Sci 1986;467:273–99.

[21] Melzack R, Wall PD. Pain mechanisms: a new theory. Science 1965;150:971–9.

[22] Melzack R. The challenge of pain. 2nd edition. New York: Basic Books; 1998.

[23] Woolf CJ. Evidence for a central component of post-injury pain hypersensitivity. Nature 1983;306:686–8.

[24] Woolf CJ, Salter MW. Neuronal plasticity: increasing the gain in pain. Science 2000;288:1765–9.

[25] Herrero JF, Laird JM, Lopez-Garcia JA. Wind-up of spinal cord neurones and pain sensation: much ado about something? Prog Neurobiol 2000;61:169–203.

[26] Seltzer Z, Beilin BZ, Ginzburg R, Paran Y, Shimko T. The role of injury discharge in the induction of neuropathic pain behavior in rats. Pain 1991;46:327–36.

[27] Yamamoto T, Shimoyama N, Mizuguchi T. Role of the injury discharge in the development of thermal hyperesthesia after sciatic nerve constriction injury in the rat. Anesthesiology 1993;79:993–1002.

[28] Skofitsch G, Jacobowitz DM. Calcitonin gene-related peptide coexists with substance P in capsaicin sensitive neurons and sensory ganglia of the rat. Peptides 1985;6:747–54.

[29] Murase K, Randic M. Actions of substance P on rat spinal dorsal horn neurones. J Physiol 1984;346: 203–17.

[30] Mantyh PW, Rogers SD, Honore P, et al. Inhibition of hyperalgesia by ablation of lamina I spinal neurons expressing the substance P receptor. Science 1997; 278:275–9.

[31] Malmberg AB, Chen C, Tonegawa S, Basbaum AI. Preserved acute pain and reduced neuropathic pain in mice lacking PKCγ. Science 1997;278:279–83.

[32] Liu H, Mantyh PW, Basbaum AI. NMDA-receptor regulation of substance P release from primary afferent nociceptors. Nature 1997;386:721–4.

[33] Woolf CJ, Thompson SW. The induction and maintenance of central sensitization is dependent on N-methyl-D-aspartic acid receptor activation: implications for the treatment of post-injury pain hypersensitivity states. Pain 1991;44:293–9.

[34] Hazelrigg SR, Cetindag IB, Fullerton J. Acute and chronic pain syndromes after thoracic surgery. Surg Clin North Am 2002;82:849–65.

[35] Ochroch EA, Gottschalk A, Augostides J, Carson KA, Kent L, Malamayan N, et al. A randomized study of long-term pain and activity during recovery from major thoracotomy using thoracic epidural analgesia. Anesthesiology 2002;97:1234–44.

[36] Sabanathan S, Eng J, Mearns AJ. Alterations in respiratory mechanics following thoracotomy. J R Coll Surg Edinb 1990;35:144–50.

[37] Spence AA, Alexander JI. Pulmonary consequences of abdominal and thoracic surgery. Int Anesthesiol Clin 1972;10:41–59.

[38] Rehder K, Cameron PD, Krayer S. New dimensions of the respiratory system. Anesthesiology 1985;62: 230–3.

[39] Hedenstierna G, Strandberg A, Brismar B, Lundquist H, Svensson L, Tokics L. Functional residual capacity, thoracoabdominal dimensions, and central blood volume during general anesthesia with muscle paralysis and mechanical ventilation. Anesthesiology 1985;62:247–54.

[40] Hatch D. Ventilation and arterial oxygenation during thoracic surgery. Thorax 1966;21:310–4.

[41] Craig DB. Postoperative recovery of pulmonary function. Anesth Analg 1981;60:46–52.

[42] Schur MS, Brown JT, Kafer ER, Strope GL, Greene WB, Mandell J. Postoperative pulmonary function in children: comparison of scoliosis with peripheral surgery. Am Rev Respir Dis 1984;130:46–51.

[43] Graham EJ, Lenke LG, Lowe TG, Betz RR, Bridwell KH, Kong Y, et al. Prospective pulmonary function evaluation following open thoracotomy for anterior spinal fusion in adolescent idiopathic scoliosis. Spine 2000;25:2319–25.

[44] Kim PK, Deutschman CS. Inflammatory responses and mediators. Surg Clin North Am 2000;80:885–94.

[45] Epstein J, Breslow MJ. The stress response of critical illness. Crit Care Clin 1999;15:17–33.

[46] Lewis KS, Whipple JK, Michael KA, Quebbeman EJ. Effect of analgesic treatment on the physiological consequences of acute pain. Am J Hosp Pharm 1994; 51:1539–54.

[47] Moraca RJ, Sheldon DG, Thirlby RC. The role of epidural anesthesia and analgesia in surgical practice. Ann Surg 2003;238:663–73.

[48] Kehlet H, Wilmore DW. Multimodal strategies to improve surgical outcome. Am J Surg 2002;183:630–41.

[49] Gottschalk A, Smith DS, Jobes DR, Kennedy SK, Lally SE, Noble VE, et al. Preemptive epidural analgesia and recovery from radical prostatectomy: a randomized controlled trial. JAMA 1998;279:1076–82.

[50] Carli F, Mayo N, Klubien K, Schricker T, Trudel J, Belliveau P. Epidural analgesia enhances functional exercise capacity and health-related quality of life after colonic surgery: results of a randomized trial. Anesthesiology 2002;97:550–9.

[51] Carli F, Halliday D. Continuous epidural blockade arrests the postoperative decrease in muscle protein fractional synthetic rate in surgical patients. Anesthesiology 1997;86:1033–40.

[52] Rigg JR, Jamrozik K, Myles PS, Silbert BS, Peyton PJ, Parsons RW, et al. Epidural anaesthesia and analgesia and outcome of major surgery: a randomised trial. Lancet 2002;359:1276–82.

[53] Rodgers A, Walker N, Schug S, McKee A, Kehlet H, van Zundert A, et al. Reduction of postoperative mortality and morbidity with epidural or spinal anaesthesia: results from overview of randomised trials. BMJ 2000;321:1493.

[54] Miller RR. Analgesics. In: Miller RR, Greenblatt DJ, editors. Drug effects in hospitalized patients: experiences of the Boston collaborative drug surveillance program, 1966–1975. New York: John Wiley & Sons; 1976. p. 133–64.

[55] Looi-Lyons LC, Chung FF, Chan VW, McQuestion M. Respiratory depression: an adverse outcome during patient controlled analgesia therapy. J Clin Anesth 1996;8:151–6.

[56] Ready LB. Acute pain: lessons learned from 25,000 patients. Reg Anesth Pain Med 1999;24:499–505.

[57] Block BM, Liu SS, Rowlingson AJ, Cowan AR, Cowan Jr JA, Wu CL. Efficacy of postoperative epidural analgesia: a meta-analysis. JAMA 2003;290:2455–63.

[58] Ballantyne JC, Carr DB, deFerranti S, Suarez T, Lau J, Chalmers TC, et al. The comparative effects of postoperative analgesic therapies on pulmonary outcome: cumulative meta-analyses of randomized, controlled trials. Anesth Analg 1998;86:598–612.

[59] Furrer M, Rechsteiner R, Eigenmann V, Signer C, Althaus U, Ris HB. Thoracotomy and thoracoscopy: postoperative pulmonary function, pain and chest wall complaints. Eur J Cardiothorac Surg 1997;12:82–7.

[60] Liu M, Rock P, Grass JA, Heitmiller RF, Parker SJ, Sakima NT, et al. Double-blind randomized evaluation of intercostal nerve blocks as an adjuvant to subarachnoid administered morphine for post-thoracotomy analgesia. Reg Anesth 1995;20:418–25.

[61] Savage C, McQuitty C, Wang D, Zwischenberger JB. Postthoracotomy pain management. Chest Surg Clin N Am 2002;12:251–63.

[62] Chan VW, Chung F, Cheng DC, Seyone C, Chung A, Kirby TJ. Analgesic and pulmonary effects of continuous intercostal nerve block following thoracotomy. Can J Anaesth 1991;38:733–9.

[63] Dauphin A, Lubanska-Hubert E, Young JE, Miller JD, Bennett WF, Fuller HD. Comparative study of continuous extrapleural intercostal nerve block and lumbar epidural morphine in post-thoracotomy pain. Can J Surg 1997;40:431–6.

[64] Debreceni G, Molnar Z, Szelig L, Molnar TF. Continuous epidural or intercostal analgesia following thoracotomy: a prospective randomized double-blind clinical trial. Acta Anaesthesiol Scand 2003;47:1091–5.

[65] Kaiser AM, Zollinger A, De Lorenzi D, Largiader F, Weder W. Prospective, randomized comparison of extrapleural versus epidural analgesia for postthoracotomy pain. Ann Thorac Surg 1998;66:367–72.

[66] Perttunen K, Nilsson E, Heinonen J, Hirvisalo EL, Salo JA, Kalso E. Extradural, paravertebral and intercostal nerve blocks for post-thoracotomy pain. Br J Anaesth 1995;75:541–7.

[67] Kittredge RD. Computed tomographic evaluation of the thoracic prevertebral and paravertebral spaces. J Comput Tomogr 1983;7:239–50.

[68] Eason MJ, Wyatt R. Paravertebral thoracic block-a reappraisal. Anaesthesia 1979;34:638–42.

[69] Nunn JF, Slavin G. Posterior intercostal nerve block for pain relief after cholecystectomy: anatomical basis and efficacy. Br J Anaesth 1980;52:253–60.

[70] Karmakar MK. Thoracic paravertebral block. Anesthesiology 2001;95:771–80.

[71] Bimston DN, McGee JP, Liptay MJ, Fry WA. Continuous paravertebral extrapleural infusion for post-thoracotomy pain management. Surgery 1999;126:650–6.

[72] Richardson J, Sabanathan S, Shah R. Post-thoracotomy spirometric lung function: the effect of analgesia: a review. J Cardiovasc Surg (Torino) 1999;40:445–56.

[73] Berrisford RG, Sabanathan SS. Direct access to the paravertebral space at thoracotomy. Ann Thorac Surg 1990;49:854.

[74] Karmakar MK, Booker PD, Franks R, Pozzi M. Continuous extrapleural paravertebral infusion of bupivacaine for post-thoracotomy analgesia in young infants. Br J Anaesth 1996;76:811–5.

[75] Richardson J, Sabanathan S, Jones J, Shah RD, Cheema S, Mearns AJ. A prospective, randomized comparison of preoperative and continuous balanced epidural or paravertebral bupivacaine on post-thoracotomy pain, pulmonary function and stress responses. Br J Anaesth 1999;83:387–92.

[76] Brichon PY, Pison C, Chaffanjon P, Fayot P, Buchberger M, Neron L, et al. Comparison of epidural analgesia and cryoanalgesia in thoracic surgery. Eur J Cardiothorac Surg 1994;8:482–6.

[77] Katz J. Cryoanalgesia for postthoracotomy pain. Ann Thorac Surg 1989;48:5.

[78] Miguel R, Hubbell D. Pain management and spirometry following thoracotomy: a prospective, randomized study of four techniques. J Cardiothorac Vasc Anesth 1993;7:529–34.

[79] Muller LC, Salzer GM, Ransmayr G, Neiss A. Intraoperative cryoanalgesia for postthoracotomy pain relief. Ann Thorac Surg 1989;48:15–8.

[80] Roberts D, Pizzarelli G, Lepore V, al-Khaja N, Belboul A, Dernevik L. Reduction of post-thoracotomy pain by cryotherapy of intercostal nerves. Scand J Thorac Cardiovasc Surg 1988;22:127–30.

[81] Soto RG, Fu ES. Acute pain management for patients undergoing thoracotomy. Ann Thorac Surg 2003; 75:1349–57.

[82] Guinard JP, Mavrocordatos P, Chiolero R, Carpenter RL. A randomized comparison of intravenous versus lumbar and thoracic epidural fentanyl for analgesia after thoracotomy. Anesthesiology 1992;77: 1108–15.

[83] Yushang C, Zhiyong Z, Xiequn X. The analysis of changes and influencing factors of early postthoracotomy pulmonary function. Chin Med Sci J 2003; 18:105–10.

[84] Peeters-Asdourian C, Gupta S. Choices in pain management following thoracotomy. Chest 1999;115: 122S–4S.

[85] Slinger PD. Pro: every postthoracotomy patient deserves thoracic epidural analgesia. J Cardiothorac Vasc Anesth 1999;13:350–4.

[86] Kahn L, Baxter FJ, Dauphin A, Goldsmith C, Jackson PA, McChesney J, et al. A comparison of thoracic and lumbar epidural techniques for post-thoracoabdominal esophagectomy analgesia. Can J Anaesth 1999; 46:415–22.

[87] Grant GJ, Zakowski M, Ramanathan S, Boyd A, Turndorf H. Thoracic versus lumbar administration of epidural morphine for postoperative analgesia after thoracotomy. Reg Anesth 1993;18:351–5.

[88] Guinard JP, Mavrocordatos P, Chiolero R, Carpenter RL. A randomized comparison of intravenous versus lumbar and thoracic epidural fentanyl for analgesia after thoracotomy. Anesthesiology 1992;77:1108–15.

[89] Thompson JS. The role of epidural analgesia and anesthesia in surgical outcomes. Adv Surg 2002;36: 297–307.

[90] Burgess FW, Anderson DM, Colonna D, Sborov MJ, Cavanaugh DG. Ipsilateral shoulder pain following thoracic surgery. Anesthesiology 1993;78:365–8.

[91] Tan N, Agnew NM, Scawn ND, Pennefather SH, Chester M, Russell GN. Suprascapular nerve block for ipsilateral shoulder pain after thoracotomy with thoracic epidural analgesia: a double-blind comparison of 0.5% bupivacaine and 0.9% saline. Anesth Analg 2002;94:199–202.

[92] Scawn ND, Pennefather SH, Soorae A, Wang JY, Russell GN. Ipsilateral shoulder pain after thoracotomy with epidural analgesia: the influence of phrenic nerve infiltration with lidocaine. Anesth Analg 2001;93:260–4.

[93] Sherman RA, Devor M, Jones D, Katz J, Marbach JJ. Phantom pain. New York: Plenum; 1997.

[94] Dajczman E, Gordon A, Kreisman H, Wolkove N. Long-term postthoracotomy pain. Chest 1991;99: 270–4.

[95] Katz J, Jackson M, Kavanagh BP, Sandler AN. Acute pain after thoracic surgery predicts long-term postthoracotomy pain. Clin J Pain 1996;12:50–5.

[96] National Institutes of Health. Pain, research, consortium: gender and pain—a focus on how pain impacts women differently than men. Bethesda, MD: NIH; 1998.

[97] Feine JS, Bushnell MC, Miron D, Duncan GH. Sex differences in the perception of noxious heat stimuli. Pain 1991;44:255–62.

[98] Fillingim RB, Maixner W. Gender differences in the responses to noxious stimuli. Pain Forum 1995;4: 209–21.

[99] Fillingim RB. Sex, gender and pain: a biopsychosocial framework. In: Fillingim RB, editor. Sex, gender, and pain. Seattle: IASP Press; 2000. p. 1–6.

[100] Fillingim RB. The influence of menstrual cycle and sex hormones an pain responses in humans. In: Fillingim RB, editor. Sex, gender, and pain. Seattle: IASP Press; 2000. p. 191–207.

[101] Wall PD. The prevention of postoperative pain. Pain 1988;33:289–90.

[102] McQuay HJ. Pre-emptive analgesia. Br J Anaesth 1992;69:1–3.

[103] Woolf CJ, Chong MS. Preemptive analgesia—treating postoperative pain by preventing the establishment of central sensitization. Anesth Analg 1993; 77:362–79.

[104] Gottschalk A. Preemptive analgesia: an ounce of prevention still may be worth a pound of cure. J Pain 2000;1:85–8.

[105] Taylor BK, Brennan TJ. Preemptive analgesia: moving beyond conventional strategies and confusing terminology. J Pain 2000;1:77–84.

[106] Moiniche S, Kehlet H, Dahl JB. A qualitative and quantitative systematic review of preemptive analgesia for postoperative pain relief: the role of timing of analgesia. Anesthesiology 2002;96:725–41.

[107] Kissin I. Preemptive analgesia: terminology and clinical relevance. Anesth Analg 1994;79:809–10.

[108] Kissin I. Preemptive analgesia: why its effect is not always obvious. Anesthesiology 1996;84:1015–9.

[109] Hogan QH. No preemptive analgesia: is that so bad? Anesthesiology 2002;96:526–7.

[110] Carr DB. Preemptive analgesia implies prevention. Anesthesiology 1996;85:1498–9.

[111] Pasqualucci A. Experimental and clinical studies about the preemptive analgesia with local anesthetics: possible reasons of the failure. Min Anestesiol 1998; 64:445–57.

[112] Murphy DF, Medley C. Preoperative indomethacin for pain relief after thoracotomy: comparison with postoperative indomethacin. Br J Anaesth 1993;70: 298–300.

[113] Obata H, Saito S, Fujita N, Fuse Y, Ishizaki K, Goto F. Epidural block with mepivacaine before surgery reduces long-term post-thoracotomy pain. Can J Anaesth 1999;46:1127–32.

[114] Neustein SM, Kreitzer JM, Krellenstein D, Reich DL, Rapaport E, Cohen E. Preemptive epidural analgesia for thoracic surgery. Mt Sinai J Med 2002;69:101–4.

[115] Doyle E, Bowler GM. Pre-emptive effect of multimodal analgesia in thoracic surgery. Br J Anaesth 1998;80:147–51.

[116] Aguilar JL, Cubells C, Rincon R, Preciado MJ, Valldeperas I, Vidal F. Pre-emptive analgesia following epidural 0.5% bupivacaine in thoracotomy. Reg Anesth 1994;19:72.

[117] Aguilar JL, Rincon R, Domingo V, Espachs P, Preciado MJ, Vidal F. Absence of an early preemptive effect after thoracic extradural bupivacaine in thoracic surgery. Br J Anaesth 1996;76:72–6.

[118] Senturk M, Ozcan PE, Talu GK, Kiyan E, Camci E, Ozyalcin S, et al. The effects of three different analgesia techniques on long-term postthoracotomy pain. Anesth Analg 2002;94:11–5.

[119] Melzack R, Coderre TJ, Katz J, Vaccarino AL. Central neuroplasticity and pathological pain. Ann N Y Acad Sci 2001;933:157–74.

[120] Levine JD, Fields HL, Basbaum AI. Peptides and the primary afferent nociceptor. J Neurosci 1993;13: 2273–86.

[121] McCrory CR, Lindahl SG. Cyclooxygenase inhibition for postoperative analgesia. Anesth Analg 2002; 95:169–76.

[122] Cohen RH, Perl ER. Contributions of arachidonic acid derivatives and substance P to the sensitization of cutaneous nociceptors. J Neurophysiol 1990;64: 457–64.

[123] Chandrasekharan NV, Dai H, Roos KL, Evanson NK, Tomsik J, Elton TS, et al. COX-3, a cyclooxygenase-1 variant inhibited by acetaminophen and other analgesic/antipyretic drugs: cloning, structure, and expression. Proc Natl Acad Sci U S A 2002;99: 13926–31.

[124] Smith WL, Langenbach R. Why there are two cyclooxygenase isozymes. J Clin Invest 2001;107: 1491–5.

[125] Pavy T, Medley C, Murphy DF. Effect of indomethacin on pain relief after thoracotomy. Br J Anaesth 1990;65:624–7.

[126] Rhodes M, Conacher I, Morritt G, Hilton C. Nonsteroidal antiinflammatory drugs for postthoracotomy pain: a prospective controlled trial after lateral thoracotomy. J Thorac Cardiovasc Surg 1992; 103:17–20.

[127] Merry AF, Wardall GJ, Cameron RJ, Peskett MJ, Wild CJ. Prospective, controlled, double-blind study of i.v. tenoxicam for analgesia after thoracotomy. Br J Anaesth 1992;69:92–4.

[128] Singh H, Bossard RF, White PF, Yeatts RW. Effects of ketorolac versus bupivacaine coadministration during patient-controlled hydromorphone epidural analgesia after thoracotomy procedures. Anesth Analg 1997;84:564–9.

[129] McCrory C, Diviney D, Moriarty J, Luke D, Fitzgerald D. Comparison between repeat bolus intrathecal morphine and an epidurally delivered bupivacaine and fentanyl combination in the management of post-thoracotomy pain with or without cyclooxygenase inhibition. J Cardiothorac Vasc Anesth 2002;16:607–11.

[130] Merry AF, Sidebotham DA, Middleton NG, Calder MV, Webster CS. Tenoxicam 20 mg or 40 mg after thoracotomy: a prospective, randomized, double-blind, placebo-controlled study. Anaesth Intensive Care 2002;30:160–6.

[131] Collins SL, Moore RA, McQuay HJ, Wiffen PJ, Edwards JE. Single dose oral ibuprofen and diclofenac for postoperative pain. Cochrane Database Syst Rev 2000;CD001548.

[132] Camu F, Van Lersberghe C, Lauwers MH. Cardiovascular risks and benefits of perioperative nonsteroidal anti-inflammatory drug treatment. Drugs 1992;44:42–51.

[133] Barbera JA, Peinado VI, Santos S. Pulmonary hypertension in chronic obstructive pulmonary disease. Eur Respir J 2003;21:892–905.

[134] Humbert M, Nunes H, Sitbon O, Parent F, Herve P, Simonneau G. Risk factors for pulmonary arterial hypertension. Clin Chest Med 2001;22:459–75.

[135] Lee A, Cooper MC, Craig JC, Knight JF, Keneally JP. Effects of nonsteroidal anti-inflammatory drugs on post-operative renal function in normal adults [update of Cochrane Database Syst Rev 2000;4: CD002765; PMID: 11034758]. Cochrane Database Syst Rev 2001;CD002765.

[136] Gilron I, Milne B, Hong M. Cyclooxygenase-2 inhibitors in postoperative pain management: current evidence and future directions. Anesthesiology 2003; 99:1198–208.

[137] Kavanagh BP, Katz J, Sandler AN, Nierenberg H, Roger S, Boylan JF, et al. Multimodal analgesia before thoracic surgery does not reduce postoperative pain. Br J Anaesth 1994;73:184–9.

[138] Kalso E, Perttunen K, Kaasinen S. Pain after thoracic surgery. Acta Anaesthesiol Scand 1992;36:96–100.

[139] Dahl JB, Hjortso NC, Stage JG, Hansen BL, Moiniche S, Damgaard B, et al. Effects of combined perioperative epidural bupivacaine and morphine, ibuprofen, and incisional bupivacaine on postoperative pain, pulmonary, and endocrine-metabolic function after minilaparotomy cholecystectomy. Reg Anesth 1994;19:199–205.

[140] Ilkjaer S, Nielsen PA, Bach LF, Wernberg M, Dahl JB. The effect of dextromethorphan, alone or in combination with ibuprofen, on postoperative pain after minor gynaecological surgery. Acta Anaesthesiol Scand 2000;44:873–7.

[141] Moiniche S, Romsing J, Dahl JB, Tramer MR. Nonsteroidal antiinflammatory drugs and the risk of operative site bleeding after tonsillectomy: a

quantitative systematic review. Anesth Analg 2003; 96:68–77.

[142] Chavez ML, DeKorte CJ. Valdecoxib: a review. Clin Ther 2003;25:817–51.

[143] Reuben SS, Connelly NR. Postoperative analgesic effects of celecoxib or rofecoxib after spinal fusion surgery. Anesth Analg 2000;91:1221–5.

[144] Reuben SS, Bhopatkar S, Maciolek H, Joshi W, Sklar J. The preemptive analgesic effect of rofecoxib after ambulatory arthroscopic knee surgery. Anesth Analg 2002;94:55–9.

[145] Russell MW, Jobes D. What should we do with aspirin, NSAIDs, and glycoprotein-receptor inhibitors? Int Anesthesiol Clin 2002;40:63–76.

[146] Shah AA, Fitzgerald DJ, Murray FE. Non-steroidal anti-inflammatory drugs (NSAIDs) and gastro-intestinal toxicity: current issues. Ir J Med Sci 1999;168: 242–5.

[147] Hennan JK, Huang J, Barrett TD, Driscoll EM, Willens DE, Park AM, et al. Effects of selective cyclooxygenase-2 inhibition on vascular responses and thrombosis in canine coronary arteries. Circulation 2001;104:820–5.

[148] Howes LG, Krum H. Selective cyclo-oxygenase-2 inhibitors and myocardial infarction: how strong is the link? Drug Saf 2002;25:829–35.

[149] Strand V, Hochberg MC. The risk of cardiovascular thrombotic events with selective cyclooxygenase-2 inhibitors. Arthritis Rheum 2002;47:349–55.

[150] Mamdani M, Rochon P, Juurlink DN, Anderson GM, Kopp A, Naglie G, et al. Effect of selective cyclooxygenase 2 inhibitors and naproxen on short-term risk of acute myocardial infarction in the elderly. Arch Intern Med 2003;163:481–6.

[151] Ray WA, Stein CM, Daugherty JR, Hall K, Arbogast PG, Griffin MR. COX-2 selective non-steroidal anti-inflammatory drugs and risk of serious coronary heart disease. Lancet 2002;360:1071–3.

[152] Wooltorton E. What's all the fuss? Safety concerns about COX-2 inhibitors rofecoxib (Vioxx) and celecoxib (Celebrex). Can Med Assoc J 2002;166: 1692–3.

[153] Layton D, Hughes K, Harris S, Shakir SA. Comparison of the incidence rates of thromboembolic events reported for patients prescribed celecoxib and meloxicam in general practice in England using Prescription-Event Monitoring (PEM) data. Rheumatology 2003;42:1354–64.

[154] Tverskoy M, Oz Y, Isakson A, Finger J, Bradley Jr EL, Kissin I. Preemptive effect of fentanyl and ketamine on postoperative pain and wound hyperalgesia. Anesth Analg 1994;78:205–9.

[155] Fu ES, Miguel R, Scharf JE. Preemptive ketamine decreases postoperative narcotic requirements in patients undergoing abdominal surgery. Anesth Analg 1997;84:1086–90.

[156] Dahl V, Raeder JC. Non-opioid postoperative analgesia. Acta Anaesthesiol Scand 2000;44:1191–203.

[157] Roytblat L, Korotkoruchko A, Katz J, Glazer M, Greemberg L, Fisher A. Postoperative pain: the effect of low-dose ketamine in addition to general anesthesia. Anesth Analg 1993;77:1161–5.

[158] Dahl V, Ernoe PE, Steen T, Raeder JC, White PF. Does ketamine have preemptive effects in women undergoing abdominal hysterectomy procedures? Anesth Analg 2000;90:1419–22.

[159] De Kock M, Lavand'homme P, Waterloos H. 'Balanced analgesia' in the perioperative period: is there a place for ketamine? Pain 2001;92:373–80.

[160] Aida S, Yamakura T, Baba H, Taga K, Fukuda S, Shimoji K. Preemptive analgesia by intravenous low-dose ketamine and epidural morphine in gastrectomy: a randomized double-blind study. Anesthesiology 2000;92:1624–30.

[161] Helmy SA, Bali A. The effect of the preemptive use of the NMDA receptor antagonist dextromethorphan on postoperative analgesic requirements. Anesth Analg 2001;92:739–44.

[162] Grace RF, Power I, Umedaly H, Zammit A, Mersiades M, Cousins MJ, et al. Preoperative dextromethorphan reduces intraoperative but not postoperative morphine requirements after laparotomy. Anesth Analg 1998; 87:1135–8.

[163] Wu CT, Yu JC, Yeh CC, Liu ST, Li CY, Ho ST, et al. Preincisional dextromethorphan treatment decreases postoperative pain and opioid requirement after laparoscopic cholecystectomy. Anesth Analg 1999; 88:1331–4.

[164] Wu CT, Yu JC, Liu ST, Yeh CC, Li CY, Wong CS. Preincisional dextromethorphan treatment for postoperative pain management after upper abdominal surgery. World J Surg 2000;24:512–7.

[165] Weinbroum AA, Lalayev G, Yashar T, Ben Abraham R, Niv D, Flaishon R. Combined pre-incisional oral dextromethorphan and epidural lidocaine for postoperative pain reduction and morphine sparing: a randomised double-blind study on day-surgery patients. Anaesthesia 2001;56:616–22.

[166] Chow TK, Penberthy AJ, Goodchild CS. Ketamine as an adjunct to morphine in postthoracotomy analgesia: an unintended N-of-1 study. Anesth Analg 1998;87:1372–4.

[167] Kararmaz A, Kaya S, Karaman H, Turhanoglu S, Ozyilmaz MA. Intraoperative intravenous ketamine in combination with epidural analgesia: postoperative analgesia after renal surgery. Anesth Analg 2003;97: 1092–6.

[168] Mao J, Price DD, Mayer DJ. Mechanisms of hyperalgesia and morphine tolerance: a current view of their possible interactions. Pain 1995;62:259–74.

[169] Price DD, Mayer DJ, Mao J, Caruso FS. NMDA-receptor antagonists and opioid receptor interactions as related to analgesia and tolerance. J Pain Symptom Manage 2000;19:S7–11.

[170] Eisenach JC, De Kock M, Klimscha W. Alpha(2)-adrenergic agonists for regional anesthesia: a clinical

review of clonidine (1984–1995). Anesthesiology 1996;85:655–74.

[171] Coursin DB, Maccioli GA. Dexmedetomidine. Curr Opin Crit Care 2001;7:221–6.

[172] Niemi G, Breivik H. Adrenaline markedly improves thoracic epidural analgesia produced by a low-dose infusion of bupivacaine, fentanyl and adrenaline after major surgery: a randomised, double-blind, cross-over study with and without adrenaline. Acta Anaesthesiol Scand 1998;42:897–909.

[173] Niemi G, Breivik H. Epinephrine markedly improves thoracic epidural analgesia produced by a small-dose infusion of ropivacaine, fentanyl, and epinephrine after major thoracic or abdominal surgery: a randomized, double-blinded crossover study with and without epinephrine. Anesth Analg 2002;94:1598–605.

[174] Niemi G, Breivik H. The minimally effective concentration of adrenaline in a low-concentration thoracic epidural analgesic infusion of bupivacaine, fentanyl and adrenaline after major surgery: a randomized, double-blind, dose-finding study. Acta Anaesthesiol Scand 2003;47:439–50.

[175] Liu Z, Tian Y, Zhang C, Jin S. Clinical study of epidural analgesia with clonidine and sumatriptan in posthysterectomy. J Tongji Med Univ 1997;17:172–6.

[176] Lund C, Qvitzau S, Greulich A, Hjortso NC, Kehlet H. Comparison of the effects of extradural clonidine with those of morphine on postoperative pain, stress responses, cardiopulmonary function and motor and sensory block. Br J Anaesth 1989;63:516–9.

[177] Curatolo M, Petersen-Felix S, Arendt-Nielsen L, Zbinden AM. Epidural epinephrine and clonidine: segmental analgesia and effects on different pain modalities. Anesthesiology 1997;87:785–94.

[178] De Kock M, Wiederkher P, Laghmiche A, Scholtes JL. Epidural clonidine used as the sole analgesic agent during and after abdominal surgery: a dose-response study. Anesthesiology 1997;86:285–92.

[179] Jahangiri M, Jayatunga AP, Bradley JW, Dark CH. Prevention of phantom pain after major lower limb amputation by epidural infusion of diamorphine, clonidine and bupivacaine. Ann R Coll Surg Engl 1994;76:324–6.

[180] Paech MJ, Pavy TJ, Orlikowski CE, Lim W, Evans SF. Postoperative epidural infusion: a randomized, double-blind, dose-finding trial of clonidine in combination with bupivacaine and fentanyl. Anesth Analg 1997;84:1323–8.

[181] Ebert TJ, Hall JE, Barney JA, Uhrich TD, Colinco MD. The effects of increasing plasma concentrations of dexmedetomidine in humans. Anesthesiology 2000;93:382–94.

[182] Arain SR, Ruehlow RM, Uhrich TD, Ebert TJ. The efficacy of dexmedetomidine versus morphine for postoperative analgesia after major inpatient surgery. Anesth Analg 2004;98:153–8.

[183] Jin F, Chung F. Multimodal analgesia for postoperative pain control. J Clin Anesth 2001;13:524–39.

[184] Katz J. Pre-emptive analgesia: importance of timing. Can J Anaesth 2001;48:105–14.

[185] Holthusen H, Backhaus P, Boeminghaus F, Breulmann M, Lipfert P. Preemptive analgesia: no relevant advantage of preoperative compared with postoperative intravenous administration of morphine, ketamine, and clonidine in patients undergoing transperitoneal tumor nephrectomy. Reg Anesth Pain Med 2002;27:249–53.

[186] Farrar MW, Lerman J. Novel concepts for analgesia in pediatric surgical patients: cyclo-oxygenase-2 inhibitors, alpha 2-agonists, and opioids. Anesthesiol Clin North Am 2002;20:59–82.

[187] Tverskoy M, Oz Y, Isakson A, Finger J, Bradley Jr EL, Kissin I. Preemptive effect of fentanyl and ketamine on postoperative pain and wound hyperalgesia. Anesth Analg 1994;78:205–9.

[188] Tryba M. [Epidural regional anesthesia and low molecular heparin: pro]. Anasthesiol Intensivmed Notfallmed Schmerzther 1993;28:179–81.

[189] Horlocker TT, Wedel DJ, Benzon H, Brown DL, Enneking FK, Heit JA, et al. Regional anesthesia in the anticoagulated patient: defining the risks (the second ASRA Consensus Conference on Neuraxial Anesthesia and Anticoagulation). Reg Anesth Pain Med 2003;28:172–97.

[190] Vandermeulen EP, Van Aken H, Vermylen J. Anticoagulants and spinal-epidural anesthesia. Anesth Analg 1994;79:1165–77.

[191] Cleeland CS, Ryan KM. Pain assessment: global use of the Brief Pain Inventory. Ann Acad Med Singapore 1994;23:129–38.

THORACIC
SURGERY
CLINICS

ELSEVIER
SAUNDERS

Thorac Surg Clin 15 (2005) 123 – 130

Chronic Pain and Thoracic Surgery

Michael A. Erdek, MD[a],*, Peter S. Staats, MD[a,b]

[a]Division of Pain Medicine, The Johns Hopkins University School of Medicine, 550 North Broadway, Suite 301, Baltimore,
MD 21205, USA
[b]160 Avenue-at-the-Commons, Shrewsbury, NJ 07702, USA

Chronic pain after thoracic surgery is a difficult problem for patients and practitioners alike. Theories for its etiology are multiple, and a review of definitions of pain, its types, and appropriate treatments is appropriate before specific consideration of pain after thoracic surgery. *Pain* has been defined by the International Association for the Study of Pain as "an unpleasant sensory and emotional experience associated with actual and potential tissue damage, or described in terms of such damage." The same organization defines *chronic pain* as "pain that persists beyond the normal time of healing." Although acute pain can be considered functional and mainly a physiologic response to tissue damage, chronic pain involves psychological and behavioral mechanisms in addition to the physiologic mechanisms [1]. It is not the duration of pain that distinguishes acute from chronic pain, but the inability of the body to restore its physiologic function to normal homeostatic levels [2]. An example of this is neuropathic pain, which is chronic, often burning pain that persists secondary to nerve injury (Box 1).

Prevalence of chronic pain

Studies attempting to ascertain the prevalence of chronic pain are beset with challenges. The intensity of pain, survey method, and definition of chronicity vary from study to study. One group attempted to review the literature to search for the prevalence of chronic benign pain among adults (all epidemiologic studies concerning pain were included, provided that the study was not focused exclusively on acute pain or pain as a consequence of a defined disease, such as cancer or rheumatoid arthritis) [1]. Fifteen studies were identified reporting the prevalence of chronic pain in a general population with subjects age 18 to 75 years. The prevalence of chronic pain ranged from 2% to 40% (median 15%). The investigators speculated as to reasons for the large variance in pain prevalence. It would be expected that studies defining chronic pain with fewer criteria for inclusion would find a higher prevalence than studies with more inclusion criteria. In addition, the investigators surmised that data collection would influence results: Clinical examination by a physician is more stringent than self-response to a questionnaire. Finally, the review noted that the prevalence of chronic pain was higher in studies in which chronic pain was not defined or the definition was unclear [1].

Neurobiology of chronic pain

The initial pain impulse usually is perceived through the *primary afferent nociceptors*, grouped into myelinated A-delta fiber mechanothermal and unmyelinated C fiber polymodal nociceptors. These nerve fibers are responsive to many mechanical, thermal and chemical stimuli [3]. Another important finding is that "silent" or "sleeping" nociceptors normally cannot be activated and become excitable only under pathologic conditions, such as inflammation [4].

---

* Corresponding author.
E-mail address: merdek@jhmi.edu (M.A. Erdek).

Box 1. Nomenclature of chronic pain

Neuroplasticity: The fact that the nervous system is not "hard-wired" and is changeable over time in the face of chronic painful stimuli

Central sensitization: Changes that occur, primarily in the dorsal horn of the spinal cord, in the face of chronic painful stimuli; these changes are thought to be mediated by *N*-methyl-D-aspartate receptors and lead to phenomena such as allodynia, hyperalgesia, and expansion of receptive fields

Peripheral sensitization: A phenomenon occurring in the peripheral nervous system at the level of the nociceptors, whereby pain perception is augmented by the release of mediators such as bradykinin, histamine, and substance P

Nociceptive pain: Pain related to acute stimuli transmitted in normal fashion through an intact nervous system; acute postoperative pain is an example of nociceptive pain

Neuropathic pain: Pain occurring as a function of injury to the peripheral or central nervous system, usually chronic in nature

Peripheral sensitization occurs when contents of damaged cells and inflammatory cells, including macrophages, lymphocytes, and mast cells, are released. Peripheral sensitization occurs when these chemicals sensitize high-threshold nociceptors and allow low-threshold stimuli not normally causing pain to be perceived as painful [3]. This phenomenon also is described as *primary hyperalgesia*.

An overview of the pharmacology related to peripheral nociception can be found in several sources [4]. Various chemicals, including bradykinin, histamine, serotonin, prostaglandins, and protons, are released into damaged tissue cells from platelets, neutrophils, lymphocytes, macrophages, and mast cells. Peptides such as substance P and calcitonin gene-related peptide are released into the periphery via the axons in neurogenic inflammation. In addition, cytokines (interleukins, interferon, and tumor necrosis factor) are released by phagocytes

and immune cells and have an important role in the inflammatory process. Nerve growth factor has a key role not only in the development of sensory and autonomic neurons, but also in the process of nociception. Inflammatory mediators, such as prostaglandins, adenosine, and serotonin, facilitate transmission of action potentials by modification of the voltage threshold of several ion channels.

Primary afferent nociceptors terminate in the dorsal horn of the spinal cord, where they synapse with second-order neurons. These second-order neurons are categorized as either nociceptive specific/high threshold or wide dynamic range/convergent [3]. The wide dynamic range neurons normally do not signal pain, but under conditions of repeated stimuli may become sensitized and hyperresponsive, leading to a phenomenon known as "wind-up" and to the development of *central sensitization*. This dorsal horn pharmacology is characterized by the action of excitatory amino acids glutamate and aspartate acting at *N*-methyl-D-aspartate (NMDA) receptors. The concept of *neuroplasticity* refers to the changes that occur at the dorsal horn and other levels of the nervous system in conjunction with the development of chronic pain. Neuroplasticity leads to the generation of spinal hypersensitivity and amplification of peripheral inputs.

Central sensitization is characterized by *allodynia* (the perception of normally nonnoxious stimuli as painful), expansion of the receptive field, and *hyperalgesia* (an increase in the magnitude of a pain response). Dorsal horn pharmacology also is characterized by modulation from the effect of inhibitory interneurons via descending pathways from the brain [3]. These mediators of endogenous "descending neuromodulation" include enkephalins, serotonin, γ-aminobutyric acid (GABA), and noradrenaline. These descending influences arise from several supraspinal structures, including the hypothalamus, periaqueductal gray matter, locus caeruleus, and nucleus raphe magnus [3].

Types of chronic pain

Nociceptive pain refers to the detection of tissue damage by specialized transducers attached to A-delta and C fibers [2]. When acute pain first occurs, it is associated with specific autonomic and somatic reflexes (eg, withdrawal from a painful stimulus), but these eventually disappear in patients with chronic pain. As a result, the intensity of chronic pain often exceeds the extent of tissue injury or other pathology.

Clinically significant acute pain involves tissue damage. As previously mentioned, the central and peripheral nervous systems are dynamic, not static, and are modulated by products of tissue damage and by changes in the central nervous system and stress-regulation systems that occur in response to such damage. Most of these modulations are of short duration, but some may persist and lead to chronic pain [2].

As opposed to nociceptive pain, *neuropathic pain* occurs as a result of a lesion or dysfunction of the nervous system itself and often is described as having a lancinating or continuous burning character [5]. Although neuropathic pain can be a devastating response to nerve injury, it is not the usual consequence, and most patients do not develop neuropathic pain after nerve injury [5].

Mechanisms of neuropathic pain

Many peripheral mechanisms in the development of neuropathic pain have been elucidated [5]. Ectopic and spontaneous discharge of injured afferent fibers has been observed. Ephaptic conduction or "cross-excitation" may occur originating from injured neurons. It also has been observed that sodium and calcium channels, which are crucial to the physiology of excitable membranes, are altered in their expression in the cell bodies and the terminal endings of peripheral nerves after nerve injury. Collateral sprouting of fibers from sensory axons into denervated areas also has been described and may play a role in neuropathic pain.

Numerous studies show that peripheral nerve injury leads to the sprouting of sympathetic fibers in the area of the dorsal root ganglion [5]. These fibers provide a basis for the employment of short-term and long-term blocks of the sympathetic nervous system in certain scenarios of chronic pain, notably *complex regional pain syndrome,* formerly called *reflex sympathetic dystrophy.*

Central mechanisms also have been implicated in the development of chronic neuropathic pain [5]. There is a considerable degree of reorganization of spinal cord pathways in response to peripheral nerve injury. Large-diameter, low-threshold A-beta fiber mechanoreceptors, which normally terminate in laminae III and IV of the dorsal horn, have been found to sprout into lamina II after nerve injury. Because laminae I and II are where small-diameter, high-threshold A-delta and C fiber nociceptors normally terminate, this reorganization might result in sensory information being erroneously interpreted

as nociceptive. It has been suggested that nerve growth factor plays a role in the development of this sprouting.

Changes in certain neurotransmitter concentrations have been shown in the model of chronic neuropathic pain [5]. GABA and adenosine levels have been decreased in the face of chronic nerve injury. It also has been generally accepted that opioids are less effective in treating neuropathic than inflammatory or nociceptive pain. One theory states that peripheral nerve injury is associated with wallerian degeneration and a loss of axonally expressed opioid receptors [5].

Chronic pain after thoracic surgery

Chronic postthoracotomy pain syndrome is defined as pain that recurs or persists along a thoracotomy scar at least 2 months after the surgical procedure; it has a reported incidence of 44% to 67% [6]. One study assessed pain levels at 1 week, 3 months, 6 months, and 12 months after elective thoracotomy [6]. These patients received intraoperative intercostal blocks with bupivacaine and postoperative parenteral opioids and nonsteroidal anti-inflammatory drugs (NSAIDs) on an as-needed basis. The incidence of chronic postthoracotomy pain in 83 patients who were followed was 80% at 3 months, 75% at 6 months, and 61% at 1 year after surgery. Normal daily life was limited by persistent postthoracotomy pain in more than 50% of patients (mostly in the vicinity of the thoracotomy scar), and sleep disturbance was reported by 25% to 30% of patients. In this study, pain levels were increased in patients with malignancy and in patients older than age 50. The development of chronic pain correlated positively with higher amounts of analgesics used in the early postoperative period. This study excluded patients using intravenous patient-controlled analgesia (PCA), an important mode of therapy in the present control of postthoracotomy pain.

Chronic postthoracotomy pain has been declared by some authors to be the most common complication after thoracotomy. One study listed several factors that might contribute to postthoracotomy pain: intercostal neuroma, rib fracture, local infection, costochondritis/costochondral dislocation, local tumor recurrence, and psychological overlay [7]. Although studies have found the incidence of chronic postthoracotomy pain as described in the previous paragraph, it has been described as severe and disabling in 3% to 5% of patients.

Types of incisions for thoracic surgery

Different thoracic incisions have been examined with regard to their potential contribution to chronic postthoracotomy pain. During open thoracotomy, the serratus anterior and latissimus dorsi may be cut (muscle splitting) or retracted (muscle sparing). Several options for entering the pleural space exist, including dividing the intercostal muscle from the superior rib edge with electrocautery, reflecting the periosteum off the superior rib edge and entering through the periosteal bed without rib resection, subperiosteal rib resection, and an intercostal approach with short-segment rib resection posteriorly [7]. Intercostal incision may damage the intercostal nerves directly, whereas rib spreading stretches anterior and posterior structures and may compress the intercostal nerves. Intercostal nerves also may be damaged by a suture closing the intercostal muscles. The aforementioned study concluded that no technique of open thoracotomy can prevent chronic postthoracotomy pain effectively, and with most evidence pointing to intercostal nerve injury as a major etiologic factor, efforts are best directed at avoiding damage to the intercostal nerves by careful intercostal incision, minimal rib spreading, and meticulous closure.

Other studies also have examined factors involved in the development of chronic postthoracotomy pain. A retrospective study assessed 85 patients' recollection of their pain at 1 day, 1 month, and 1 year after thoracotomy [8]. Although the level of pain decreased in most patients as time elapsed subsequent to surgery, 35 patients still reported pain at 1 year. Stepwise regression analysis revealed female gender and pain at postoperative day 1 were predictive for subsequent postthoracotomy pain.

The issue of posterolateral versus muscle-sparing thoracotomy was addressed in a prospective, randomized study of 60 patients [9]. The group undergoing the muscle-sparing procedure showed a significantly lower visual analog scale for pain and narcotic use in the first week after surgery. In addition, the operating time was longer in the posterolateral group (the increased closure time in this group made up for the faster exposure).

One trial of 280 consecutive patients undergoing elective thoracotomy for pulmonary resection closed the first half of this group with pericostal sutures (placed on top of the fifth rib and on top of the seventh rib) and the second half with intracostal sutures (placed on top of the fifth rib and through the small holes drilled in the bed of the sixth rib) [10]. The mean pain scores of the pericostal group were statistically significantly lower at 2 weeks, 1 month, 2 months, and 3 months (with the 2- and 3-month scores being very low for both groups).

Although video-assisted thoracoscopic surgery (VATS) was designed with a primary goal of reducing pain-related operative morbidity associated with classic open thoracotomy, comparative studies have shown there is no difference in chronic pain after thoracotomy in an open fashion versus VATS [7]. Intercostal nerve injury and rib insult can occur from insertion of trocars or excessive torquing of instruments during VATS.

Role of preemptive analgesia on postthoracotomy pain

The rationale for preemptive analgesia is administration of analgesia before surgical insult to reduce the sensitization that might be produced by a nociceptive impulse to the nervous system. One study contacted patients who previously had participated in a randomized trial comparing preemptive multimodal analgesia with placebo 1.5 years after thoracotomy with regard to presence of long-term pain [11]. The original study, which provided demand morphine PCA without background infusion, showed no efficacy of preemptive analgesia versus placebo in reducing the intensity of acute postoperative pain. This follow-up study of 30 patients successfully contacted 77% of them and found that 52% continued to have postthoracotomy pain on a daily or weekly basis. The pain typically was described as a dull, aching, or burning pain located in the chest wall, with a mean pain score of 3.3 ($\pm$ 1.6) on a 10-point verbal reporting scale. When the data are stratified according to treatment group, 58% of patients experiencing long-term pain were in the preemptive analgesia group, whereas 55% of patients who were pain-free came from the preemptive group.

This study confirmed that early postoperative pain was the only factor that significantly predicted the development of long-term pain [11]. There was no difference in psychological profiles between patients who did and did not report pain. The authors of this study reported several limitations in their study, including not examining patients for recurrence of malignant disease and a relatively small sample size.

Another study reported 30 subjects who underwent placebo-controlled randomization to either preoperative or postoperative intravenous morphine, intramuscular diclofenac, and intercostal nerve blocks from T2 to T11 for thoracotomy [12]. Morphine PCA and diclofenac were provided in the postoperative period, with assessments of pain provided every 6 hours for the first 48 hours. Results showed no difference between groups in consumption of PCA morphine, visual analog scores, time to discharge from the hospital, or development of postthoracotomy pain. The group that received preemptive analgesia showed a statistically significantly lower visual analog score during vital capacity breath. This study posited potential sources of postthoracotomy pain, including surgical incision, disruption of ribs and intercostal nerves, pleural inflammation, pulmonary parenchymal damage, and the presence of postoperative intercostal drains [12]. Patients in this study did not receive thoracic epidural analgesia (TEA), a current mainstay in the treatment of perioperative thoracotomy pain. One reason these authors posed for the relative lack of efficacy of preemptive analgesia compared with some beneficial results shown in animal studies is that clinical postoperative pain is clearly a different entity from the nociception inflicted during animal studies [12].

Another study addressed the issue of preemptive analgesia by evaluating three different analgesic techniques in 69 patients with regard to postthoracotomy pain in prospective, randomized fashion [13]. Patients were randomized to preoperative initiation of TEA with bupivacaine and morphine, postoperative initiation of the same TEA solution, or intravenous PCA with morphine. Epidural catheters were placed at the T7-8 interspace and confirmed by administration of contrast material under fluoroscopy. Preoperative TEA was associated with significantly less pain than postoperative TEA and intravenous PCA during rest, coughing, and movement. In this study, the superiority of postoperative TEA to intravenous PCA could be observed only during rest. Both epidural groups experienced less pruritus and vomiting than the intravenous PCA group.

The same study also examined persistence of pain at 2 and 6 months postoperatively. The preoperative TEA group had a statistically significantly lower incidence of pain than the intravenous PCA group at both time periods, but one might question the clinical significance of the difference in the pain levels (1.4 ± 1.2 versus 0.6 ± 0.8 on a 10-point scale) [13]. The study seemed to corroborate the finding of other studies with regard to long-term postthoracotomy pain—that despite its frequent incidence (62%), the intensity of the pain seems to be low. Although there is some evidence showing that preemptive analgesia may lead to a small decrease in postthoracotomy pain symptoms, a convincing study showing clearly clinically significant data remains to be performed.

Thoracic epidural analgesia and postthoracotomy pain

Postthoracotomy pain comprises several factors, including wound pain, stretching of the thorax, and manipulation of the lungs and the pleura. A nonrandomized study of 114 patients examined the effect of TEA on postoperative and long-term pain after thoracotomy [14]. A total of 89 patients received TEA, and 22 patients, secondary to technical difficulties or patient refusal, received intravenous PCA with oxycodone and intercostal nerve block with bupivacaine (3 patients were excluded from final analysis due to reoperation within 1 week). All patients received oral analgesics in the postoperative period. Epidural catheters remained in place for approximately 5 days, which correlated roughly with the mean number of days of chest tube drainage.

Patients in this study were assessed with regard to visual analog scales for pain at rest and when coughing. At 3 months, 11% of TEA patients and 29% of intravenous PCA patients complained of chronic pain, defined as a visual analog score greater than 3/10 and at least as "moderate" on the verbal rating scale. At 6 months, these figures were 12% for the TEA group and 23% for the intravenous PCA group. At 6 months, one fifth of all patients were taking oral analgesics on a daily basis. Because of the small number of patients treated with intravenous PCA, the fact that the treatment allocation was not randomized, and the fact that the pain therapy was not standardized, no statistical comparisons were made. Also in this study, nearly one catheter in four came out inadvertently during the treatment period. This seems like quite a high number, and with the use of meticulous techniques of securing catheters in place and daily rounds by a dedicated pain service to ensure catheter integrity, one would suspect this could be improved on.

Other issues: pleurodesis and poststernotomy pain

The use of talc in the treatment of spontaneous pneumothorax and pleural effusion also may lead to chronic pain [15]. Talc poudrage may lead to thickening of the parietal pleura resulting from infiltration by Langerhans giant cells forming a foreign-body reaction to a crystalline material. This low-grade mononuclear cell inflammatory reaction apparently results in the development of fibrinous pleural adhesions. The authors of a case study recommended the use of video-assisted thoracoscopic pleurectomy and abrasion as an alternative treatment that might reduce the incidence of chronic thoracic pain in this particular group of patients [15].

A retrospective study was done to evaluate chronic poststernotomy pain in patients who had undergone thymectomy and coronary artery bypass graft (CABG) surgery [16]. This study described several possible etiologies for chronic poststernotomy pain, including osteomyelitis of the sternum, fracture or incomplete healing of the bone, sternocostal chondritis, costal fracture, injury of the brachial plexus, entrapment of nerves due to sternal wires, or hypersensitivity reaction against the metal wires. Questionnaires were returned by 62 thymectomy patients and 625 CABG patients (87% response rate). In the thymectomy group, 27% of the patients reported chronic poststernotomy pain at least 6 months after surgery. In the CABG group, 28% of patients had poststernotomy pain at least 2 years after surgery. Thymectomy patients' pain was primarily around the sternotomy scar site, whereas CABG patients' pain also was found in the arm, shoulder, and leg. In general, younger patients seemed to be at higher risk for long-lasting pain [16]. Although these are two different operations with two different patterns of pain, the incidence of chronic poststernotomy pain in these populations was similar.

Treatment of chronic pain after thoracic surgery

Treatment of chronic pain after thoracic surgery is often multifaceted and consists of pharmacologic, behavioral, and procedural modalities.

Pharmacologic treatment

The pharmacologic treatment of chronic pain consists of drugs that work via several different mechanisms [17]. A first-line pharmacologic treatment is inhibition of inflammation via institution of cyclooxygenase (COX) inhibitor therapy. The COX-1 isoform is constitutive (necessary for normal physiologic function of stomach, kidney, and platelets), whereas the COX-2 isoform is inducible and involved in inflammation [17]. The advent of COX-2 selective inhibitors, such as celecoxib, rofecoxib, and valdecoxib, has been met with interest, although they are not entirely COX-2 selective and still have some COX-1 activity. These drugs produce no physical dependence or tolerance, and there is marked individual variation in analgesic efficacy and side effects [17].

The tricyclic antidepressants (TCAs) are a viable option for the treatment of neuropathic postthoracotomy pain. TCAs include the tertiary amines, such as amitriptyline; the secondary amines, such as nortriptyline (which may have fewer side effects); and the serotonin selective reuptake inhibitors. Balanced reuptake inhibition of noradrenaline and serotonin is found with TCAs such as imipramine and amitriptyline, whereas desipramine inhibits reuptake of noradrenaline greater than that of serotonin.

The membrane-stabilizing drugs originally designed as anticonvulsants are another excellent option for the treatment of neuropathic pain. These drugs block ion channels, such as those of sodium and calcium, and may suppress the neuronal release of glutamate [18].Gabapentin is one of those most commonly employed; it is titrated in stepwise fashion, often on a weekly basis. Other options of this class include topiramate, lamotrigine, tiagabine, and oxycarbazepine.

The *number needed to treat* (NNT) is defined as the number of patients needed to treat with a certain drug to obtain one patient with at least 50% relief [18]. In a review of placebo-controlled trials for other types of neuropathic pain (diabetic neuropathy, postherpetic neuralgia, and central poststroke pain), NNT in the two to three range have been found for the TCAs. The ion channel blockers have NNT in the two to four range for similar types of neuropathic pain.

A third option for the treatment of postthoracotomy neuropathic pain is the application of the local anesthetic lidocaine in the form of a topical 5% patch [19]. To maintain effectiveness of the therapy, manufacturers suggest that it be used in a 12-hours-on, 12-hours-off fashion.

A controversial therapy is the topical application of capsaicin cream, which works by its depletion of substance P [20]. Capsaicin is often painful when applied, and some authors have advocated the institution of epidural analgesia before its use to maintain patient comfort during therapy.

An additional modality of pharmacologic therapy is the use of opioids. There is growing recognition that selected patients with chronic non–cancer-related pain can be provided opioid drugs for prolonged periods without overt evidence of tolerance and without intolerable toxicity, such as decreased mental status [17]. Long-term opioid therapy for chronic pain often involves a long-acting or sustained-release form (eg, methadone, transdermal fentanyl, or sustained-release oxycodone or morphine) combined with an immediate-release form to cover "breakthrough" or incident-related pain.

Increasing numbers of practitioners are requiring opioid "contracts" or urine drug assays as a condition for ongoing prescription of opioid therapy.

The evidence of involvement of excitatory amino acids in neuropathic pain has prompted studies on drugs with an NMDA-antagonistic effect [18]. The evidence to support the use of drugs such as ketamine, dextromethorphan, and memantine has not been strong to date, however.

Behavioral treatment

Multidisciplinary pain management involves health care providers from several disciplines, each of whom specializes in different features of the pain experience [21]. This team approach may involve a pain management specialist, a physiatrist, a psychologist or psychiatrist, a physical or occupational therapist, and a pharmacist. The care team tailors the care plan according to the individual needs of the patient, with a focus on achieving measurable treatment goals established beforehand with the patient. Realistic treatment goals for patients may include reduction of pain; improvement in physical functioning, mood, and sleep; the development of active coping skills; and a return to work.

Behavioral methods used to treat chronic pain include relaxation techniques, hypnosis, biofeedback, cognitive-behavioral therapy, and education [21]. Cognitive-behavioral therapy has four basic components: education, skills acquisition, cognitive and behavioral rehearsal, and generalization and maintenance. Biofeedback information may be provided to the patient by electromyography, electroencephalography, galvanometry, and temperature.

Interventional treatment

A first-line interventional therapy for the management of chronic thoracic pain is neural blockade. Intercostal nerve blocks may be done posteriorly at the angle of the rib to interrupt transmission via the intercostal nerve with a short-acting local anesthetic, such as lidocaine, or a longer acting anesthetic, such as bupivacaine or ropivacaine. The needle for the intercostal nerve block is placed just under the rib where the nerve courses, but not so deep as to enter the pleural space. The practitioner is well advised to exercise care in avoiding large amounts of local anesthetic in the intercostal region, given the relatively high amount of systemic vascular absorption observed at these sites.

The blocks also may be done more proximal to the spinal cord itself in the form of selective thoracic nerve root blocks. Here the radicular pain is treated by injecting a small amount of local anesthetic (potentially with steroid for a longer lasting effect) near the neural foramen at the nerve root exit site. Given the risks of complications, such as pneumothorax, intercostal intravascular injection, and subarachnoid injection, the use of fluoroscopic guidance is advisable. A patient who responds favorably to a diagnostic selective thoracic nerve root block may undergo pulsed radiofrequency ablation of a given thoracic nerve root.

The epidural injection of local anesthetics also can be provided, and the addition of steroids may provide relief of longer duration. Local anesthetics may be delivered by a single-shot technique or via an indwelling catheter. These injections may provide relief by somatic blockade of nociceptive afferent impulses and by interruption of the sympathetic nervous system in an effort to modulate sympathetically mediated pain. Some authors have advocated the use of intrathecal opioid therapy for chronic pain refractory to more conventional oral routes of analgesia, but outcome studies for its efficacy in nonmalignant pain such as persistent postthoracotomy pain are lacking.

Transcutaneous electrical nerve stimulation may provide relief [22]. A patch is applied over the affected area, often with the assistance of a physical therapist, to alleviate some of the persistent intercostal pain associated with chronic postthoracotomy neuralgia.

Although a detailed discussion of spinal cord stimulation is beyond the scope of this article, it is worth mentioning as an advanced method of interventional therapy for refractory postthoracotomy pain. In addition to the aforementioned pulsed radiofrequency ablation technique, a positive response to selective nerve root block may be addressed by spinal cord stimulation and electrode stimulation of the given nerve root itself. A patient usually undergoes so-called trial stimulation with a temporary percutaneous electrode for a period of several days, with the opportunity to manipulate the parameters of stimulation, such as frequency, amplitude, and pulse width. The goal of trial stimulation is to provide a sensation of vibration over the painful area that results in a diminution of the pain perceived in that area by the patient. A successful response to trial stimulation may lead to implantation of electrode leads on a more permanent basis in the operating room. These are connected to either an implantable pulse generator battery or a radiofrequency receiver, which is coupled to an external source of power.

Suggestions for referral to a pain specialist

Many patients with chronic postthoracotomy pain can be managed by a physician without necessity for a referral. Certain patients become difficult to manage, however, without a consultation with a specialist in pain management. If the referring physician finds that the use of traditional methods such as NSAIDs and opioids is unsuccessful, he or she may choose to attempt titration of an agent such as a membrane stabilizer or TCA. When the physician exceeds his or her comfort level with any of these means, it is reasonable to seek referral. Many pain management specialists who practice in tertiary or quaternary referral centers, owing to sheer referral volume, may function in a consultative fashion with the patient's referring or primary care physician, rather than assuming the care of that patient.

Summary

The development of chronic pain after thoracic surgery is a particularly undesirable yet common complication. As the study of the pathophysiology of chronic pain with regard to the plasticity of the central nervous system advances, new insights are being gained into not only the potential origins of chronic postthoracotomy pain, but also its potential treatment options. Pain that is originally nociceptive in nature in the acute postoperative period after thoracotomy may become neuropathic in time, requiring a different paradigm for its treatment.

The ongoing research into the development of chronic pain, including that observed after thoracic surgery, portends the development of further advances in options for its control. The employment of multidisciplinary strategies of pharmacologic, behavioral, and interventional procedural techniques provides the current foundation for the management of this challenging condition.

References

[1] Verhaak PF, Kerssens JJ, Dekker J, Sorbi MJ, Bensing JM. Prevalence of chronic benign pain disorder among adults: a review of the literature. Pain 1998; 77:231–9.

[2] Loeser JD, Melzack R. Pain: an overview. Lancet 1999;353:1607–9.

[3] Siddall PJ, Cousins MJ. Neurobiology of pain. Int Anesthesiol Clin 1997;35:1–26.

[4] Besson JM. The neurobiology of pain. Lancet 1999; 353:1610–5.

[5] Bridges D, Thompson SW, Rice AS. Mechanisms of neuropathic pain. Br J Anaesth 2001;87:12–26.

[6] Perttunen K, Tasmuth T, Kalso E. Chronic pain after thoracic surgery: a follow-up study. Acta Anaesthesiol Scand 1999;43:563–7.

[7] Rogers ML, Duffy JP. Surgical aspects of chronic post-thoracotomy pain. Eur J Cardiothorac Surg 2000;18:711–6.

[8] Gotoda Y, Kambara N, Sakai T, Kishi Y, Kodama K, Koyama T. The morbidity, time course and predictive factors for persistent post-thoracotomy pain. Eur J Pain 2001;5:89–96.

[9] Ackali Y, Demir H, Tezcan B. The effect of standard posterolateral versus muscle-sparing thoracotomy on multiple parameters. Ann Thorac Surg 2003;76:1050–4.

[10] Cerfolio R, Price T, Bryant A, Bass C, Bartolucci A. Intracostal sutures decrease the pain of thoracotomy. Ann Thorac Surg 2003;76:407–12.

[11] Katz J, Jackson M, Kavanagh BP, Sandler AN. Acute pain after thoracic surgery predicts long-term post-thoracotomy pain. Clin J Pain 1996;12:50–5.

[12] Doyle E, Bowler GM. Pre-emptive effect of multimodal analgesia in thoracic surgery. Br J Anaesth 1998;80:147–51.

[13] Senturk M, Ozcan PE, Talu GK, et al. The effects of three different analgesia techniques on long-term postthoracotomy pain. Anesth Analg 2002;94:11–5.

[14] Tiippana E, Nilsson E, Kalso E. Post-thoracotomy pain after thoracic epidural analgesia: a prospective follow-up study. Acta Anaesthesiol Scand 2003;47:433–8.

[15] Milton R, Cale AR. Chronic pain due to talc pleurodesis for spontaneous pneumothorax. Ann Thorac Surg 2003;76:1740–1.

[16] Kalso E, Mennander S, Tasmuth T, Nilsson E. Chronic post-sternotomy pain. Acta Anaesthesiol Scand 2001;45:935–9.

[17] Portenoy RK. Current pharmacotherapy of chronic pain. J Pain Symptom Manage 2000;19:S16–20.

[18] Sindrup SH, Jensen TS. Efficacy of pharmacological treatment of neuropathic pain: an update and effect related to mechanism of drug action. Pain 1999;83:389–400.

[19] Dworkin R, Backonja M, Rowbotham M, et al. Advances in neuropathic pain. Arch Neurol 2003;60:1524–34.

[20] Ellison N, Loprinzi C, Kugler J, et al. Phase III placebo-controlled trial of capsaicin cream in the management of surgical neuropathic pain in cancer patients. J Clin Oncol 1997;15:2974–80.

[21] Ashburn MA, Staats PS. Management of chronic pain. Lancet 1999;353:1865–9.

[22] Carrol E, Badura A. Focal intense brief transcutaneous electric nerve stimulation for treatment of radicular and postthoracotomy pain. Arch Phys Med Rehabil 2001;82:262–4.

THORACIC
SURGERY
CLINICS

ELSEVIER
SAUNDERS

Thorac Surg Clin 15 (2005) 131 – 142

Anesthetic Considerations for Special Thoracic Procedures

Erin A. Sullivan, MD

*Department of Anesthesiology, University of Pittsburgh Medical Center Presbyterian Hospital, 200 Lothrop Street, PUH C-224,
Pittsburgh, PA 15213, USA*

The anesthetic considerations and perioperative management for special thoracic surgical procedures are reviewed in this article. These procedures include video-assisted thoracoscopic surgery (VATS), endobronchial surgery, surgery for massive hemoptysis, and surgery in patients with anterior mediastinal masses.

Video-assisted thoracoscopic surgery

In 1921, the Swedish physician Jacobeus [1] reported the first series of thoracoscopic procedures as a technique to diagnose and treat pulmonary tuberculosis and pleural effusions. The advent of modern thoracic anesthesia and thoracic surgical techniques has been paramount to the development of VATS. This minimally invasive surgical technique, initially performed solely for diagnostic purposes, has been advocated for a variety of diagnostic and therapeutic procedures (Box 1). Compared with conventional thoracotomy, VATS decreases the impairment of early postoperative pulmonary function, decreases postoperative pain, and may allow for a more rapid recovery, reducing total length of hospital stay and total cost of care [2–4]. Although VATS offers many advantages for patients who otherwise would be considered as too high risk for conventional thoracotomy, it does present some potential complications. Complications associated with VATS include infection, hemorrhage, hemodynamic instability, prolonged air leak, "down lung" syndrome (increased secretions, atelectasis, and

pneumonia that develop postoperatively after one-lung ventilation), tumor seeding, re-expansion pulmonary edema, cardiac dysrhythmias, chronic pain, and nerve injury [5,6]. The potential for conversion of a VATS procedure to an open thoracotomy always exists and should be considered when formulating the anesthetic plan. The incidence of conversion from VATS to a thoracotomy has been reported to range from 1% to 20% [7,8]. Indications for conversion to thoracotomy are listed in Box 2.

Preoperative evaluation

The preoperative assessment and management of patients scheduled for thoracic surgery are thoroughly described in another article in this issue. Because patients scheduled for VATS often present with similar comorbidities and indications for surgery as patients scheduled for open thoracotomy, and there is not a reliable means to predict whether a VATS will be converted to an open procedure, the preoperative evaluation of these groups of patients is similar [9]. History, physical examination, and review of relevant laboratory and radiographic studies should be performed.

Options for pain management should be discussed with the patient, including intercostal nerve block, intravenous patient-controlled analgesia, thoracic paravertebral block, and thoracic epidural anesthesia. Although many anesthesiologists do not use thoracic epidural anesthesia for most VATS procedures, the anesthesiologist should discuss this mode of pain management with the patient preoperatively in the event that the surgeon's assessment of the probability of conversion to an open thoracotomy is 50% or greater. Under this circumstance, the thoracic epidural

---

E-mail address: esulliva@pitt.edu

Box 1. Indications for diagnostic and therapeutic thoracoscopy

Pulmonary parenchymal and pleural disease

    Biopsy, staging (malignancies)
    Tuberculosis
    Mesothelioma
    Interstitial fibrosis
    Solitary nodules
    Evaluation of traumatic thoracic injury
    Pleurodesis
    Drainage of pleural effusions
    Lung volume reduction surgery
    Pulmonary wedge resection, lobectomy
    Resection of bullae, blebs, and
      granulomas
    Decortication
    Empyemectomy
    Diaphragmatic disease

Esophageal disease

    Biopsy, staging (malignancies)
    Vagotomy
    Heller myotomy
    Zenker's diverticulum
    Antireflux procedures
    Minimally invasive esophagectomy

Mediastinal masses

    Lymphoma, metastatic disease
    Thymectomy
    Chylothorax

Cardiovascular procedures

    Patent ductus arteriosus ligation
    Internal mammary artery dissection
    Pericardial window, stripping
    Thoracoscopic mid–coronary artery
      bypass graft surgery

Miscellaneous

    Sympathectomy (hyperhydrosis,
      complex regional pain syndrome)
    Transthoracic anterior vertebral surgery

    Removal of intrathoracic foreign bodies
      (sheared catheters, surgical sponge)

From Shah JS, Bready LL. Anesthesia for thoracoscopy. In: Benumof JL, Joshi GP, editors. Anesthesia for minimally invasive surgery: laparoscopy, thoracoscopy, hysteroscopy. Philadelphia: WB Saunders; 2001. p. 154; with permission.

catheter may be placed either before the beginning of surgery in anticipation of conversion to an open thoracotomy or after the patient is awake in the postanesthesia care unit. A thorough discussion of the benefits and risks of thoracic epidural anesthesia, including the possibility that a catheter placed before surgery in anticipation of conversion to an open thoracotomy may not be used for the management of perioperative pain if the procedure is performed via VATS.

Intraoperative management

    Many of the same principles that apply to a patient undergoing open thoracotomy also apply to VATS (see other articles in this issue). Historically, thoracoscopy was performed under local anesthesia with intravenous sedation. Today, VATS most commonly is performed using a general anesthetic technique with controlled ventilation and a device to provide effective lung isolation. Standard monitors, including an electrocardiogram, pulse oximetry, noninvasive blood pressure cuff, and capnography, are employed. Some studies have reported the use of only non-

Box 2. Indications for conversion from thoracoscopy to thoracotomy

    Unsatisfactory operative lung
      deflation/isolation
    Extensive pulmonary resection or
      pneumonectomy required
    Extensive pleural adhesions
    Centrally located pulmonary lesion
    Lesion too large for thoracoscopic
      resection
    Excessive bleeding
    Surgical complications resulting from
      attempted thoracoscopy

invasive monitoring during VATS; however, these studies involved relatively healthy patients undergoing simple procedures [10]. Depending on the patient's preexisting comorbidities and the complexity of the procedure, it may be appropriate to use invasive monitors, such as an arterial line, central venous pressure line, or pulmonary artery catheter. The data obtained from pulmonary artery catheter monitoring during thoracoscopy may be altered by hypoxic pulmonary vasoconstriction, one-lung ventilation, surgical manipulation, and catheter position [11,12]. Transesophageal echocardiography also may be an extremely useful and accurate intraoperative monitor for assessment of cardiac filling and function during VATS procedures that do not involve the esophagus.

VATS can be performed using local, regional, or general anesthesia; as previously stated, anesthesia depends on the patient's cardiopulmonary status and the complexity of the surgical procedure itself [13,14]. Various regional anesthetic techniques have been used successfully either alone or in combination, including thoracic paravertebral blocks, intercostal nerve blocks plus ipsilateral stellate ganglion block, thoracic epidural anesthesia, and field blocks [15]. Regional anesthetic techniques require careful patient selection and VATS of brief duration. Patients who are uncooperative or have a potentially difficult airway should not be considered for VATS using regional anesthesia alone. Potential complications resulting from this anesthetic approach include failure of the regional technique to produce satisfactory surgical conditions and the temptation to counteract this by oversedating the patient with intravenous anesthetic agents, hypoxemia and hypercapnia as a result of oversedation and paradoxical respirations, and hemodynamic compromise secondary to the creation of an open pneumothorax and mediastinal shift. All of these complications require conversion to general anesthesia, sometimes on an emergent basis. Emergent management of a difficult airway, particularly in the lateral decubitus position, may result in significant patient morbidity or death due to an inability to ventilate or intubate.

Most anesthesiologists use a general anesthetic technique with controlled ventilation and a lung separation device for patients undergoing VATS. Effective lung isolation and deflation of the operative lung is essential for the success of the VATS procedure because the surgeon must work within the confines of a closed thoracic cavity. To facilitate satisfactory operative lung deflation, it may be helpful to ventilate the patient with oxygen before lung isolation rather than an air/oxygen mixture, particularly if the patient has poor pulmonary elastic recoil or chronic obstructive pulmonary disease. Denitrogenation of the lungs with 100% oxygen before attempted lung isolation facilitates lung deflation by absorption of residual oxygen. Tidal volumes should be adjusted to 5 to 7 mL/kg to minimize mediastinal shifting that may inhibit further the surgeon's ability to perform VATS successfully. Because the application of continuous positive airway pressure to the operative lung might be detrimental to the success of VATS, small increments of positive end-expiratory pressure may be applied to the nonoperative lung if the patient's oxygenation is compromised during one-lung ventilation (details of lung separation are discussed in a separate article). This maneuver may have detrimental effects on oxygenation in some patients, however, if it significantly increases shunt flow to the operative lung.

Carbon dioxide (CO_2) insufflation into the pleural space during one-lung ventilation is used occasionally to expedite collapse of the nondependent lung for VATS; however, it is not a procedure without significant risk. Cardiovascular compromise, including profound hypotension and bradycardia, may occur when the insufflation of CO_2 exceeds 1 L/min or when the intrathoracic pressure exceeds 5 mm Hg. These changes resolve rapidly when insufflation is discontinued and the CO_2 is released from the nondependent hemithorax. Other complications of CO_2 insufflation include CO_2 or air embolism and subcutaneous emphysema. Treatment of CO_2 embolism includes immediate discontinuation of insufflation; relieving the pneumothorax; and treating hemodynamic instability with volume infusion, with vasopressors, and by placing the patient in Trendelenburg position with the left side down [16].

Depending on the surgical procedure and the likelihood of conversion to an open thoracotomy, a regional anesthetic technique, such as thoracic epidural anesthesia, may be combined with the general anesthetic. Selection of specific anesthetic agents should be individualized and based on the preexisting condition of the patient and the anticipated length of the procedure. The goal for a general anesthetic approach is to provide satisfactory intraoperative anesthesia and analgesia using agents that facilitate tracheal extubation at the conclusion of surgery and minimize the occurrence of postoperative respiratory depression [17].

Postoperative management

Postoperative management of VATS patients is similar to management of thoracotomy patients. Although thoracoscopy is reported to be less painful and to cause less respiratory dysfunction compared with open thoracotomy, one must maintain a vigilant approach with regard to postoperative pain management and pulmonary therapy.

The degree of postoperative pain experienced by VATS patients is highly variable and depends on the surgical procedure performed. Procedures involving uncomplicated thoracoscopic pulmonary resection tend to produce pain limited to the intercostal port insertion sites and the chest tubes. In many instances, this pain may be managed effectively with intravenous patient-controlled analgesia (ie, morphine, hydromorphone), intravenous nonsteroidal medications (unless otherwise contraindicated), or oral analgesic medications. At the other end of the pain spectrum are procedures involving the pleura, such as pleural stripping or instillation of pleural sclerosing agents to minimize the reoccurrence of spontaneous pneumothorax or pleural effusions. These procedures are extremely painful and require more aggressive modalities of pain management, such as thoracic epidural analgesia. Inadequate pain management for these patients ultimately leads to postoperative respiratory failure, particularly for patients with limited pulmonary reserve.

Because general anesthesia by itself impairs pulmonary function, it is just as important to provide satisfactory postoperative pulmonary therapy for patients who have had a thoracoscopic procedure versus thoracotomy. Judicious and appropriate use of bronchodilators, chest physiotherapy, and incentive spirometry and early patient ambulation help to minimize the risk of operative morbidity and promote a timely functional recovery.

Endobronchial surgery

Endobronchial tumors produce a gradual obstruction of the main stem bronchi leading to severe dyspnea and collapse of the affected lung. Several therapies are currently available for the palliative treatment of these life-threatening lesions: laser therapy, insertion of bronchial stents, and a new experimental technique called photodynamic therapy (PDT).

Laser therapy

In 1974, the CO_2 laser first was reported as a useful surgical technique during bronchoscopy [18]. Today the laser commonly is used for the resection of airway tumors and other lesions, such as laryngeal papillomas, subglottic stenoses, and vascular malformations. Cancer tissue is reported to be more vulnerable to laser destruction than normal tissue, making laser therapy a viable option for palliation of endobronchial tumors. The criteria established for laser resection of endobronchial tumors includes extension of the lesion into the bronchial wall, but not beyond the cartilage, and an axial length of less than 4 cm [19].

Lasers are useful for the palliative treatment of obstructive malignancies of the esophagus [20], trachea, and main stem bronchi. In contrast to external radiation and chemotherapy, laser therapy does not produce systemic toxicity, and it is not dose limited. Symptomatic relief occurs almost immediately with laser therapy, but may take several weeks with chemotherapy and external radiation [21,22].

Hazards of laser therapy

The hazards associated with laser therapy include atmospheric contamination, perforation of a vessel or structure, embolism, and energy transfer to an inappropriate location. From January 1989 to June 1990, 21 laser injuries were reported to the US Food and Drug Administration—2 minor, 12 serious, and 7 fatal [23]. Of these reported injuries, 24% resulted from gas embolism; in 24%, there was perforation of an organ or vessel; 19% involved eye exposure or injury; in 14%, there was an airway fire; 9% of injuries resulted in other burns; and there was a 9% incidence of miscellaneous injury [23].

Smoke and plume (fine particulate matter that is small enough to penetrate to the level of the alveoli) are released as a by-product of laser tissue vaporization and may be teratogenic, mutagenic, and a vector for viral infection [24]. The mutagenicity of laser condensate has been reported in vitro to be half that of electrocautery [25]. Although some studies have reported that smoke plume serves as a vector for viral infection via transmission of viral DNA particles (mostly condylomas and skin warts), this topic remains controversial, particularly with regard to transmission of human immunodeficiency virus (HIV). One study described the detection of non-infectious DNA fragments found in a CO_2 laser plume from HIV-infected tissue pellets [26], whereas another study concluded that HIV was not detected in electrosurgical smoke plume at all [27]. Other studies have indicated that although laser plume does not appear to contain viable tumor cells, it may contain viable bacterial spores [28,29].

The most effective means of preventing dissemination of the laser plume is to use an efficient smoke evacuator at the surgical site [30]. In addition, smoke evacuators may help to eliminate laser plume that otherwise would cause visual obstruction of the surgeon and reduce the potential for ignition. High-efficiency surgical masks that filter small particles of plume ($\geq$0.3 μm) also are effective in minimizing the dissemination of potentially harmful laser plume and should be worn by all operating room personnel.

Another hazard associated with laser therapy for endobronchial lesions is the inadvertent perforation of a large blood vessel or bronchus. Airway hemorrhage occurs most often during laser therapy of an endobronchial lesion that completely occludes a main stem bronchus. In this instance, the direction of the main stem bronchus is distorted, and the possibility for bronchial and vascular perforation exists. Because blood vessels measuring larger than 3 mm in diameter are not coagulable by laser, life-threatening hemorrhage may occur, resulting in hypoxemia, hypoventilation, and hemodynamic compromise. Other complications resulting from inadvertent perforation of the trachea or bronchi include pneumothorax, pneumomediastinum, and tracheo-esophageal fistula.

Venous gas embolization has been reported during neodymium:yttrium-aluminum-garnet (Nd:YAG) resection of endobronchial lesions [31–33]. Two of these reviews reported several deaths resulting from cardiovascular collapse described as severe brady-cardia, shock, myocardial infarction, and cardiac arrest [32,33]. Possible etiologies of venous gas embolism during Nd:YAG surgery may include entrainment of helium (used as a coolant gas) or air/oxygen (from a jet ventilation device or vigorous bag mask ventilation) into a pulmonary vein during airway hemorrhage.

The wavelengths of all currently available medical lasers are transmitted through air and reflected by smooth metal surfaces. Inadvertent trigger of the laser at the wrong time may result in damage to the eyes, tissue burns, ignition of surgical drapes, and, of particular concern, airway burns.

It is imperative that all operating room personnel and the patient are provided with proper eye protection during laser surgery. Eye injury from CO_2 lasers may result in serious corneal injury, and the Nd:YAG laser may cause retinal damage. The patient's eyes should be protected first by taping the eyelids closed, then by covering the eyes with saline-soaked pads. Operating room personnel should be provided with special eyewear designed for the wavelength of the laser in use. For CO_2 lasers, any clear glass or plastic lenses suffice because they are opaque to far-infrared. Contact lenses are *not* sufficient protection. Nd:YAG lasers require specially coated lenses that are opaque to near-infrared. All

windows into the operating room should be covered during laser procedures because lasers other than the far-infrared CO_2 produce beams that pass through glass. Specific warning signs should be posted on the outside door of the operating room to prevent other personnel from entering while the laser is in use.

Perhaps the most feared complication of laser use during airway surgery is an airway fire. The estimated incidence of endotracheal tube fires is small (< 0.5%) [34]. Many of these fires, when handled appropriately, result in minimal or no harm to the patient; however, catastrophic consequences are possible.

An oxygen-rich atmosphere can potentiate the ignition of any hydrocarbon material, including tissue, plastic, and rubber. Fires may result from direct laser illumination, reflected laser light, or smoke plume. Most endotracheal fires initially are confined to the external surface of the endotracheal tube causing local thermal destruction. If a fire remains unrecognized and progresses to the oxygen-rich environment on the interior of the endotracheal tube, combustion occurs, blowing heat and toxic by-products of combustion distal into the pulmonary parenchyma. A similar circumstance occurs during inadvertent puncture and deflation of the tracheal cuff of the endotracheal tube. Specific management of airway fires is discussed later in this section.

Anesthetic implications of laser therapy

Deep intravenous sedation combined with topical airway anesthesia and general anesthesia have been used for laser therapy of the airway. Likewise, laser therapy has been delivered with the assistance of flexible fiberoptic bronchoscopy and rigid bronchos-copy. General anesthesia is preferred for rigid bronchoscopy and has been recommended for flexi-ble fiberoptic bronchoscopy. Although topical air-way anesthesia and intravenous sedation may be used for laser procedures that are performed with flexible fiberoptic bronchoscopy, any movement by the patient can cause the laser beam to be misdirected and result in serious injury [34,35]. For some patients with central airway obstruction, awake fiberoptic intubation or a general anesthetic induction technique that initially preserves spontaneous ventilation may be necessary to maintain airway patency. This is particularly true for patients with a variable intra-thoracic obstruction because the use of neuromuscu-lar blocking agents potentially could convert a partial airway obstruction into a complete airway obstruction owing to the loss of muscular tone [34]. Nevertheless, airway manipulation with any type of instrument in patients with central airway lesions, whether with a rigid bronchoscope or flexible fiberoptic broncho-scope with or without an endotracheal tube, must be exercised with great care to avoid exacerbating an intraluminal obstruction or bleeding.

The mixture of airway gases is an important issue during laser therapy. Combustion of excess oxidizers can lead to serious events described previously. Most clinicians recognize the need to reduce the fraction of inspired oxygen to less than 0.4 or to the minimal oxygen concentration consistent with adequate patient oxygenation. Nitrous oxide is also an oxidizer capable of combustion. Adding nitrous oxide to oxygen may be just as dangerous as administering a high concentration of oxygen alone [36]. The use of an oxygen/air mixture seems to be acceptable.

The use of a helium/oxygen mixture has been reported to prevent the ignition and fires of non-wrapped unmarked polyvinyl chloride endotracheal tubes [37]. Helium also has a lower density allowing the use of a smaller endotracheal tube without turbulence and high flow resistance. The use of helium prevents an accurate measurement of anes-thesia gases by most mass spectrometry units because they have no collector plates for helium. In this instance, erroneously high values for other gases, such as oxygen, carbon dioxide, nitrogen, nitrous oxide, and the volatile anesthetic gases, are observed.

A polyvinyl chloride endotracheal tube with an internal diameter large enough to accommodate a flexible fiberoptic bronchoscope and to provide adequate ventilation of the lungs is used when performing laser therapy under general anesthesia. Because the laser beam is directed distal to the tip of the endotracheal tube for procedures involving central airway obstruction, there is only a small chance that the tube material would ignite if the recommended concentrations of inspired gases are used. External ignition of an endotracheal tube during laser therapy is due to the transfer of heat between the laser itself and the tube; internal ignition is due to laser perforation of the tube with support of combustion by the gases entrained inside of the tube. As a safety measure, inflation of the endotracheal tube cuff with saline reduces the risk of fire from a misdirected laser because saline absorbs the laser's energy [38]. Alternatively, many endotracheal tubes are designed specifically for use during airway laser surgery. Although these special endotracheal tubes may offer some advantage, reports of airway fires resulting in serious airway injury have been docu-mented [39,40]. The use of an oil-based ointment for lubrication of all endotracheal tubes used during la-ser therapy should be avoided because this lubricant may be combustible.

Rigid bronchoscopy has been widely used as an alternative technique to endotracheal intubation for laser therapy of endobronchial lesions. Rigid bron-choscopy provides good visibility and allows for easier retrieval of debris that may accumulate in the airway. The rigid bronchoscope maintains a patent airway and substantially decreases the risk of fire because it is constructed of metal that is nonignitable and nonflammable. The metal is capable of reflecting the laser beam and producing indirect tissue damage. The same precautions for administration of gases used during general endotracheal anesthesia for laser therapy also apply to administration of general anesthesia with rigid bronchoscopy. Although the steel bronchoscope is not combustible, use of high oxygen concentrations may cause carbonized tissue to ignite.

Rigid bronchoscopy requires the administration of general anesthesia and neuromuscular blockade. Ventilation and oxygenation of the patient are achieved using many techniques, including controlled positive-pressure ventilation, the Sanders injection system, and high-frequency positive-pressure (jet) ventilation. For assisted/controlled positive-pressure ventilation, a rigid bronchoscope equipped with an eyepiece to occlude the proximal end and a side-arm adapter attached to the anesthetic breathing system may be used to deliver volatile anesthetic agents. This technique has the disadvantage of having to interrupt the ventilation of the patient and delivery of the volatile anesthetic agent whenever the eyepiece is removed to prevent environmental contamination with the volatile agent and to avoid anesthetic gas inhalation by the endoscopist. A study conducted by Duckett et al [41] showed a significantly higher arterial partial pressure of CO_2 using this technique compared with a Sander injection system and total intravenous anesthesia. The Sanders injection system and high-frequency jet ventilation allow for ventila-tion through a rigid bronchoscope without interrup-tion. Because volatile anesthetics cannot be delivered using these techniques, total intravenous anesthesia with propofol is frequently used. When using total intravenous anesthesia for laser procedures, one must ensure that the intravenous anesthetic is carefully titrated to provide optimal surgical conditions (eg, adequate general anesthesia).

Because laser beams can cause retinal damage, protective colored eyeglasses are required to be worn by all operating room personnel and the patient. These colored eyeglasses may make it difficult to read some colored anesthesia monitor displays, increase the time needed to perform simple tasks, and increase the likelihood of medication errors [42].

Management of airway fires

If an airway fire should occur during laser therapy, the surgeon and anesthesiologist must act quickly, decisively, and in a controlled fashion with clear communication being of the utmost importance. The laser should be discontinued immediately followed by termination of ventilation, removal of the oxygen source, and extubation of the trachea. These procedures serve to decrease inhalation of the toxic products of combustion and decrease the amount of oxidizing agents and fuel present to perpetuate the fire. The flaming material should be extinguished. Subsequently the patient should be ventilated with 100% oxygen via bag mask along with maintenance of general anesthesia. Rigid or flexible bronchoscopy should follow to evaluate the airway for damage and to remove any debris. If there is any evidence of airway damage detected during bronchoscopy, the patient's trachea should be reintubated. If the damage to the airway is severe, a low tracheotomy may be indicated. Postoperatively the patient may require prolonged endotracheal intubation and mechanical ventilation. Steroids may help to decrease airway edema.

Tracheal and bronchial stents

Tracheal and bronchial stents are used to prevent airway obstruction caused by internal or external compression of the trachea and bronchi. These stents may provide either temporary or definitive therapy for many obstructive conditions, including endobronchial tumors, mediastinal masses, and tracheal or bronchial strictures. Previously the only options available for treatment of these lesions were laser excision, dilation, and conventional surgical excision.

There are two types of stents: metallic and Silastic (Dumon). Rigid bronchoscopy is the conventional approach for stent placement; however, self-expanding metallic stents may be placed using flexible fiberoptic bronchoscopy. Although the metallic stents are more stable and not as prone to dislodgment as the Silastic stents, they are much more difficult to remove.

Optimal anesthetic management for tracheal and bronchial stents is achieved with general anesthesia and neuromuscular blockade, although some practitioners use flexible fiberoptic bronchoscopy and deep intravenous sedation. General anesthesia with neuromuscular blockade offers the advantage of a motionless surgical field. Care must be exercised when anesthetizing patients with severe symptoms of airways obstruction, as described in the section on anesthetic implications of laser therapy.

Photodynamic therapy

PDT is a new treatment available for palliation of obstructive esophageal and tracheobronchial malignancies and several other forms of cancer. PDT requires the use of a photoactive drug (photosensitizer) and light (visible or infrared) [43]. The photosensitizer tends to accumulate preferentially in the tumor. On exposure to a light source (visible or infrared), the photosensitizer absorbs the light, and a series of chemical reactions occurs leading to the direct or indirect production of cytotoxic species (free radicals and singlet oxygen) [44]. This cytotoxic reaction with the subcellular organelles and macromolecules leads to selective necrosis and apoptosis of the cancer cells that host the photosensitizer. One advantage of PDT is that it does not involve the generalized destruction of noncancerous cells. PDT also acts on the vascular supply to the tumor by reducing blood flow and subsequently causing tumor necrosis. Only tumors that are located superficially and can be reached by direct light or light delivered through an optical fiber are susceptible to this therapy.

PDT can be performed using topical airway anesthesia plus intravenous sedation or with general anesthesia similar to that used for laser therapy. Because combustion is not an issue during PDT, the patient may be ventilated with 100% oxygen.

Surgery for massive hemoptysis

Massive hemoptysis occurs in less than 0.5% of all patients who are admitted to the hospital for pulmonary dysfunction [45]. Greater than 90% of patients presenting with massive hemoptysis also have a history of chronic pulmonary infection. Some common infectious etiologies include tuberculosis and bronchiectasis. Neoplasms account for most noninfectious causes of bronchial hemorrhage. Chronic inflammation of the airways promotes vascularization of the high-pressure bronchial arteries that subsequently may erode or perforate, causing massive hemoptysis [46].

Cardiovascular etiologies include mitral stenosis, arteriovenous malformations, pulmonary embolism, and pulmonary artery perforation/rupture secondary to the placement of a pulmonary artery catheter [47]. Pulmonary artery catheter–related rupture of a pulmonary artery has a reported incidence of 0.1% to 0.2% [48,49]. This event may present as either hemoptysis or hemothorax. Rao et al [48] reported a series of 4684 patients who underwent pulmonary artery catheterization; 4 of these patients experienced pulmonary artery rupture. Of these four incidents, three occurred during cardiac surgery and full anti-coagulation, and one resulted from excessive inflation of the pulmonary catheter balloon. Mortality from massive hemoptysis usually results from hypoxia rather than exsanguination and is more likely if the patient is anticoagulated. The differential diagnosis for massive hemoptysis is listed in Box 3.

Anesthetic management of massive hemoptysis

Surgery is indicated in a patient who has required multiple blood transfusions, who has persistent

---

Box 3. Causes of massive hemoptysis

Infection

   Tuberculosis
   Bronchiectasis
   Lung abscess
   Necrotizing pneumonia

Neoplasm

   Bronchogenic carcinoma
   Metastatic carcinoma
   Mediastinal tumor
   Endobronchial polyp

Cardiovascular disease

   Mitral stenosis
   Pulmonary arteriovenous malformation
   Pulmonary embolism
   Pulmonary vasculitis

Miscellaneous

   Pulmonary artery catheterization
   Cystic fibrosis
   Pulmonary contusion/laceration
   Reperfusion of pulmonary vasculature
      after pulmonary embolectomy
   Tracheal-innominate artery fistulas
   Postsurgical complications

From Benumof JL. Anesthesia for emergency thoracic surgery. In: Anesthesia for thoracic surgery. Philadelphia: WB Saunders; 1995; with permission.

---

hemoptysis, or who has deterioration of pulmonary function [49]. Relative contraindications to surgery include inoperable pulmonary carcinoma, failure to localize the site of hemorrhage, and the presence of severe bilateral pulmonary disease. For patients with a relative contraindication for surgery or patients who refuse surgery, selective bronchial artery emboliza-tion may be attempted.

Although a chest x-ray may help to localize the site of bleeding, it may not be precise. Bronchoscopy is a much more precise technique for determining the cause and the source of bleeding. Insertion of a rigid bronchoscope facilitates ventilation and suctioning of the airway. Flexible fiberoptic bronchoscopy may be used when the patient is not actively bleeding or when bleeding is confined to the upper lobes. Bronchoscopy may be a diagnostic and a therapeutic intervention. Topical iced saline and vasoconstrictors may be administered via the bronchoscope. In some instances, this may be sufficient to stop the bleeding. More recently, selective intrabronchial spraying of fibrin precursors has been administered through the suction port of a flexible fiberoptic bronchoscope [50,51].

The goals for successful anesthetic management of a patient with massive hemoptysis include proper airway management with successful isolation of the bleeding lung, volume resuscitation, and maintenance of satisfactory arterial blood gases. Standard monitors are applied, and large-bore intravenous catheters should be placed to facilitate volume resuscitation. Invasive monitors, such as an arterial line and central venous catheter, may be indicated. Supplemental oxygen should be administered, and the patient should be positioned initially with the bleeding lung in the dependent position to minimize spillage and contamination of the other lung. Although coughing may exacerbate bleeding, this reflex should not be obliterated in the awake patient with an unsecured airway because this potentiates the aspiration of blood. After the patient's airway is secured, coughing may be suppressed in an attempt to decrease bleeding; suctioning the airway of an intubated patient diminishes the need for an intact cough reflex.

It may be necessary to perform an awake fiber-optic intubation to secure the patient's airway safely, although copious amounts of blood can make fiber-optic visualization difficult [35,52]. This intubation may be accomplished using a single-lumen endo-tracheal tube followed by placement of a bronchial blocker to facilitate lung isolation. Alternatively a main stem bronchial intubation of the unaffected lung may be performed with the assistance of the fiber-optic bronchoscope. Ideally a double-lumen endotracheal tube should be used to facilitate surgical exposure and provide for selective suctioning of the affected lung and differential pulmonary ventilation if necessary. If the patient is hemodynamically unstable, it is probably safer to secure the patient's airway with a single-lumen endotracheal tube and use a bronchial blocking device because double-lumen endotracheal tubes may be more difficult to place, particularly in the setting of massive hemoptysis. If the patient presents at the time of surgery with a single-lumen endotracheal tube already in place, one has the option of either using a bronchial blocking device placed with the assistance of a fiberoptic bronchoscope or changing the tube to a double-lumen endotracheal tube as long as the patient is hemodynamically stable. After resection of the bleeding pulmonary segment, the patient should remain intubated and mechanically ventilated.

Surgery for anterior mediastinal masses

Patients with anterior mediastinal masses frequently require anesthesia for diagnostic procedures and therapeutic surgery. These patients pose special problems for the anesthesiologist because they may present with symptoms that are obvious (eg, superior vena cava obstruction) or occult (eg, cardiac and major airways compression). These less obvious symptoms frequently may become apparent only after the induction of or emergence from general anesthesia and if not recognized immediately can lead to significant patient morbidity and mortality.

Perhaps the most common anesthesia complication related to anterior mediastinal masses is tracheobronchial obstruction. Airway obstruction caused by anterior mediastinal masses has been attributed to alterations in pulmonary and chest wall mechanics associated with changes in patient position or to the onset of neuromuscular blockade that obliterates the normal muscle tone that normally maintains airway patency. During the preoperative evaluation of patients with anterior mediastinal masses, it is important to determine if the patient exhibits positional dyspnea because this may be a symptom of airway compression. Likewise, it is important to review the patient's CT scan or MRI to determine the extent of the mass and the degree of compression or obstruction of the surrounding structures. An echocardiogram performed in the upright and supine positions may help to delineate whether there is significant compression of the heart. This information is helpful to the anesthesiologist for determining the optimal and safest anesthetic technique for the surgical procedure.

Anesthetic management

The anesthetic management of a patient with an anterior mediastinal mass is influenced by the potential for total airway obstruction by the mass during induction and emergence from anesthesia and the chemosensitivity or radiosensitivity of the tumor [53]. If a patient presents with positional dyspnea for a biopsy of an anterior mediastinal mass that exhibits severe airway obstruction as depicted on CT or MRI, consideration should be given to performing the procedure under local anesthesia if it is feasible to maintain spontaneous ventilation and normal neuromuscular tone and reduce the possibility of total airway obstruction. Additionally, if the mass is believed to be either chemosensitive or radiosensitive, consideration should be given to providing these therapies before a therapeutic surgical procedure that requires general anesthesia to shrink the size of the tumor and perhaps reduce the potential for airway obstruction during induction and emergence.

A potential disadvantage of preoperative radiation is that the histologic appearance may be altered, making an accurate diagnosis difficult. Ferrari and Bedford [54] described a series of 44 patients 18 years old or younger with anterior mediastinal masses who had general anesthesia for a diagnostic procedure before receiving radiation or chemotherapy. Although there were no fatalities, seven patients experienced severe airway compromise, and the authors concluded that the benefits of obtaining an accurate histologic diagnosis and initiating an appropriate therapeutic regimen outweighed the risks of airway obstruction. Some anesthesiologists would disagree with these findings because the reported incidence of life-threatening complications due to airway obstruction by an anterior mediastinal mass is 16% to 20% [55,56].

If general anesthesia is required for the surgical procedure, it is suggested that a careful evaluation of the patient's airway should be performed with the patient awake using a flexible fiberoptic bronchoscope, a small amount of intravenous sedation, and topical airway anesthesia [55]. The anesthesiologist has the option of securing the patient's airway with an endotracheal tube during this examination. Alternatively, if the patient is unable to cooperate with awake fiberoptic bronchoscopy, an asleep fiberoptic bronchoscopy employing an inhalation induction of general anesthesia may be conducted with a volatile agent, such as sevoflurane, which allows for maintenance of spontaneous ventilation while the patient's airway is secured. Spontaneous ventilation allows for maintenance of the normal transpulmonary pressure gradient during inspiration; airway patency is preserved even in the presence of extrinsic compression [57]. Neuromuscular blocking agents should be avoided because they may exacerbate airway compression secondary to the loss of muscular tone.

If airway obstruction occurs during general anesthesia, it usually can be relieved by one of several techniques: (1) rigid bronchoscopy; (2) inserting an anode (reinforced) endotracheal tube past the obstruction; (3) direct laryngoscopy, which lifts the laryngeal structures to simulate normal muscle tone that may have been caused by a neuromuscular blocking agent [58]; (4) change the position of the patient from supine to lateral decubitus or prone [59]; or (5) if the procedure is performed via median sternotomy, opening the chest relieves the extramural compression of the airway [60].

Airway obstruction and pulmonary edema requiring reintubation may occur in the postoperative period as a result of expansion of the tumor caused by edema secondary to surgical manipulation [61]. Negative-pressure pulmonary edema may result from vigorous attempts at inspiration against the obstructed airway.

As previously discussed, airway obstruction may occur even after awake fiberoptic intubation. Some clinicians have advocated the use of femorofemoral bypass or at least femorofemoral cannulation before the induction of general anesthesia ensues in patients with greater than 50% compression of the trachea or main stem bronchi [62]. Other risk factors that would warrant the preinduction placement of femorofemoral cannulas include positional dyspnea and a mediastinal mass greater than 50% of thoracic diameter.

Summary

Significant advances have been achieved in surgical and anesthetic techniques for the treatment of patients presenting with a variety of complex intrathoracic lesions. Despite the technologic advances, these patients continue to pose a challenge for anesthesiologists to provide safe and effective clinical care. A thorough understanding of the patient's underlying pathology inclusive of a detailed preoperative evaluation and effective communication between the surgical and anesthesia teams would help to ensure a favorable outcome.

References

[1] Jacobeus H. Cauterization of adhesions in pneumothorax: treatment of tuberculosis. Surg Gynecol Obstet 1921;32:49.

[2] Hazelrigg SR, Nunchuck SK, Landreneau RJ. Cost analysis for thoracoscopy: thoracoscopic wedge resection. Ann Thorac Surg 1993;56:633–5.

[3] Ferson PF, Landreneau RJ, Dowling RD, et al. Comparison of open versus thoracoscopic lung biopsy for diffuse infiltrative pulmonary disease. J Thorac Cardiovasc Surg 1993;106:194–9.

[4] Rubin JW, Finney NR, Borders BM, et al. Intrathoracic biopsies, pulmonary wedge excision and management of pleural disease: is video-assisted closed chest surgery the approach of choice? Am Surg 1994;60: 860–3.

[5] Inderbitzi RG, Grillet MP. Risk and hazards of video-thoracoscopic surgery: a collective review. Eur J Cardiothorac Surg 1996;10:483–9.

[6] Krasna MJ, Deshmukh S, McGlaughlin JS. Complications of thoracoscopy. Ann Thorac Surg 1996;1066–9.

[7] Jancovici R, Lang-Lazdunski L, Pons F, et al. Complications of video-assisted thoracic surgery: a five year experience. Ann Thorac Surg 1996;61: 533–7.

[8] Walker WS, Pugh GC, Craig SR, et al. Continued experience with thoracoscopic major pulmonary resection. Int Surg 1996;81:255.

[9] Horswell JL. Anesthetic techniques for thoracoscopy. Ann Thorac Surg 1993;56:624–9.

[10] Lewis RJ, Caccavale RJ, Sisler GE, et al. One hundred consecutive patients undergoing video-assisted thoracic operations. Ann Thorac Surg 1992;54:421–6.

[11] Nadeau S, Noble W. Misinterpretation of pressure measurements from the pulmonary artery catheter. Can Anaesth Soc J 1986;33:352.

[12] Tuman K, Carroll G, Ivankovich A. Pitfalls in interpretation of the pulmonary artery catheter data. J Cardiothorac Anesth 1989;3:625.

[13] Plummer S, Hartley M, Vaughan R. Anaesthesia for telescopic procedures in the thorax. Br J Anaesth 1998;80:223.

[14] Nezu K, Kushibe K, Tojo T, et al. Thoracoscopic wedge resection of blebs under local anesthesia with sedation for treatment of a spontaneous pneumothorax. Chest 1997;111:230.

[15] Mulder D. Pain management principles and anesthesia techniques for thoracoscopy. Ann Thorac Surg 1993; 56:630.

[16] Harris RJ, Benveniste G, Pfitzner J. Cardiovascular collapse caused by carbon dioxide insufflation during one-lung anaesthesia for thoracoscopic dorsal sympathectomy. Anaesth Intensive Care 2002;30:86–9.

[17] Weiss S, Aukburg S. Thoracic anesthesia. In: Longnecker D, Tinker J, Morgan G, editors. Principles and practices of anesthesiology. 2nd edition. St. Louis: Mosby-Year Book; 1998.

[18] Strong MS, Vaughan CW, Polany J, et al. Broncho-

scopic carbon dioxide laser surgery. Ann Otol 1974; 83:769.

[19] Boyce JR. Laser therapy for bronchoscopy. Anesth Clin North Am 1989;7:597–609.

[20] Lightdale CJ, Heier SK, Marcon NE, et al. Photodynamic therapy with porfimer sodium versus thermal ablation therapy with Nd:YAG laser for palliation of esophageal cancer: a multicenter randomized trial. Gastrointest Endosc 1995;42:507–12.

[21] Gelb AF, Epstein JB. Laser in treatment of lung cancer. Chest 1984;86:662–6.

[22] Unger M. Bronchoscopic utilization of the Nd-YAG laser for obstructing lesions of the trachea and bronchi. Surg Clin North Am 1984;64:931–8.

[23] US Food and Drug Administration. Special report: laser safety. Laser Nurs 1990;4:3.

[24] Kokosa J, Eugene J. Chemical composition of laser-tissue interaction smoke plume. J Laser Appl 1989; 2:59.

[25] Tomita Y, Mihashi S, Nagata K, et al. Mutagenicity of smoke condensates induced by CO2-laser and electrocauterization. Mutat Res 1981;89:145.

[26] Baggish MS, Poiesz BJ, Joret D, et al. Presence of human immunodeficiency virus DNA in laser smoke. Lasers Surg Med 1991;11:197.

[27] Johnson GK, Robinson WS. Human immunodeficiency virus-1 (HIV-1) in the vapors of surgical power instruments. J Med Virol 1991;33:47.

[28] Voohries RM, Lavyne MH, Strait TA, et al. Does the CO2 laser spread viable brain-tumor cells outside the surgical field? J Neurosurg 1984;60:819.

[29] Byrne PO, Sisson PR, Oliver PD, et al. Carbon dioxide laser irradiation of bacterial targets *in vitro*. J Hosp Infect 1987;9:265.

[30] Smith JP, Moss CE, Bryant CJ, et al. Evaluation of a smoke evacuator used for laser surgery. Lasers Surg Med 1989;9:276.

[31] Dullye KK, Kaspar MD, Ramsay MAE, et al. Laser treatment of endobronchial lesions. Anesthesiology 1997;86:1387–90.

[32] Dumon F, Shapshay S, Bourcereau J, et al. Principles for safety in application of neodymium-YAG laser in bronchology. Chest 1984;86:163–8.

[33] Vorc'h G, Fischler M, Personne C, et al. Anesthetic management during Nd:YAG laser resection for major tracheobronchial obstructing tumors. Anesthesiology 1984;61:636–7.

[34] Brodsky JB. Bronchoscopic procedures for central airway obstruction. J Cardiothorac Vasc Anesth 2003; 17:842.

[35] Conacher ID, Paes LL, McMahon CC, et al. Anesthetic management of laser surgery for central airway obstruction: a 12-year case series. J Cardiothorac Vasc Anesth 1998;12:153–6.

[36] Wolf GL, Simpson JI. Flammability of endotracheal tubes in oxygen and nitrous oxide enriched atmosphere. Anesthesiology 1987;67:236.

[37] Pashayan AG, Gravenstein JS, Cassis NJ, et al. The helium protocol for laryngotracheal operations with

[38] Lejeune FE, Guice C, LeTard F, et al. Heat sink protection against lasering endotracheal tubes. Ann Otol Rhinol Laryngol 1982;9:606–7.

[39] Ossoff RH. Laser safety in otolaryngology-head and neck surgery: anesthetic and educational considerations for laryngeal surgery. Laryngoscope 1989;99:1.

[40] Emergency Care Research Institute. Laser-resistant endotracheal tubes and wraps. Health Devices 1990; 19:112.

[41] Duckett JE, McDonnel TJ, Unger M, et al. General anaesthesia for Nd:YAG laser resection of obstructing endobronchial tumours using the rigid bronchoscope. Can Anaesth Soc J 1985;32:67–72.

[42] Boucek C, Freeman JA, Bircher NG, et al. Impairment of anesthesia task performance by laser protection goggles. Anesth Analg 1993;77:1232–7.

[43] Dougherty TJ. Photodynamic therapy. Photochem Photobiol 1993;58:895–900.

[44] Girotti AW. Photosensitized oxidation of cholesterol in biological systems: reaction pathways, cytotoxic effects and defense mechanisms. J Photochem Photobiol B Biol 1994;22:171–2.

[45] Benumof JL. Anesthesia for emergency thoracic surgery. In: Anesthesia for thoracic surgery. Philadelphia: WB Saunders; 1995.

[46] Wedel M. Massive hemoptysis. In: Moser KM, Spragg RG, editors. Respiratory emergencies. 2nd edition. St. Louis: CV Mosby; 1982. p. 194.

[47] Reich DL, Thys DM. Mitral valve replacement complicated by endobronchial hemorrhage: spontaneous, traumatic, or iatrogenic? J Cardiothorac Anesth 1988;2:359–62.

[48] Rao TLK, Gorski DW, Laughlin S, et al. Safety of pulmonary artery catheterization. Anesthesiology 1982;57A:116.

[49] McDaniel DD, Stone JG, Faltas AN, et al. Catheter-induced pulmonary artery hemorrhage. J Cardiovasc Surg 1981;82:1–4.

[50] Benumof JL. Anesthesia for emergency thoracic surgery. In: Anesthesia for thoracic surgery. Philadelphia: WB Saunders; 1995.

[51] Bense L. Intrabronchial selective coagulation treatment of hemoptysis: report of three cases. Chest 1990; 97:990.

[52] Klafta JM, Olson JP. Emergent lung separation for management of pulmonary artery rupture. Anesthesiology 1997;87:1248–50.

[53] Neuman G, Weingarten AE, Abramowitz RM, et al. The anesthetic management of the patient with an anterior mediastinal mass. Anesthesiology 1984;60:144.

[54] Ferrari LR, Bedford BF. General anesthesia prior to treatment of anterior mediastinal masses in pediatric cancer patients. Anesthesiology 1990;72:991.

[55] Tinker TD, Crane DL. Safety of anesthesia for patients with anterior mediastinal masses: I (correspondence). Anesthesiology 1990;73:1060.

[56] Zornow MH, Benumof JL. Safety of anesthesia for

patients with anterior mediastinal masses: II (correspondence). Anesthesiology 1990;73:1061.

[57] Silbert KS, Biondi JW, Hirsch NP. Spontaneous respiration during thoracotomy in a patient with mediastinal mass. Anesth Analg 1987;66:904.

[58] DeSoto H. Direct laryngoscopy as an aid to relieve airway obstruction in a patient with a mediastinal mass. Anesthesiology 1987;67:116.

[59] Prakash UBS, Abel MD, Hubmay RD. Mediastinal mass and tracheal obstruction during general anesthesia. Mayo Clin Proc 1988;63:1004.

[60] Fletcher R, Nordstrom L. The effects on gas exchange of a large mediastinal tumor. Anaesthesia 1986; 41:1135.

[61] Price SL, Hecker BR. Pulmonary oedema following airway obstruction in Hodgkin's disease. Br J Anaesth 1987;59:518.

[62] Shamberger RC. Preanesthetic evaluation of children with anterior mediastinal masses. Semin Pediatr Surg 1999;8:61.

THORACIC
SURGERY
CLINICS

ELSEVIER
SAUNDERS

Thorac Surg Clin 15 (2005) 143 – 157

Anesthetic Considerations for Lung Volume Reduction Surgery and Lung Transplantation

Philip M. Hartigan, MD[a,b,*], Alessia Pedoto, MD[a,b]

[a]Department of Anesthesiology, Perioperative and Pain Medicine, Brigham and Women's Hospital, 75 Francis Street, Boston, MA 02115, USA
[b]Department of Anesthesia, Harvard Medical School, Boston, MA 02115, USA

Lung volume reduction surgery

Lung volume reduction surgery (LVRS) is a therapeutic option for select patients with severe chronic obstructive pulmonary disease (COPD) unresponsive to maximal medical treatment and may be used as a bridge to lung transplantation (Table 1). Improvement in pulmonary function has been attributed to four mechanisms: enhanced elastic recoil, correction of ventilation/perfusion (V/Q) mismatch, improved efficiency of respiratory musculature, and improved right ventricular filling [1]. The National Emphysema Treatment Trial found that significant survival benefit (compared with optimal medical therapy) could be shown in the subgroup of patients with heterogeneous, upper lobe–predominant disease and low baseline exercise tolerance [2]. It is evident that the tenuous survival benefit of LVRS hinges on the tight containment of perioperative complications and that anesthetic management may be instrumental to this.

The principal risk for anesthetic complications occurs during induction and one-lung ventilation (OLV). Positive-pressure ventilation employed throughout the case is potentially hazardous, however, to patients with severe obstructive lung disease. Hazards include dynamic pulmonary hyperinflation, cardiovascular instability, alveolar barotrauma, disruption of surgical

staple lines, and chronic ventilator dependency. Rapid postoperative extubation is an emphasized priority and often the major anesthetic challenge [3].

Pathophysiology of chronic obstructive pulmonary disease

COPD is a slowly progressive disease that includes chronic bronchitis (characterized by airway inflammation and sputum production), and emphysema (a permanent destructive enlargement of the airspaces distal to the terminal bronchioles). Destruction of normal lung parenchyma causes a reduction of elastic recoil, with an increased work of breathing and impaired gas exchange. As the disease develops nonuniformly, normal lung parenchyma becomes underexpanded, causing an increase in V/Q mismatch. Superimposed bronchospasm and secretions can contribute to airway obstruction, resulting in expiratory airflow limitation, air trapping, and hyperinflation. Total lung capacity and residual volume increase, whereas forced expiratory volume in 1 second (FEV_1) decreases. Pulmonary hypertension can develop gradually in cases of severe COPD [4]. The severity correlates with the degree of airflow obstruction and the impairment of gas exchange. Proposed mechanisms include irreversible vascular remodeling (from direct effects of smoking and chronic inflammation, with a decrease in nitric oxide [NO] and prostaglandins and an increase in endothelin-1 production) and chronic hypoxic vasoconstriction [5]. Right ventricular function adapts through hypertrophy if pulmonary hypertension develops slowly. Ultimately, right

---

* Corresponding author. Department of Anesthesiology, Perioperative and Pain Medicine, Brigham and Women's Hospital, 75 Francis Street, Boston, MA 02115.

E-mail address: phartigan@partners.org (P.M. Hartigan).

Table 1
Indications for lung volume reduction surgery

Inclusion criteria	Exclusion criteria
End-stage emphysema, refractory to medical treatment	Age >75
Severe dyspnea	Cigarette smoking previous 3–6 mo
FEV$_1$ <35% of predicted	Severe obesity/cachexia
Hyperinflated lungs by chest x-ray, plethysmography	Severe comorbidity
Able to complete pulmonary rehabilitation program	Severe pulmonary hypertension
	Inability to participate in rehabilitation
	Severe hypercapnia (PaCO$_2$ ≥55 mm Hg)
	Ventilator dependency

Data from Fein AM. Lung volume reduction surgery: answering the crucial question. Chest 1998;113(Suppl): 277S–82S.

ventricular compensatory changes result in a reduction in compliance, preload dependence, and increased vulnerability to ischemia. Acute exacerbations in right ventricular afterload, particularly in settings of hypoxia and hypotension, may result in right ventricular failure.

Lung hyperinflation may compromise cardiovascular function by increasing intrathoracic pressures and decreasing venous return. A "tamponade-like" effect can occur, with reduction of preload and impairment of right ventricular diastolic function. Elevated mean alveolar pressure associated with auto-positive end-expiratory pressure (PEEP) may compress intra-alveolar vessels, increasing pulmonary vascular resistances and right ventricular output impedance. With progressive right ventricular dysfunction, left shifting of the interventricular septum can impair cardiac output further (ventricular interdependence).

Hypercapnia and hypoxia contribute to an increased baseline catecholamine tone, leading to intravascular volume depletion. Peripheral edema may occur in the absence of frank heart failure, probably because of increased sympathetic tone, which also leads to a decrease in renal blood flow. The renin-angiotensin-aldosterone system is activated, with absorption of bicarbonate, sodium, and water, and vasopressin secretion is increased [6].

Adverse effects of anesthesia on respiratory function

The potential negative respiratory effects of anesthesia are legion (Table 2). The most significant effect is the 15% to 20% (approximately 500 mL) decrease in functional residual capacity (FRC), which occurs promptly on supine induction and lasts for "some hours" after emergence [7]. The consequences of FRC reduction include atelectasis, intrapulmonary shunt, increased airways resistance, decreased pulmonary compliance, and increased work of breathing. The precise mechanism is incompletely understood and seems to be independent of the anesthetic agents used (excepting ketamine) or the presence or absence of spontaneous breathing, controlled ventilation, or paralysis [7]. Fluoroscopic studies in patients with COPD during anesthesia reveal that the FRC reduction is not simply attributable to a cephalad shift in the diaphragm [8,9], as long suggested by the work of Froese and Bryan [10]. Paradoxically, COPD may protect against this FRC reduction during anesthesia, possibly through air trapping or auto-PEEP [9].

Gas exchange is additionally impaired by general anesthesia as a result of a broadening of the V/Q ratio dispersion, and this effect is more pronounced in patients with COPD [11]. In particular, carbon dioxide elimination decreases because of an increase in ventilation of dead space and areas of high V/Q ratio. Adequate ventilation during the OLV phase is particularly difficult. Hypoxic pulmonary vasoconstriction is attenuated by clinical concentrations of vasodilators and inhaled anesthetic agents. All inhalational agents, opioids, and most intravenous agents decrease respiratory drive in a dose-dependent

Table 2
Respiratory effects of anesthesia

↓ FRC
↑ Dead space
↑ V/Q mismatch
↓ Hypoxic pulmonary vasoconstriction
↓ Respiratory drive in response to:
  Hypercapnia
  Hypoxemia
  Acidosis
↓ Upper airway muscle tone → upper airway obstruction
↑ Tendency to bronchospasm
↑ Volume of secretions
↑ Viscosity of secretions
Altered respiratory mechanics
  ↑ Atelectasis/shunt
  ↓ Compliance
  ↓ Airway caliber/ ↑ airflow resistance
  ↑ Work of breathing
  ↑ Risk of air trapping

Data from Hartigan PM, Body SC. Anesthetic considerations for lung volume reduction surgery. In: Fessler H, Reilly J, Sugarbaker D, editors. Lung volume reduction surgery for emphysema (Lung biology in health and disease, vol. 184). New York: Marcel Dekker; 2004. p. 219–45.

manner. This effect is more pronounced and prolonged in patients with COPD. Pharyngeal muscle tone is depressed by anesthesia, predisposing to upper airway obstruction after extubation. Distal airway obstruction can occur from the effects of a decreased FRC on small airways, accumulated secretions, and bronchospasm, with COPD predisposing to the latter two factors. In addition, thoracic surgery may induce a degree of reflex diaphragmatic dysfunction, independent of pain. It is controversial whether the mechanical benefits of LVRS immediately counteract these residual negative respiratory effects.

The combined effects of anesthesia, thoracic surgery, and severe COPD derange gas exchange, make positive-pressure ventilation hazardous, and complicate separation from the ventilator. Postoperative respiratory failure can be precipitated easily by small amounts of residual anesthetic agents or paralytics, bronchospasm, splinting, hypercarbia, acidosis-induced diaphragm dysfunction, or mucous plugging.

Preoperative considerations

Reversible components of COPD should be aggressively medically optimized before surgery with bronchodilators and steroids (inhaled or systemic). Smoking cessation for 18 hours produces a significant decrease in nicotine and carboxyhemoglobin levels, normalizes the oxyhemoglobin dissociation curve, and reduces tissue hypoxia. Longer time is required, however, for the beneficial effect on mucus production, mucociliary transport, and small airway resistance [12]. Respiratory infections should be treated before surgery because of the associated increase in airway reactivity and mucus production and higher incidence of postoperative complications [13]. In cases of recent upper respiratory tract infection, postponing surgery should be considered. Despite the minimally invasive approaches now broadly employed, LVRS is associated with significant cardiac stress. Tachycardia, hypercapnia, pulmonary hypertension, systemic hypotension, and postoperative hypoxemia are common. Age and smoking history are risk factors for coronary artery disease (CAD) present in this population. Preoperative screening is compromised by pulmonary limitations on exertion. Despite efforts at selection, a high prevalence of CAD has been shown angiographically in the LVRS patient population [14], and intraoperative myocardial infarction has been reported [15]. β-Blockers and antianginal drugs should not be withheld for fear of bronchospasm or cardiac depression [3].

Bronchodilators should be continued up to the time of surgery. Anxiolytics or sedatives should be administered with caution, to avoid depression of respiratory drive and worsening of preexisting hypoxia and hypercapnia [12].

Monitors

Whether the procedure is performed via median sternotomy or a thoracoscopic approach, intra-arterial blood pressure monitoring is indicated before induction to provide rapid-response hemodynamic monitoring and blood gas sampling capability. Central venous catheters are widely employed for central drug delivery and as a rough monitor of right heart function and intravascular volume. If an evaluation of right heart function or myocardial ischemia is sought, transesophageal echocardiography (TEE) is of greater value than a pulmonary artery catheter. Central venous pressures are falsely elevated by intrinsic and extrinsic PEEP, particularly in patients with severe COPD because of the high compliance of their lungs. If the pulmonary artery catheter floats to the nondependent, operative lung, pulmonary artery pressures and cardiac output determinations may be confounded by distortions in blood flow at the catheter tip resulting from atelectasis during OLV. Because of an increase in dead space, the gradient between end-tidal carbon dioxide and $PaCO_2$ is increased by an unpredictable amount, and arterial blood gases are needed to define the gradient.

Most anesthesia ventilators are incapable of detecting or measuring auto-PEEP. In-line flow-volume loop monitors are commercially available that can detect, but not measure, auto-PEEP. Failure of the expiratory flow to return to zero before initiation of a new breath indicates the presence of auto-PEEP (Fig. 1). Rotary flowmeters, inserted into the expiratory limb of the anesthesia breathing circuit, are useful, economical substitutes to visualize the presence or absence of end-expiratory flow (reflecting auto-PEEP).

Induction

Hypotension after induction is encountered frequently and has many potential contributing causes. The first to exclude is air trapping (auto-PEEP), by providing a prolonged expiratory phase with a disconnected circuit. Maintaining spontaneous ventilation does not eliminate auto-PEEP, especially if the patient becomes tachypneic or an endotracheal tube is in place. LVRS patients often behave as if they have reduced intravascular volume and exhibit

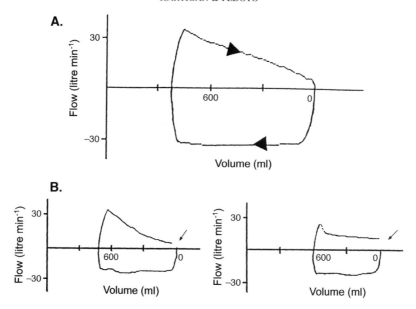

Fig. 1. (*A*) Normal flow-volume curve obtained by an on-line flow sensor. Direction of flow is marked by arrows. (*B*) Flow-volume curves during thoracic surgery obtained from patients with moderate (*left*) and severe (*right*) obstructive airways disease. Dynamic hyperinflation and auto-PEEP are indicated by the failure of end-expiratory flow to return to zero. (*Adapted from* Bardoczky G, D'Hollander JD, Yernault A, Van Meuylem A, Moures JM, Rocmans P. On-line expiratory flow-volume curves during thoracic surgery: occurrence of auto-PEEP. Br J Anaesth 1994;72:25–8; with permission.)

exaggerated decreases in blood pressure in response to impediments to venous return. Most induction agents have vasodilating effects. The epidural test dose may cause or contribute to the hypotension, particularly if the catheter is malpositioned in the subarachnoid space. Tension pneumothorax should be considered, especially in patients with bullous disease. Myocardial ischemia may occur either as a cause or as a consequence of hypotension during induction. Management usually depends on the etiology. Because impaired venous return is the common mechanism of the most common causes, augmentation of cardiac filling with vasopressors, fluids, and prolonged expiration should be the initial response. Preemptive vasopressors or fluid boluses with induction also are effective.

Lung isolation

Lung isolation may be accomplished with any of the usual techniques. Collapse of the operative lung is often slow because of the reduced elastic recoil of emphysematous lungs. For this reason, most practitioners favor a double-lumen tube, which can accommodate a pediatric bronchoscope for distal suctioning of the operative bronchus. Because of the principle of flow limitation, however, suctioning is of limited value in accelerating atelectasis. The flow

resistance characteristics of double-lumen tubes have been reviewed [16] and may contribute to air trapping, particularly during OLV [17].

Anesthetic agents and techniques

Choices of anesthetic agents are largely directed by the goal of early extubation. Narcotics (excluding remifentanil) should be used sparingly. Although potent volatile agents are used widely in thoracic surgery for their ease of titration and bronchodilating properties, their elimination is significantly delayed in patients with severe obstructive lung disease. End-tidal anesthetic agent levels may be grossly misleading owing to increased dead space in LVRS patients. Consequently, total intravenous anesthesia (TIVA) (usually some combination of propofol and remifentanil) is most widely used for LVRS. As a continuous infusion, TIVA allows for dense depression of airway reflexes and predictable rapid recovery. TIVA agents do not inhibit hypoxic pulmonary vasoconstriction (HPV) directly and are thought by many to yield improved oxygenation during OLV [18,19]. Clinical studies on this matter have yielded mixed results, however [19,20]. Ketamine has powerful analgesic and bronchodilating properties and has been employed as a useful adjunct in TIVA; however, hallucinations and pulmonary hypertension may occur at higher doses. Intraoperative use of a thoracic epidural, as hemodynamically tolerated, can reduce TIVA requirements.

One-lung ventilation in patients with severe chronic obstructive pulmonary disease

The most vexing problem in LVRS is how to achieve safe mechanical ventilation, particularly during the OLV phase. Ventilator settings must be adjusted to accommodate the competing priorities for adequate oxygenation, ventilation, and prevention of barotrauma.

Oxygenation is rarely an issue when a high fraction of inspired oxygen (FIO_2) is employed, owing in part to the inescapable presence of auto-PEEP in this population (Fig. 2) [20]. A high FIO_2 additionally may reduce pulmonary vascular resistance and right ventricular strain. Hypoxia should prompt a bronchoscopic evaluation of tube position and secretions. Intermittent continuous positive airway pressure (CPAP) or reinflation of the collapsed lung improves oxygenation, but impairs the progress of surgery [16]. Adding extrinsic PEEP to the dependent lung often is employed, but is unlikely to improve oxygenation. Slinger et al [21] showed that the response to PEEP depends on the patient's end-expiratory pressure relative to the lower inflection point of the patient's static compliance curve. Because patients with severe obstructive disease are

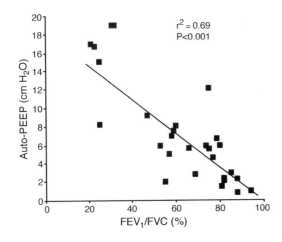

Fig. 2. Relationship during one-lung ventilation between the degree of airflow obstruction (forced expiratory volume in 1 second/forced vital capacity [FEV_1/FVC]) and dynamic hyperinflation (auto-PEEP). (*From* Ducros L, Moutafis M, Castelain M, Liu N, Fischler M. Pulmonary air trapping during two-lung and one-lung ventilation. J Cardiothorac Vasc Anesth 1999;13:35; with permission.)

generally at or beyond that inflection point, owing to unavoidable auto-PEEP during OLV, the addition of extrinsic PEEP is nonbeneficial from an oxygenation standpoint. Adding extrinsic PEEP to patients with preexisting auto-PEEP (70% of auto-PEEP levels) does not increase the total PEEP [22] and has no detrimental effect.

Recognition that the consequences of permissive hypercapnia are relatively benign (for limited periods), whereas the consequences of barotrauma are dire, has led to a gradual shift in consensus on optimal OLV strategies. LVRS patients are at particular risk of barotrauma during OLV and two-lung ventilation. Air trapping, with disruption of bullae, or vulnerable staple lines may lead to persistent air leaks with significant morbidity and mortality. Most practitioners have adopted a "lung-protective" ventilatory strategy, with small tidal volumes (5–7 mL/kg) and long expiratory times. Data in humans that "traditional" OLV strategies (10 mL/kg) [23] are injurious are indirect. The acute respiratory distress syndrome (ARDS) trial [24], which showed reduced mortality with a lung-protective ventilatory strategy, heightened awareness of the potential for, and consequences of, ventilator-induced lung injury. In the isolated, perfused rabbit lung model, compared with a lung-protective strategy, traditional OLV was associated with clinical indicators of early acute lung injury, including deteriorations in compliance, edema, and the elaboration of thromboxane B_2 [25].

Permissive hypercapnia is well tolerated in the short-term. Lengthy surgical duration resulting in advanced hypercapnia and respiratory acidosis may result in pulmonary hypertension, right ventricular strain, tachycardia, dysrhythmias, and myocardial depression or ischemia [26]. Emergence and extubation may be delayed by hypercarbia and acidosis-induced diaphragmatic and cerebral dysfunction. In the authors' experience, it is common to allow the pH to drift down to 7.25 during OLV. When the pH drops to less than 7.2, it is important to communicate with the surgeon, assess the anticipated time remaining until two-lung ventilation can be resumed, and consider more aggressive ventilation in the interim. Sodium bicarbonate is not of value in this scenario, where the ability to eliminate carbon dioxide through ventilation is limited. The unpredictable gradient between end-tidal carbon dioxide and $PaCO_2$ emphasizes the need for periodic arterial blood gas determinations.

Determination of the optimal balance point between carbon dioxide elimination and risk of barotrauma is hampered by an inability to determine the threshold for barotrauma. The volume in any given patient that results in disruption of the most vulnerable lung unit is not assessable. Peak inspiratory pressures are highly imperfect reflections of the degree of volume stress. Although pressure control ventilation is popular in thoracic surgery, there are no good data that barotrauma risk is reduced by use of pressure control versus volume control mode at comparable levels of carbon dioxide removal.

Emergence strategies

Rapid extubation at the end of the procedure is challenging because of the respiratory effects of anesthesia and surgery and the severity of preexisting disease. Failure or delay in extubation can be caused by the presence of drugs with depressant/sedating effects, neuromuscular agents, inadequate pain control, secretions, bronchospasm, or hypercapnia/acidosis. Strategies to avoid these events are largely common sense, but not always straightforward to execute (Table 3). Attention to detail and timing is crucial to success. A bolus of remifentanil can be useful to provide profound blunting of airway reflexes and bronchospasm during the exchange of endotracheal tubes and "toilet" bronchoscopy at the termination of the case.

The presence of increased dead space, V/Q inequality, and air trapping causes end-tidal levels of anesthetics to underestimate the amount of residual volatile anesthetic [3]. TIVA does not eliminate delayed emergence completely, but is widely considered to be more predictable. The degree to which

Table 3
Causes and strategies to avoid delayed/failed extubation after lung volume reduction surgery

Causes	Strategies
Secretions	Terminal "toilet" bronchoscopy
Bronchospasm	In-line nebulized bronchodilator treatment at end of surgery
	Deep remifentanil anesthesia during terminal bronchoscopy
Respiratory depression	Avoid systemic narcotics (except remifentanil)
	Avoid inhalational agents (use TIVA)
Weakness	Full reversal of neuromuscular blockade
Pain/splinting	Dense thoracic epidural blockade at end of surgery
Hypercapnic/acidosis	Limit degree of "permissive hypercapnia" during one-lung ventilation (fast surgery), and cautiously increase ventilation during terminal two-lung phase

hypercapnia and acidosis contribute to delayed emergence is unclear. Delay in extubation to achieve more physiologic values of pH is occasionally necessary and preferable to aggressive ventilation, which risks barotrauma and air leaks. If a thoracic epidural is employed, it should be dosed appropriately so that the patient breathes comfortably on emergence, without requiring supplemental systemic narcotics.

Postoperative pain management

Restrained use of narcotics (excluding remifentanil) generally is recommended in view of the sensitivity of LVRS patients to respiratory depression. Enduring postoperative analgesia is essential to prevent splinting, which can precipitate respiratory failure postoperatively. Although the thoracoscopic or midline sternotomy approaches commonly used for LVRS are less painful than thoracotomy incisions, aggressive regional techniques are widely employed for their narcotic-sparing effects. Intercostal, paravertebral, and thoracic epidural blocks all have been employed with success. Of these, thoracic epidural analgesia is most widely used because it can be titrated and maintained for a longer duration. Comparative studies of regional techniques in LVRS patients are absent.

Nonsteroidal anti-inflammatory drugs appear to enhance the analgesic effect of epidural drugs for incisional pain [27] and may aid the management of shoulder pain. Side effects, such as bleeding, platelet dysfunction, renal toxicity, and gastric ulceration, must be considered. Cyclooxygenase type 2 inhibitors are a promising alternative, with fewer side effects.

Postoperative respiratory management

After extubation, LVRS patients require close monitoring for postoperative respiratory failure, bronchospasm, oversedation, obstruction, stridor, mucus plugs, and hypotension. Nebulized bronchodilator treatments should be employed before or immediately after extubation. The head of the bed should be steeply inclined to optimize pulmonary mechanics. Serial arterial blood gases may be necessary to evaluate temporal trends toward impending respiratory failure. Should the patient require reintubation, care to avoid hyperinflation and subsequent barotrauma and air leaks is imperative. The premise that respiratory drive is depressed by supplemental oxygen in carbon dioxide–retaining COPD patients has been discredited [28,29], and the last thing one should do is to withhold oxygen from a somnolent, hypoventilating LVRS patient in the postanesthesia care unit, in an effort to encourage deeper breathing. A trial of noninvasive mechanical ventilation with pressure support can sometimes prevent reintubation.

Lung transplantation

Greater survival benefit is provided by lung transplantation compared with LVRS, with 5-year survival statistics now approaching 60%, according to the International Society of Heart and Lung Transplantation. Severe COPD is the most common indication, followed by idiopathic pulmonary fibrosis, cystic fibrosis, α_1-antitrypsin deficiency, and primary pulmonary hypertension. Current North American proportions for each diagnostic category with 1-year survival statistics for each are listed in Table 4.

Most pulmonary transplants are single-lung (SLTx) or bilateral, sequential double-lung transplants (DLTx). SLTx usually is preferred when ventilation and perfusion would be distributed mainly to the transplanted lung (eg, pulmonary fibrosis, nonbullous emphysema, and primary pulmonary hypertension). DLTx is performed when predominant ventilation or perfusion would remain in the untransplanted lung (eg, severe COPD and bullous emphysema) or when there is risk of contamination of the transplanted lung (cystic fibrosis, bronchiectasis, severe bronchiolitis obliterans).

Regional and institutional preferences affect the choice of operation. Survival advantages of DLTx over SLTx have been reported for some groups [30], whereas other regions regard DLTx as an inefficient

use of limited donor organs. Combined heart-lung transplantation is now uncommon and limited to patients with coexistent severe cardiac (usually congenital) and pulmonary disease. In an effort to expand donor and recipient pools, inroads have been made in the use of living donor, lobar, and split-lung transplantation and the use of non–heart-beating donors and "extended" donors and recipients, who by conventional criteria would be excluded [31]. Research is actively seeking ways to improve graft preservation and donor lung assessment.

Specific anesthetic considerations for lung transplantation vary with the procedure, the recipient's diagnosis (pathophysiology), and the perceived cardiopulmonary reserve. These are the first three things that the anesthesiologist needs to know. They largely determine the technique of lung isolation, the anticipated physiologic responses to OLV and pulmonary artery cross-clamping, and the anticipated need for cardiopulmonary bypass (CPB).

Overview of anesthetic management

SLTx is most common and usually is performed without CPB. Critical junctures include the induction of general anesthesia and the phases of OLV, pulmonary artery cross-clamp, and graft reperfusion. Failure to maintain satisfactory gas exchange and pulmonary and systemic hemodynamic stability during these phases mandate extracorporeal support. If CPB is employed, intraoperative gas exchange and hemodynamic issues are simplified, but the risk of complications of CPB is incurred. Strategies for mechanical ventilation are largely dictated by the pathophysiology (restrictive versus obstructive) and can affect hemodynamics and gas exchange.

The same critical junctures and issues apply to DLTx, which is more frequently performed with CPB. If CPB is to be avoided, the more diseased (less perfused) lung generally is transplanted first. When DLTx patients have suppurative disease, adequate gas exchange depends on aggressive secretion removal. The decision to employ CPB depends on the perceived cardiopulmonary reserve and institutional preferences, acknowledging that objective quantification of cardiopulmonary reserve is elusive.

General goals include hemodynamic stability and adequate gas exchange during the aforementioned critical junctures, avoidance of pulmonary hypertension and right ventricular failure, and early postoperative extubation. General principles of lung isolation, OLV, pain control for thoracic surgery, and early extubation strategies are discussed elsewhere in this issue.

Table 4
Lung transplants in North America; January 2002–January 2003*

Recipient's diagnosis	n	%	1-Year survival (%)
Emphysema/COPD	426	36.4	82.70
Idiopathic pulmonary fibrosis	208	17.8	69.40
Cystic fibrosis	183	15.6	81.70
α-1-Antitrypsin deficiency	88	7.5	73.10
Primary pulmonary hypertension	50	4.3	72.10
Retransplant/graft failure	29	2.5	59.50
Other	134	11.5	Not reported
Not reported	53	4.4	Not reported

* Incidence and 1-year survival data, by diagnosis.
From International Society of Heart and Lung Transplantation Website, www.ishlt.org; with permission.

Preoperative evaluation

Typically the anesthesiologist's first contact with the recipient occurs in a preparation room, shortly before a specified induction time, predetermined by the surgeon and harvesting team to limit graft ischemia time. The thorough cardiopulmonary evaluation performed when the recipient initially was listed is often many months out-of-date. Interval changes in exertion capacity, oxygen and steroid dependency, wheezing, orthopnea, or symptoms of respiratory infection should be evaluated at this time. Perceived deterioration of pulmonary function or right ventricular "reserve" may prompt a change of plans to include extracorporeal circulatory support. The usual litany of anesthetic preoperative issues must be addressed, including airway evaluation, coexisting diseases, and laboratory data. Despite time pressures, truncation of these details for expediency invites preventable complications.

Significant CAD generally excludes patients from lung transplantation. Not all centers routinely employ coronary angiography in all candidates. Noninvasive determination of CAD in patients with end-stage pulmonary disease may be problematic, and most patients possess multiple risk factors. Exercise testing is limited by pulmonary disease, dipyridamole scanning is affected by certain bronchodilators, and dobutamine thallium scanning has limited specificity and unknown sensitivity in this population [32]. An association between idiopathic pulmonary fibrosis and CAD has been reported [33]. Diagnosis of significant CAD may prompt exclusion from transplantation, pretransplant coronary stenting, or concurrent surgical revascularization with lung transplantation. The incidence of significant (>50% stenosis) CAD in lung transplant recipients older than age 50 was 17% in one study [34], and mortality due to CAD among lung transplant recipients may be 5% to 8% [31].

Steroids and bronchodilators should be continued up to the time of surgery. Anxiolytics are often appropriate for a young patient with cystic fibrosis or primary pulmonary hypertension, but should be employed with caution in older, COPD patients. β-Adrenergic blockers should not be withheld for fear of bronchospasm. The effect of a steroid bolus on blood glucose levels should be anticipated in diabetic patients.

Monitors

Intra-arterial blood pressure monitoring is mandatory for all transplants and generally should be established before induction. For DLTx, many prefer the femoral site because radial arterial waveforms often become damped by the rib cage retraction of clamshell incisions.

Pulmonary artery catheters are widely employed. Pulmonary artery pressures commonly are found to be surprisingly elevated compared with the remote, preoperative, right heart catheterization data owing to disease progression. Monitoring of pulmonary artery pressures and cardiac output during the critical phases of OLV, pulmonary artery cross-clamping, and graft reperfusion may help guide interventions and provide early detection of problems. Personnel must be cognizant of potential pitfalls in pulmonary artery catheter interpretation in this setting. Central vascular pressures may be elevated by intrinsic or extrinsic PEEP, and pulmonary artery occlusion pressures may be spuriously depressed by balloon inflation, while the contralateral pulmonary artery is cross-clamped [35,36]. The tip of the pulmonary artery catheter should be positioned just distal to the pulmonic valve, or the surgeon should be reminded to palpate the pulmonary artery to exclude the presence of a catheter before cross-clamping. Modified pulmonary artery catheters allowing for measurement of continuous cardiac output, mixed venous oximetry, or right ventricular ejection fraction have been employed and have their advocates. Continuous arterial blood gas monitoring technology is now available and may be particularly advantageous during the critical phases of lung transplantation.

TEE is the most powerful monitor to evaluate right ventricular function. The morphology of the right ventricle precludes full evaluation by a two-dimensional probe, but continuous views of right ventricular regional wall motion, cavity size, and septal position offer a good estimate of right ventricular function. In addition, TEE may be useful to help guide intravascular fluid management, evaluate the pulmonary arterial and venous anastomoses, guide the weaning from CPB (if applicable), detect air emboli, exclude a patent foramen ovale, and estimate pulmonary artery pressures from tricuspid regurgitant jets.

Induction

The principal disasters to be avoided during induction include aspiration, failure to intubate or ventilate, hypotension, bronchospasm, pulmonary hypertension, and right ventricular decompensation. Aspiration is potentially fatal to patients with end-stage lung disease facing transplantation and immunosuppression. Increasingly, antireflux surgery is being performed electively on transplant-listed patients. The emergent nature of transplants usually results in nonfasted patients, mandating all the usual preventive maneuvers against aspiration of gastric contents. If a nonreassuring airway examination precludes a straightforward rapid-sequence induction, awake fiberoptic-guided intubation of the topically anesthetized airway may be necessary. Raising the head of the bed reduces the risk of passive regurgitation and improves respiratory mechanics during this process.

The causes and prevention of induction-related hypotension and bronchospasm in patients with severe obstructive disease were discussed in the LVRS section. Pulmonary hypertension is often unmonitored during induction and is a particular concern in patients with idiopathic pulmonary hypertension. Patients with cystic fibrosis are at risk of mucous plugging and benefit from aggressive bronchoscopic pulmonary "toilet" using DNase (Pulmozyme, Genentech, Inc., South San Francisco, California) immediately after induction and intermittently throughout the case. Findings on the initial bronchoscopic examination should be shared with the anesthesia team because they may be relevant to the choice of lung isolation techniques. The presence of a surgeon and perfusion team at induction is indicated for tenuous lung transplant recipients, in case there is an emergent need for a chest tube or for CPB.

One-lung ventilation phase

When lung transplantation is attempted without CPB, anesthetic management may help avoid CPB by prolonging the surgical window of satisfactory gas exchange. In an effort to avoid hypoxemia, all the usual maneuvers, including CPAP, PEEP, intermittent reinflation, and bronchoscopy to remove secretions and ensure correct tube position, should be employed. Because bronchial blockers preclude bronchoscopic examination and suctioning of the operative bronchus, double-lumen tubes are the most commonly used technique for lung isolation. A left-sided, double-lumen tube works for DLTx, but may need to be withdrawn slightly at the time of left bronchial anastomosis. Other things being equal, one may expect lower PaO_2 values when the surgical position is supine compared with lateral [37]. Low-dose (<5 ppm) inhaled NO potentially may improve oxygenation [38], whereas higher doses (10–20 ppm) may be effective in reducing pulmonary hypertension. As such, inhaled NO may be a valuable tool in avoidance of CPB. Occasional recruitment maneuvers (sustained inspirations to 40 cm H_2O) more

recently were shown to improve one-lung oxygenation [39].

Ventilatory settings must be adjusted in accordance with the pathophysiology. In general, as discussed for LVRS, a balance must be sought between adequate gas exchange and minimal lung injury. In contrast to LVRS, the OLV phase of lung transplantation is more prolonged and includes a period of pulmonary artery cross-clamp. In addition, many transplant patients may have more marginal "right ventricular reserve," making the perils of permissive hypercapnia potentially greater. The threshold for concern regarding barotrauma is influenced by the presence or absence of bullae and whether the ventilated lung is newly transplanted, with a fresh anastomosis, or is destined to be sacrificed. Much of the art of this process involves finding the appropriate balance, prolonging the surgical window, and anticipating when or if there will be a need for CPB so that it might be instituted in an unfrantic manner. When the pH approaches 7.1, pulmonary artery pressures approach systemic levels, and there is evidence of right ventricular dysfunction, it is time to consider either more aggressive ventilation (eg, higher pressures and tidal volumes, faster rate) or CPB. Evidence-based guidance on this critical decision point is currently absent.

Pulmonary hypertension and right ventricular failure

Pulmonary hypertension is fairly common and results from fixed (intimal and smooth muscle hypertrophy) and reversible causes. Vasoactive drugs, hypoxia, hypercarbia, acidosis, pain, and agitation all can exacerbate pulmonary hypertension. Chronic pulmonary hypertension leads to right ventricular hypertrophy, dependence on diastolic perfusion, and increased susceptibility to ischemia. If pulmonary hypertension leads to right ventricular failure, ventricular interaction may lead to systemic hypotension, right ventricular ischemia, and perpetuation of the vicious cycle [40]. Vulnerable periods during lung transplantation include induction of anesthesia, initiation of positive-pressure ventilation, the OLV phase, and the time of pulmonary artery cross-clamping. Management requires inotropes, inodilators, and selective pulmonary vasodilators (inhaled NO), guided by TEE (or alternatively CPB). If right ventricular ischemia is suspected, inotropes with vasoconstricting effects, such as norepinephrine, may be advantageous, despite their potential to exacerbate pulmonary hypertension [41]. Pulmonary hypertension in patients with idiopathic pulmonary hypertension should be resolved immediately by the unclamping of a single new lung.

Pulmonary artery cross-clamp phase

The effect of pulmonary artery cross-clamping on right ventricular function may be difficult to predict and manage. Although oxygenation improves, the abrupt increase in pulmonary vascular resistance may precipitate right ventricular failure. Test clamping the pulmonary artery before ligation and examining the hemodynamic and TEE response is variously practiced, but is, as yet, of unproven predictive value, and right ventricular failure may take time to evolve. Acute right ventricular failure is probable in patients with severe pulmonary hypertension and preexisting right ventricular dysfunction. These patients should be transplanted on CPB. Patients with normal or hypertrophic (preconditioned), well-functioning right ventricular free walls, low pulmonary artery pressures, or relatively little perfusion to the lung being transplanted are likely to tolerate cross-clamping well. The gray zone in between is vast. Reliable predictors of adequate cardiopulmonary reserve for lung transplantation remain unknown. The pulmonary artery cross-clamp phase of the second lung during DLTx may be complicated by increased vasoreactivity of the transplanted lung.

Pulmonary venous anastomosis

The atrial clamp employed for the venous anastomosis potentially may obstruct right coronary arterial flow, emphasizing the importance of observing the ECG (and TEE if available) during this phase. Several case reports have shown the utility of TEE for early diagnosis of pulmonary venous anastomotic stenoses [42]. Threshold values defining a need to redo anastomoses have not been defined clearly, but Michel-Cherqui et al [42] found in a series of 18 patients that pulmonary vein diameters less than 0.5 cm were associated with accelerated flow and that a diameter of 0.25 cm was associated with graft dysfunction requiring reoperation.

Graft recruitment and reperfusion

Before reperfusion, the anesthesiologist should assess bronchoscopically the bronchial anastomosis and remove secretions or blood. Residual pulmoplegia, air, and metabolites can be expelled partially from the graft vasculature by retrograde flow with the left atrial clamp removed. Gentle recruitment maneuvers can aid in the expulsion of the aforementioned

residua and should reveal a pink, fully inflated graft. Overdistention of the graft is to be avoided, and PEEP is advocated to discourage alveolar derecruitment and edema.

Unclamping the pulmonary artery resumes antegrade perfusion and completes graft washout. The pathophysiology of this event is poorly understood. Systemic hypotension is common and may be a result of washout of pulmoplegia (high potassium, cold solution), by-products of anaerobic metabolism, inflammatory mediators, or air. Coronary air emboli may be suspected from ECG changes, arrhythmias, or regional wall motion abnormalities on TEE. If CPB is employed, a period of reperfusion with gentle ventilation allows for hemodynamic stability during the washout phase.

Barring early graft dysfunction, myocardial ischemia, or anastomotic stenoses, the initial hypotension is self-limited and generally can be weathered with vasopressors, inotropes, and intravascular volume expansion. TEE may prove diagnostically valuable at this stage. Improvements in gas exchange, pulmonary artery pressures, pulmonary compliance, and right ventricular function are expected early in the reperfusion stage. Pulmonary hypertension and right ventricular failure might result from reactive pulmonary vasoconstriction and should be treated as described previously.

Cardiopulmonary bypass

Debate continues over the role of CPB in lung transplantation surgery [43,44]. CPB is necessary for heart-lung transplants and for cases of severe pulmonary hypertension with right ventricular dysfunction or unequivocal intolerance of OLV. It is unnecessary for most SLTx and DLTx procedures. The conundrum is when and if to use CPB for patients whose acid-base status and pulmonary artery pressures are marginal or deteriorating or are anticipated to deteriorate during the course of surgery. Predictors of the need for CPB have been sought, but the decision remains an individualized clinical judgment [45,46]. The anesthesiologist rightfully should be involved in this judgment because he or she would have insights as to whether the patient might improve with corrective maneuvers. Such maneuvers might include the manipulation of ventilatory parameters or the use of inhaled NO, inotropes, vasoactive agents, or bronchodilators.

Known benefits of CPB include improved surgical exposure and avoidance of hemodynamic and gas exchange derangements during critical periods. Possible disadvantages include the risk of coagulopathy;

increased fluid and transfusion requirements; and the potential for pulmonary, renal, and neurologic complications of CPB. Waiting too long to impose CPB and cannulating emergently in an unstable patient increase the risk of vascular injury or mishap and may allow irreversible right ventricular damage to become established. Inhaled NO has proved useful in unstable patients when the goal is to avoid CPB [47].

A theoretical advantage of CPB is that it facilitates a slow, controlled reperfusion of the graft, with washout of pulmoplegia, air, mediators, cold, and byproducts of anaerobic metabolism, while maintaining hemodynamic stability [48]. A theoretical disadvantage is that CPB may act synergistically or additively to the ischemia/reperfusion (I/R) process to aggravate early allograft dysfunction [44,49,50].

In the absence of randomized controlled outcome studies, the CPB decision remains a matter of judgment and institutional preference for many "gray-zone" scenarios. At the authors' institution, the trend has been an increasing use of CPB for DLTx patients. CPB also allows for alleviation of overperfusion of the first graft during implantation of the second during DLTx. An emerging option is the intraoperative use of extracorporeal membrane oxygenation (ECMO) to avoid CPB during lung transplantation. Ko et al [51] described the use of ECMO in 15 lung transplants in which the need for CPB was anticipated. ECMO did not increase blood transfusion requirements, and because heparin-bound cannulas were used, heparin requirements were limited to 5000 U. Femoral venoarterial cannulation allowed for excellent surgical exposure and extension of ECMO support into the postoperative period when necessary. Ko et al [51] further speculated that patients with pulmonary hypertension might benefit from the diversion of some blood flow from the graft during the first 24 hours to prevent possible flow-related endothelial injury.

Closure phase

Generally the period between implantation and transport to the ICU is a "honeymoon" period. Significant edema has not yet accumulated in the allograft to reduce compliance or impair gas exchange. If CPB was employed, the usual considerations for weaning and heparin reversal apply. Aprotinin is widely advocated for patients who require CPB [52], but no consensus exists on the appropriate dose for transplant patients. In anticipation of pulmonary edema, fluid and diuretic therapy should aim for a negative fluid balance in the first 24 hours. Extubation may occur in the operating

room in select cases or within hours after transfer to the ICU. Occasionally the chest cannot be closed immediately if the grafts are edematous or large for the recipient. COPD patients after SLTx often experience hyperinflation of the remaining native lung. In extreme cases, this hyperinflation can cause mediastinal shift and circulatory compromise requiring differential lung ventilation via a double-lumen tube. Generally, this phenomenon is mild until the ICU period, when edema of the transplanted lung exaggerates the compliance difference between the lungs.

The close of the case usually requires changing to a single-lumen endotracheal tube for bronchoscopy and transient postoperative ventilation. Airway exchange catheter stylets may be useful for patients with difficult airways or edema, but caution must be exercised to prevent disruption of bronchial anastomoses.

The extent of the transplant incisions requires aggressive pain control. As discussed elsewhere in this issue, thoracic epidural analgesia has many advantages and remains the gold standard. If CPB (and anticoagulation) is not anticipated and if time permits, catheter placement may be performed preoperatively. When in doubt, when time does not permit, or when patients are anticoagulated (eg, idiopathic pulmonary hypertension), patients may be managed with moderate-dose narcotics intraoperatively and have thoracic epidural analgesia established after emergence (either before or after extubation). Because of the risk of renal failure with cyclosporine, nonsteroidal anti-inflammatory drugs are relatively contraindicated.

Reimplantation response: can the anesthesiologist help?

The pulmonary reimplantation response, characterized by early (4–72 hours) development of pulmonary hypertension, pulmonary capillary leak, alveolar infiltrates, edema, and decreased compliance and gas exchange, occurs in 60% of lung transplants [53,54]. Its most severe form, often termed *primary graft failure*, occurs in approximately 15% of lung transplants and is a leading cause of early (30 days) mortality [53]. The postulated mechanism, I/R injury, presumes the exclusion of acute rejection, infection, cardiogenic pulmonary edema, volume overload, or surgical complications such as torsion or stenosis of the venous anastomosis. Primary graft failure has been correlated with the subsequent development of obliterative bronchiolitis [55].

The mechanism of I/R injury is incompletely understood. In general, resumption of oxygen delivery to ischemically impaired pulmonary endothelium leads to the generation of reactive oxygen species, which further injure the lung and trigger release of proinflammatory mediators, which attract neutrophils and initiate neutrophil adherence and activation. Subsequent expression of neutrophil enzymes, such as myeloperoxidase, induces further damage. Pulmonary hypertension is a consequence of hypoxic pulmonary vasoconstriction and decreased production of NO in ischemically damaged pulmonary endothelium. Logic strongly suggests that processes that exacerbate the ischemic insult or the pulmonary inflammatory response would predispose to or worsen I/R injury. Relevant factors likely include graft ischemic time, preservation technique, operative manipulation, CPB, level of flow and oxygen content of reperfusate, technique of ventilation, and administration of inhaled NO.

Currently, evidence for the specific role of each of the aforementioned factors in lung transplant recipients is lacking, inconsistent, or controversial [53,54, 56–59]. Much research remains to be done. In the meantime, efficiency by the anesthesia team and coordination with surgical and harvesting teams to minimize graft ischemia time are emphasized. Reduction in FIO_2 to the lowest level that provides satisfactory saturations during reperfusion potentially may mitigate I/R injury and is widely practiced. Gentle recruitment of and "lung-protective" ventilation of newly transplanted lungs also has been mentioned as a logical, but incompletely proved anesthetic maneuver potentially to prevent or reduce I/R injury. Skilled anesthetic management of the OLV phase in marginal candidates might help avoid CPB, which has been postulated to exacerbate I/R injury [44]. Administration of inhaled NO by anesthesiologists during the reperfusion period is widely practiced, but controversial.

The line of reasoning and supportive evidence that inhaled NO might ameliorate I/R injury after lung transplantation are compelling [58]. NO potently inhibits neutrophil adhesion and aggregation [60,61], reduces myeloperoxidase activity [62], reduces microvascular permeability [63], scavenges oxygen radicals [60,61], inhibits expression of certain inflammatory mediators [64], alleviates reactive pulmonary hypertension [65], and improves V/Q matching and oxygenation in acutely injured lungs [66]. Ischemic pulmonary endothelium is deficient in NO production, rendering it vulnerable to I/R injury. Reperfusion is associated with dramatic decreases in endogenous NO in the donor lung [67]. Exogenous administration provides NO and induces production of constitutive NO synthase proteins [68]. Allograft

function is improved in NO-treated canine donor lungs [69]. The effects on pulmonary vascular tone and V/Q matching make inhaled NO widely used for symptomatic treatment of patients with established reimplantation responses. Several authors have reported beneficial clinical responses in that setting [70–73]. Whether the anti-inflammatory properties of NO can prevent or ameliorate I/R cascades is less widely accepted.

Two clinical trials using historic controls suggest that NO may prevent I/R injury [74,75]. In the only prospective randomized controlled trial to date, Meade et al [76] found no difference in physiologic variables or outcomes between lung transplant recipients who received NO and recipients who did not. That study has been criticized as underpowered, and the NO was initiated 10 minutes after reperfusion [77].

Questions and cautions remain regarding the efficacy, dose, and timing of inhaled NO for prevention of I/R injury. NO itself potentially may induce oxidative damage by combining with superoxide during the initial phase of reperfusion [78,79]. NO may cause methemoglobinemia [72], and higher oxides of NO are airway irritants. Valino et al [80] reported that NO may adversely affect surfactant function. Consensus on the intraoperative utility of NO to prevent the reimplantation response awaits further studies.

Summary

Anesthetic considerations for lung transplantation and LVRS have been reviewed, with an emphasis on critical intraoperative junctures and decision points. Cognizance of these issues promotes coordinated and optimal care and provides the potential to improve outcome in this particularly high-risk population.

References

[1] Fein AM. Lung volume reduction surgery: Answering the crucial question. Chest 1998;113(Suppl):277S–82S.

[2] National Emphysema Treatment Trial Research Group. A randomized trial comparing lung-volume-reduction-surgery with medical therapy for severe emphysema. N Engl J Med 2003;348:2059–73.

[3] Hartigan PM, Body SC. Anesthetic considerations for lung volume reduction surgery. In: Fessler H, Reilly J, Sugarbaker D, editors. Lung volume reduction surgery for emphysema (Lung biology in health and disease, vol. 184). New York: Marcel Dekker; 2004. p. 219–45.

[4] Barbera JA, Peinado VI, Santos S. Pulmonary hyper-

tension in chronic obstructive pulmonary disease. Eur Respir J 2003;21:892–905.

[5] Meyers BF, Patterson GA. Chronic obstructive pulmonary disease: 10. bullectomy, lung volume reduction surgery, and transplantation for patients with chronic obstructive pulmonary disease. Thorax 2003;58:634–8.

[6] Palange P. Renal and hormonal abnormalities in chronic obstructive pulmonary disease. Thorax 1998; 53:989–91.

[7] Nunn JF. Respiratory aspects of anaesthesia. In: Nunn's Applied Respiratory Physiology. 4th edition. Oxford: Butterworth Heinmann; 1993. p. 348–417.

[8] Kleinman B, Frey K, Van Drunen M, Sheikh T, DiPinto D, Mason R, et al. Motion of the diaphragm in patients with chronic obstructive pulmonary disease while spontaneously breathing versus during positive pressure breathing after anesthesia and neuromuscular blockade. Anesthesiology 2002;97:298–305.

[9] Warner D. Diaphragm function during anesthesia: still crazy after all these years. Anesthesiology 2002; 97:295–7.

[10] Froese A, Bryan A. Effects of anesthesia and paralysis on diaphragmatic mechanics in man. Anesthesiology 1974;41:242–55.

[11] Gunnarsson L, Tokics L, Lundquist H, Brismar B, Strandberg A, Berg B, et al. Chronic obstructive pulmonary disease and anaesthesia: formation of atelectasis and gas exchange impairment. Eur Respir J 1991; 4:1106–16.

[12] Boysen P. Evaluation of the patient with pulmonary disease. In: Rogers M, Tinker J, Covino B, editors. Principles and practice of anesthesiology. St Louis: Mosby-Year Book; 1993. p. 232–42.

[13] DeSoto H, Patel R, Solimon I. Changes in oxygen saturation following general anesthesia in children with upper respiratory infection signs and symptoms undergoing two otolaryngological procedures. Anesthesiology 1988;68:276–9.

[14] Thurnheer R, Muntwyler J, Stammberger U, Bloch KE, Zollinger A, Weder W, et al. Coronary artery disease in patients undergoing lung volume reduction surgery for emphysema. Chest 1997;112:122–8.

[15] Hogue C, Stamos T, Winters KJ, Moulton M, Krucylak PE, Cooper JD. Acute myocardial infarction during lung volume reduction surgery. Anesth Analg 1999; 88:332–4.

[16] Slinger P, Lesiuk L. Flow resistance of disposable double-lumen, single-lumen, and Univent tubes. J Cardiothorac Vasc Anesth 1998;12:142–4.

[17] Ducros L, Moutafis M, Castelain M, Liu N, Fischler M. Pulmonary air trapping during two-lung and one-lung ventilation. J Cardiothorac Vasc Anesth 1999;13: 35–9.

[18] Hillier J, Gilbe C. Anaesthesia for lung volume reduction surgery. Anaesthesia 2003;58:1210–9.

[19] Abe K, Shimizu T, Takashina M, Shiozaki H, Yoshiya I. The effects of propofol, isoflurane, and sevoflurane on oxygenation and shunt fraction during one-lung ventilation. Anesth Analg 1998;87:1164–9.

[20] Von Dossow V, Welte M, Zaune U, Martin E, Walter M, Ruckert J, et al. Thoracic epidural analgesia combined with general anesthesia: the preferred anesthetic technique for thoracic surgery. Anesth Analg 2001;92:848–54.

[21] Slinger P, Kruger M, McRae K, Winton T. Relation of the static compliance curve and positive end-expiratory pressure to oxygenation during one-lung vantilation. Anesthesiology 2001;95:1096–102.

[22] Gay G, Rodarte J, Hubmayer R. The effects of positive end-expiratory pressure on isovolumic flow and dynamic hyperinflation in patients receiving mechanical ventilation. Am Rev Respir Dis 1989;139:621–6.

[23] Benumof J. Conventional and differential lung management of one-lung ventilation. In: Anesthesia for thoracic surgery. 2nd edition. Philadelphia: Saunders; 1995. p. 406–31.

[24] Amato M, Barbas C, Medeiros D, Magaldi R, Schettino G, Lorenzi-Filho G, et al. Effect of protective-ventilation strategy on mortality in the acute respiratory distress syndrome. N Engl J Med 1998; 338:347–54.

[25] De Abreu M, Heintz M, Heller A, Szechenyi R, Albrecht M, Koch T. One-lung ventilation with high tidal volumes and zero positive end-expiratory pressure is injurious in the isolated rabbit lung model. Anesth Analg 2003;96:220–8.

[26] Morisaki H, Serita R, Innami Y, Kotake Y, Takeda J. Permissive hypercapnia during thoracic anesthesia. Acta Anesthesiol Scand 1999;43:845–9.

[27] Gilron I, Milne B, Hong M. Cyclooxygenase-2 inhibitors in postoperative pain management: current evidence and future directions. Anaesthesiology 2003; 99:1198–208.

[28] Aubier M, Murciano D, Milic-Emili J. Effects of administration of oxygen on ventilation and blood gasses in patients with chronic obstructive pulmonary disease and respiratory failure. Am Rev Respir Dis 1980;122:747–54.

[29] Hanson C, Marshall B, Frasch H, Marshall C. Causes of hypercarbia with oxygen therapy in patients with chronic obstructive pulmonary disease. Crit Care Med 1996;24:23–8.

[30] Cassivi SD, Meyers BF, Battafarano RJ, Guthrie TJ, Trulock EP, Lynch JP, et al. Thirteen-year experience in lung transplantation for emphysema. Ann Thorac Surg 2002;74:1663–9.

[31] McRae K, Keshavjee S. The future of lung transplantation. In: Slinger PD, editor. Progress in thoracic anesthesia (a Society of Cardiovascular Anesthesiologists monograph). Baltimore: Lippincott Williams & Wilkins; 2004. p. 91–119.

[32] Henzlova MJ, Padilla ML, Freilich A, Gass AL, Courtney MC, Diamond AJ, et al. Dobutamine thallium 201 perfusion imaging in candidates for lung transplantation. J Heart Lung Transplant 1995;14: 251–6.

[33] Kizer JR, Zisman DA, Blumenthal NP, Kotloff RM, Kimmel SE, Strieter RM, et al. Association between

pulmonary fibrosis and coronary artery disease. Arch Intern Med 2004;164:551–6.

[34] Snell GI, Richardson M, Griffiths A, Williams T, Esmore D. Coronary artery disease in potential lung transplant recipients >50 years old: the role of coronary intervention. Chest 1999;116:874–9.

[35] Benumof JL. Monitoring. In: Anesthesia for thoracic surgery. 2nd edition. Philadelphia: Saunders; 1995. p. 232–99.

[36] Wittnich C, Trudel J, Zidulka A, Chu-Jeng C. Misleading "pulmonary wedge pressure" after pneumonectomy: its importance in postoperative fluid therapy. Ann Thorac Surg 1986;42:192–6.

[37] Bardoczky GI, Szegedi LL, d'Hollander AA, Moures JM, de Franquen P, Yernault JC. Two-lung and one-lung ventilation in patients with chronic obstructive pulmonary disease: the effects of position and FiO2. Anesth Analg 2000;90:35–41.

[38] Sticher J, Scholz S, Boning O, Schermuly R, Schumacher C, Walmrath D, et al. Small-dose nitric oxide improves oxygenation during one-lung ventilation: an experimental study. Anesth Analg 2002;95:1557–62.

[39] Tussman G, Bohm H, Sipman F, Maisch S. Lung recruitment improves the efficiency of ventilation and gas exchange during one-lung ventilation anesthesia. Anesth Analg 2004;98:1604–9.

[40] Hohn L, Schweizer A, Morel D, Spiliopoulos A, Licker M. Circulatory failure after anesthesia induction in a patient with severe primary pulmonary hypertension. Anesthesiology 1999;91:1943–5.

[41] Ghignone M, Girling B, Prewitt R. Volume expansion versus norepinephrine in treatment of a low cardiac output complicating an acute increase in right ventricular afterload in dogs. Anesthesiology 1984;60:132–5.

[42] Michel-Cherqui M, Brusset A, Liu N, Raffin L, Schlumberger S, Ceddaha A, et al. Intraoperative transesophageal echocardiographic assessment of vascular anastomoses in lung transplantation. Chest 1997;111:1229–35.

[43] Marczin N, Royston D, Yacoub M. Pro: lung transplantation should be routinely performed with cardiopulmonary bypass. J Cardiothorac Vasc Anesth 2000; 14:739–45.

[44] McRae K. Con: lung transplantation should not be routinely performed with cardiopulmonary bypass. J Cardiothorac Vasc Anesth 2000;14:746–50.

[45] Hirt S, Haverich A, Wahlers T, Schaefers H, Alken A, Borst H. Predictive criteria for the need of extracorporeal circulation in single-lung transplantation. Ann Thorac Surg 1992;54:676–80.

[46] Triantafillou A, Pasque M, Huddleston C, Pond C, Cerza R, Forstot R, et al. Predictors, frequency, and indications for cardiopulmonary bypass during lung transplantation in adults. Ann Thorac Surg 1994;57: 1248–51.

[47] Myles P, Venema H. Avoidance of cardiopulmonary bypass during bilateral sequential lung transplantation using inhaled nitric oxide. J Cardiothorac Vasc Anesth 1995;9:571–4.

[48] Meyers BF, Patterson GA. Technical aspects of adult lung transplantation. Semin Thorac Cardiovasc Surg 1998;10:213–20.

[49] Aeba R, Griffith B, Kormos R, Armitage J, Gasior T, Fuhrman C, et al. Effect of cardiopulmonary bypass on early graft dysfunction in clinical lung transplantation. Ann Thorac Surg 1994;57:715–22.

[50] DeSanto LS. The effect of cardiopulmonary bypass and extracorporeal membrane oxygenation on early pulmonary allograft function. Int J Artif Organs 2000; 23:727–9.

[51] Ko W, Chen Y, Lee Y. Replacing cardiopulmonary bypass with extracorporeal membrane oxygenation in lung transplantation operations. Artif Organs 2001; 25:607–12.

[52] Gu Y, Haan J, Brenken U, DeBoer W, Prop J, Van Oeveren W. Clotting and fibrinolytic disturbance during lung transplantation: effect of low-dose aprotinin. J Thorac Cardiovasc Surg 1996;112:599–606.

[53] Levine S, Angel L. Primary graft failure: who is at risk? Chest 2003;124:1190–2.

[54] Christie JD, Bavaria JE, Palevsky HI, Litsky L, Blumenthal NP, Kaiser LR, et al. Primary graft failure following lung transplantation. Chest 1998;114:51–60.

[55] Fiser S, Tribble C, Long S, Kaza A, Kern J, Jones D, et al. Ischemia-reperfusion injury after lung transplantation increases risk of late bronchiolitis obliterans syndrome. Ann Thorac Surg 2002;73:1041–8.

[56] Khan SU, Salloum J, O'Donovan PB, Mascha EJ, Mehta AC, Matthay MA, et al. Acute pulmonary edema after lung transplantation: the pulmonary reimplantation response. Chest 1999;116:187–94.

[57] de Perrot M, Lui M, Waddell TK, Keshavjee S. Ischemia-reperfusion-induced lung injury. Am J Respir Crit Care Med 2003;167:490–511.

[58] Lang J, Lell W. Pro: inhaled nitric oxide should be used routinely in patients undergoing lung transplantation. J Cardiothorac Vasc Anesth 2001;15:785–9.

[59] McQuitty C. Con: inhaled nitric oxide should not be used routinely in patients undergoing lung transplantation. J Cardiothorac Vasc Anesth 2001;15:790–2.

[60] Kubes P, Suzuki M, Granger D. Nitric oxide: an endogenous modulator of leukocyte adhesion. Proc Natl Acad Sci U S A 1991;88:4651–5.

[61] Gaboury J, Woodman R, Granger D, Reinhardt P, Kubes P. Nitric oxide prevents leukocyte adherence: role of superoxide. Am J Physiol 1993;265:H862–7.

[62] Okabayashi K, Triantafillou A, Yamashita M, Aoe M, DeMeester S, Cooper J, et al. Inhaled nitric oxide improves lung allograft function after prolonged storage. J Thorac Cardiovasc Surg 1996;112:293–9.

[63] Kurose I, Kubes P, Wolf R, Anderson DC, Paulson J, Miyasaka M, et al. Inhibition of nitric oxide production: mechanisms of vascular albumin leakage. Circ Res 1993;73:164–71.

[64] Karamsetty M, Klinger J. NO: more than just a vasodilator in lung transplantation. Am J Respir Cell Mol Biol 2002;26:1–5.

[65] Frostell C, Fratacci M, Wain J, Jones R, Zapol W.

Inhaled nitric oxide: a selective pulmonary vasodilator reversing hypoxic pulmonary vasoconstriction. Circulation 1991;83:2038–47.

[66] Rossaint R, Falke K, Lopez F, Slama K, Pison U, Zapol W. Inhaled nitric oxide for the adult respiratory distress syndrome. N Engl J Med 1993;328:399–405.

[67] Pinsky D, Naka Y, Chowdhury N, Liao H, Oz M, Michler R, et al. The nitric oxide/cyclic GMP pathway in organ transplantation: critical role in lung preservation. Proc Natl Acad Sci U S A 1994;91:12086–90.

[68] Cardella JA, Keshavjee S, Bai X, Yeoh J, Granton J, Meade M, et al. Increased expression of nitric oxide synthase in human lung transplants after nitric oxide inhalation. Transplantation 2004;77:886–90.

[69] Fujino S, Nagahiro I, Triantafillou A, Boasquevisque C, Yano M, Cooper J, et al. Inhaled nitric oxide at the time of harvest improves early lung allograft function. Ann Thorac Surg 1997;63:1383–90.

[70] MacDonald P, Mundy J, Rogers P, Harrison G, Branch J, Glanville A, et al. Successful treatment of life-threatening acute reperfusion injury after lung transplantation with inhaled nitric oxide. J Thorac Cardiovasc Surg 1995;110:861–3.

[71] Date H, Triantafillou A, Trulock E, Pohl M, Cooper J, Patterson G. Inhaled nitric oxide reduces human lung allograft dysfunction. J Thorac Cardiovasc Surg 1996; 111:913–9.

[72] Adatia I, Lillihei C, Arnold J, Thompson J, Plazzo R, Fackler J, et al. Inhaled nitric oxide in the treatment of postoperative graft dysfunction after lung transplantation. Ann Thorac Surg 1994;57:1311–8.

[73] Kemming G, Merkel M, Schallerer A, Habler OP, Kleen MS, Haller M, et al. Inhaled nitric oxide (NO) for the treatment of early allograft failure after lung transplantation. Intensive Care Med 1998;24:1173–80.

[74] Thabut G, Brugiere O, Leseche G, Stern J, Fradj K, Herve P, et al. Preventive effect of inhaled nitric oxide and pentoxifylline on ischemia-reperfusion injury after lung transplantation. Transplantation 2001;71: 1295–300.

[75] Ardehali A, Laks H, Levine M, Shipner R, Ross D, Watson L, et al. A prospective trial of inhaled nitric oxide in clinical lung transplantation. Transplantation 2001;72:112–5.

[76] Meade M, Granton J, Matte-Martyn A, McRae K, Weaver B, Cripps P, et al. A randomized trial of inhaled nitric oxide to prevent ischemia-reperfusion injury after lung transplantation. Am J Respir Crit Care Med 2003;167:1483–9.

[77] Glanville A. Inhaled nitric oxide after lung transplantation: no more cosmesis? Am J Respir Crit Care Med 2003;167:1463–4.

[78] Freeman B. Free radical chemistry of nitric oxide: looking at the dark side. Chest 1994;105(3 Suppl): 79S–84S.

[79] Eppinger M, Ward P, Jones M, Bolling S, Deeb G. Disparate effects of nitric oxide on lung ischemia-reperfusion injury. Ann Thorac Surg 1995;60:1169–76.

[80] Valino F, Casals C, Guerrero R, Alvarez L, Santos M, Saenz A, et al. Inhaled nitric oxide affects endogenous surfactant in experimental lung transplantation. Transplantation 2004;77:812–8.

ELSEVIER
SAUNDERS

Thorac Surg Clin 15 (2005) 159 – 180

THORACIC
SURGERY
CLINICS

Progress in Postoperative ICU Management

Charl J. De Wet, MBChB[a], Kevin McConnell, MD[b],
Eric Jacobsohn, MBChB, MHPE, FRCPC[a,c],*

[a]Department of Anesthesiology and Division of Cardiothoracic Surgery, Washington University School of Medicine,
660 South Euclid Avenue, Campus Box 8054, St. Louis, MO 63110, USA
[b]Department of Surgery, Washington University School of Medicine, 660 South Euclid Avenue, St. Louis, MO 63110, USA
[c]Cardiothoracic Intensive Care Unit, Washington University School of Medicine, 660 South Euclid Avenue,
St. Louis, MO 63110, USA

Uncomplicated thoracic surgical patients infrequently require routine postoperative intensive care. Immediate extubation of most uncomplicated lung resections and esophageal surgery is well established, and most of these patients subsequently are cared for in high-dependency or step-down units. However, many complicated thoracic surgical patients (eg, complicated esophagectomies and lung transplantation) and patients with complications from the initial surgical procedure (eg, respiratory failure/acute respiratory distress syndrome [ARDS] after esophagectomy, postpneumonectomy pulmonary edema (PPPE), and severe sepsis) require ICU admission for early postoperative care.

The critical care of a complicated postoperative thoracic surgical patient has undergone significant developments since the 1990s. As critical care outcomes research has flourished, so has the application of evidence-based principles to critical care. The authors show many of these principles by presenting the case of a complicated, thoracic surgical patient, then explore many of these new developments in critical care.

Case presentation

A 53-year-old man with past medical history significant for gastroesophageal reflux disease, alcoholism, obesity, and non–insulin-dependent diabetes mellitus is diagnosed with stage I esophageal cancer and undergoes an Ivor-Lewis esophagectomy. He had a negative preoperative dobutamine stress echocardiogram. Preoperatively a thoracic epidural is placed at the T4-5 level. His intraoperative course is notable for an estimated blood loss of 700 mL. Intraoperatively, he is administered 500 mL of hetastarch (Hespan), 750 mL of 5% albumin, and 3 L of Ringer's lactate. Postoperatively, he was admitted to the step-down unit. To ensure good perfusion to the new anastomosis, a liberal fluid regimen was prescribed. He received an infusion of Ringer's lactate at 250 mL/h, and his mean arterial pressure at all times was maintained at greater than 70 mm Hg. He had excellent analgesia from the thoracic epidural and was aggressively mobilized on postoperative day (POD) 1.

He did well until POD 4, when he was noted to have a temperature of 39.3°C, tachypnea, intermittent confusion, and decreased urinary output. On clinical examination, weight was 110 kg, height was 172 cm, blood pressure was 90/40 mm Hg, and heart rate was 115 beats/min (sinus). Examination revealed coarse bilateral crackles and use of accessory muscles, and the chest x-ray showed bilateral diffuse pulmonary infiltrates. The ECG and troponin were negative

* Corresponding author. Department of Anesthesiology and Division of Cardiothoracic Surgery, Washington University School of Medicine, 660 South Euclid Avenue, Campus Box 8054, St. Louis, MO 63110.

E-mail address: jacobsoe@msnotes.wustl.edu (E. Jacobsohn).

for ischemia. Resuscitation was begun with 5% albumin and Ringer's lactate. He was admitted to the ICU.

In addition to ongoing goal-directed resuscitation, immediate pan-cultures were done (blood, sputum/ bronchoalveolar lavage, urine, wound), and empirical vancomycin, cefepime, metronidazole, and flucona- zole were started. He was intubated because of worsening respiratory distress and worsening oxy- genation. Initially, he was placed on an inspired fraction of oxygen (FIO_2) of 100%, and positive end- expiratory pressure was titrated to compliance and was set at 12 cm H_2O. He had a severely reduced compliance. The ventilator tidal volume was set initially at 8 mL/kg ideal body mass (700 mL), but the peak ventilator pressures were 42 cm H_2O, de- spite an inspiratory-to-expiratory ratio of 1:1. Al- though he was well sedated with propofol and was not triggering the ventilator, he was administered one dose of intermediate-acting neuromuscular blockade. There was no change in the peak airway pressure, and the tidal volume was reduced to 550 mL. The peak ventilator pressures were now in the range of 29 to 32 cm H_2O. A lung protective ventilatory strategy was continued, but the patient required 100% oxygen to maintain a saturation of 92%. The initial sedation was continued with propofol and fentanyl.

A pulmonary artery catheter (PAC) was placed, and the initial hemodynamics were consistent with distributive shock and pulmonary hypertension sec- ondary to lung injury: cardiac index, 4.7 L/min/m^2; pulmonary artery pressure, 45/26 mm Hg; pulmonary capillary wedge pressure, 12 mm Hg, pulmonary artery pressure, 40/25 mm Hg, central venous pres- sure, 5 mm Hg; calculated systemic vascular resis- tance, 400 dynes $\cdot$ cm^{-5} $\cdot$ s^{-1}. In addition to judicious ongoing crystalloid and colloid resuscitation, a nor- epinephrine infusion was started at 0.05 µg/kg/min, but the patient remained hypotensive despite escala- tion of the dose to 0.15 µg/kg/min. A vasopressin infusion was started at 0.04 IU/min, and the dose of norepinephrine was titrated down to 0.03 µg/kg/min. The patient also was started on dexamethasone, 4 mg intravenously every 6 hours, and an adrenocortico- tropic hormone (ACTH)–stimulation test was done. The initial laboratory studies were notable for an elevated glucose level, white blood cell count, mild disseminated intravascular coagulation, and slight increase in the transaminases. The hemoglobin was 7.7 g/dL.

The patient was transfused 2 U of packed red blood cells, and an insulin infusion was initiated to maintain glucose in the range of 90 to 150 mg/dL. A CT scan of the chest and abdomen did not reveal an anastomosis leak. The immediate Gram stain of the sputum revealed many leukocytes and mixed organ- isms. With the working diagnosis of pneumonia, ARDS, and severe sepsis, it was decided to start activated protein C. Despite the hemodynamics and hemoglobin being optimized, he continued to require 100% oxygen to maintain a saturation of 88%. He was started on inhaled prostacyclin as a selective pulmonary artery vasodilator for refractory hypox- emia. He had an immediate improvement; the FIO_2 was weaned to 60%, and the pulmonary artery pres- sure decreased to 35 mm Hg.

On POD 6 (after 24 hours in the ICU), the sputum and blood culture were positive for gram-positive cocci in clumps. The vancomycin was continued, oxacillin was added, and all other antibiotics were discontinued. Twenty-four hours later, the cultures were finalized, revealing oxacillin-sensitive *Staphy- lococcus aureus;* vancomycin was discontinued. Over the next 48 hours, the vasopressor requirement dimin- ished, and the norepinephrine was tapered off. The PAC was removed 24 hours after being placed. The ACTH-stimulation test showed appropriate adrenal response, and the dexamethasone was discontinued. The gram-positive coverage was continued for a total of 8 days.

The oxygenation improved steadily, and the inhaled prostacyclin was tapered over 48 hours. The sedation was titrated to the Ramsey sedation scale, and daily interruptions in sedation were made. Early enteral nutrition was started on POD 5 through the small bowel feeding tube that had been placed intra- operatively. The pulmonary mechanics gradually improved, and by POD 7, all sedative infusions were discontinued. Weaning from mechanical ventilation progressed well according to an established proto- col and with frequent intensivist reassessment. The patient was extubated 8 days after admission to the ICU.

New developments in the management of sepsis

Sepsis remains the second most common cause of mortality in patients treated in ICUs. Delays in the diagnosis of sepsis are common, particularly in some patient populations that do not present with the classic findings of sepsis. Tachypnea and confusion are often early signs of sepsis. Early diagnosis, source control, and treatment form the cornerstones of current management. There have been many impor- tant developments in the treatment of sepsis since the late 1990s, and these are addressed in a publication endorsed by several international critical care and other professional societies [1].

Antibiotic therapy and source control

Delays in diagnosis and delays in instituting appropriate, broad-spectrum antimicrobial coverage increase mortality [2]. Gram-positive bacteria and fungal organisms now are recognized as increasingly common causes of sepsis [3]. Obvious sources of infection should be drained or removed as soon as possible, including vascular access catheters, such as tunneled or surgically implanted catheters. Blood cultures should be obtained, preferably before administering appropriate antibiotic coverage. Two or more blood cultures are recommended and should be obtained peripherally. Cultures from other body fluids should be obtained based on the clinical scenario. The sensitivity and benefits of imaging studies to search for a source of the infection should be weighed against the risk of transporting a hemodynamically unstable patient and potential interruption of other therapies. Jimenez and Marshall [4] showed that hospital mortality from sepsis with inadequate initial choice of antibiotics is double that when the initial antibiotic choice is adequate. Appropriate doses of broad-spectrum antibiotics, including loading doses when appropriate, should be administered within 60 minutes of the diagnosis of sepsis [1]. The choice of antibiotics is dictated by the clinical scenario and unit-specific or hospital-specific antibiograms. Although controversial, some experts still suggest the use of two antibiotics for *Pseudomonas*. Neutropenic patients should receive broad-spectrum antibiotics for the entire course of neutropenia.

The duration of antibiotic coverage is controversial and should be guided by clinical response and culture results. The initial broad-spectrum choice should be reviewed at least every 48 hours. All efforts should be made to restrict the antibiotic spectrum as soon as possible to limit the appearance of drug-resistant organisms (resistant gram-negative organisms, vancomycin-resistant enterococcus) and other antibiotic-associated complications (fungal superinfections and *Clostridium difficile* colitis). Chastre et al [5] showed that in patients with microbiologically proven ventilator-associated pneumonia who had received appropriate initial empirical therapy (with the possible exception of patients with nonfermenting gram-negative bacillus infections), there was comparable effectiveness with 8 days versus 15 days of antibiotic treatment. The 8-day group had less antibiotic use, and in patients who developed recurrent infections,

multiresistant pathogens emerged less frequently in patients who had received 8 days of antibiotics.

Early goal-directed therapy and use of vasopressors

Resuscitation should begin as soon as the syndrome of sepsis is recognized. A study by Rivers et al [6] showed that early goal-directed therapy (EGDT) in sepsis that strives to detect patients at high risk for hemodynamic compromise using variables other than traditional vital signs improves the likelihood of survival (Fig. 1). EGDT strives to normalize oxygen delivery and to minimize oxygen consumption in patients with severe sepsis and septic shock. Rivers et al [6] used infusions of fluids and transfusions of red blood cells to increase oxygen delivery. Resuscitation end points chosen for assessment of the adequacy of oxygen delivery were the normalization of mixed venous oxygen saturation, lactate, base deficit, and pH. Patients in the group that received EGDT received more fluid, inotropic support, and blood transfusions *during the first 6 hours* based on hemodynamic data that also included central venous oxygen saturation and lactate measurements than did control patients, who received standard resuscitation therapy based on "traditional" signs of adequate perfusion, such as urine output, blood pressure, and central venous pressure. During the interval from 7 to 72 hours, patients in the group receiving EGDT had a higher central venous oxygen concentration, a lower mean lactate concentration, a lower mean base deficit, and a higher mean pH than the control group. Mortality was 30.5% in the group receiving EGDT compared with 46.5% in the control group ($P = .009$).

Based on this work, Dellinger [7] proposed a decision tree to initiate monitoring based on traditional end points, such as blood pressure, and subsequent titration based on central venous pressures and pulmonary artery pressures for management decisions in septic shock. This approach has been criticized, however, by the authors of EGDT, who point out that the key difference between the two groups was in the timing and physiologic titration of therapy, which was based on central venous oxygen saturation and not on the global management of these patients: Over the first 6 hours, the EGDT group received more inotropic support; however, over the total 72-hour period, the mean difference in total red blood cell transfusion was only 72 mL, the total fluid given essentially equalized, and there was no difference in dobutamine use. These authors point out that the EGDT group required significantly less vasopressors, pulmonary artery catheterization, and mechanical ventilation over the total 72 hours. In a

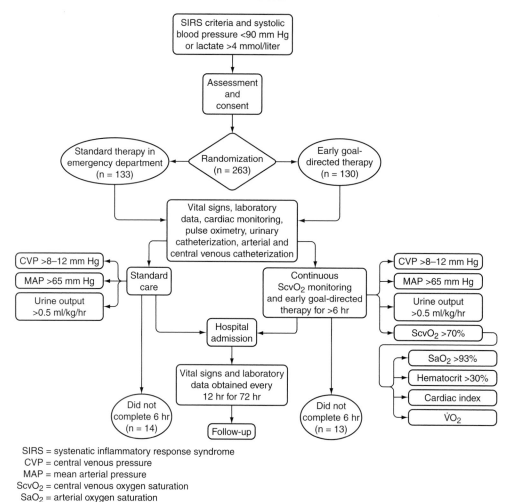

Fig. 1. Decision tree for early goal-directed therapy for resuscitation in septic shock. CVP, central venous pressure; MAP, mean arterial pressure; SaO2, arterial oxygen saturation; ScvO2, central venous oxygen saturation; SIRS, systemic inflammatory response syndrome. (*From* Rivers E, Nguyen B, Havstad S, et al. Early goal-directed therapy in the treatment of severe sepsis and septic shock. N Engl J Med 2001;345:1368–77; with permission.)

subset analysis, they also found that in patients with a lactate of greater than 4 mmol/L despite a mean arterial pressure of greater than 110 mmHg, the control group had a 40% higher mortality [8]. The study was criticized, however, for the fact that almost 10% of patients did not receive antibiotics within 6 hours of the initial diagnosis of sepsis [9].

The choice of vasoactive agents is controversial. There has been renewed interest regarding the use of vasopressin in vasodilated shock states [10–12]. Many septic patients have been shown to have relative vasopressor deficiency, and *replacement* doses of vasopressin have been shown to reduce significantly the requirement for catecholamine support. Although

high endogenous levels of vasopressin in nonshock states do not produce hypertension, in shock states vasopressin stimulation of vascular V1 receptors seems to be an important mechanism of blood pressure augmentation. Literature supports vasopressin as an option to increase blood pressure in septic shock and to taper more traditional vasopressors (norepinephrine) already in place. Septic shock–associated exhaustion of neurohypophyseal stores resulting from intense and prolonged stimulation and impairment of baroreflex-mediated stimulation of vasopressin release may lead to inappropriately low levels of serum vasopressin. Low doses of vasopressin, targeted to achieve serum vasopressin levels similar to those present in cardiogenic shock, have been shown to produce a significant increase in mean arterial pressure in septic shock, often leading to the discontinuation of traditional vasopressors.

The effect of this strategy on clinical outcome is unknown because no randomized, prospective clinical outcome trials exist. If vasopressin is used, it seems most appropriate in patients requiring moderate-to-high-dose vasopressors, especially when blood pressure remains inadequate. Dosing should be limited to 0.01 to 0.04 U/min because higher doses put the patient at a greater risk for splanchnic and coronary artery ischemia and a decrease in cardiac output. Any vasopressor support, especially vasopressin therapy, has to be started judiciously, however, ideally with some assessment of cardiac output. Vasopressin has no inotropic effects; there is a potential for cardiac output to decrease. Escalating doses of vasopressin can have serious deleterious effects in the presence of low or inadequately increased cardiac output. It is important to recognize patients who do not have an appropriate cardiac output response in sepsis to establish the cause of the inappropriate cardiac output response and to start dobutamine therapy when appropriate. The aim of dobutamine is not to increase cardiac output to some *predefined, elevated* level because two large prospective trials failed to show benefit from increasing oxygen delivery to supranormal levels [13,14]. Rather, dobutamine should be titrated to normalize cardiac output and ensure adequacy of peripheral perfusion as evidenced by lack of acidosis. There is currently no evidence-based rationale to choose colloids over crystalloids for purposes of resuscitation. Fluid management in the ICU is discussed more fully later.

Activated protein C

The current understanding of the pathophysiology of sepsis encompasses a triad of abnormal coagulation, inflammation, and reduced fibrinolysis, leading to microvascular thrombosis and end-organ dysfunction [15]. Extreme clinical manifestations of disseminated intravascular coagulation, such as purpura fulminans or digital ischemia, have long been identified as a poor prognostic sign of septic shock. Subclinical manifestations of disseminated intravascular coagulation are present, however, in essentially all patients with septic shock (some combination of increased D dimers, decreased protein C, thrombocytopenia, and increased prothrombin time), and consumptive coagulopathy is likely an important facet of pathophysiology in septic shock. The activation of protein C from its inactive form is an important

mechanism for modulating sepsis-induced consumptive coagulopathy and the resultant microvascular occlusion and end-organ dysfunction (Fig. 2) [16].

Recombinant human activated protein C is an anticoagulant that has anti-inflammatory effects and promotes fibrinolysis. It has proved effective in the treatment of sepsis [17]. In patients with *severe* sepsis (PROWESS trial), the administration of activated protein C resulted in a 19.4% reduction in the relative risk of death and an absolute risk reduction of 6.1% [17]. Activated protein C inactivates factors Va and VIIIa, preventing the generation of thrombin. The efficacy of an anticoagulant agent in patients with sepsis has been attributed to feedback between the coagulation system and the inflammatory cascade. Inhibition of thrombin generation by activated protein C decreases inflammation by inhibiting platelet activation, neutrophil recruitment, and mast-cell degranulation. Activated protein C has direct anti-inflammatory properties, including blocking of the production of cytokines by monocytes and blocking cell adhesion. Activated protein C also has been shown to modulate the abnormal fibrinolytic response during severe sepsis. Although the role of activated protein C seems to be established in severe sepsis, there is controversy about its potential role and efficacy in less severe forms of sepsis. As a result of the less severe sepsis subgroup analysis in the PROWESS trial, the US Food and Drug Administration required a phase IIIB study to assess the use of the drug in less severe sepsis [18]. There was a planned enrollment of 11,000 patients, making this the largest sepsis drug study ever performed. At the first interim analysis and after enrolling only 25% of the planned patients, the trial was discontinued by the company on the basis of futility (personal communication to investigators, 2004). A concerning issue that remains is why activated protein C was successful, whereas two other anticoagulants—antithrombin III and tissue factor pathway inhibitor—failed as treatments of sepsis in large, well-designed studies. A possible explanation for the failure of these two anticoagulant agents is that they work at different sites in the coagulation cascade. Also, activated protein C has antiapoptotic actions that may contribute to its efficacy.

A major risk associated with activated protein C is hemorrhage [17,19,20]; 3.5% of patients had serious bleeding (intracranial hemorrhage, a life-threatening bleeding episode, or a requirement for ≥ 3 U of blood) compared with 2% of patients who received placebo ($P < .06$). With open-label use of activated protein C after the trial, 13 of 520 patients (2.5%) had intracranial hemorrhage. Caution is advised in the use

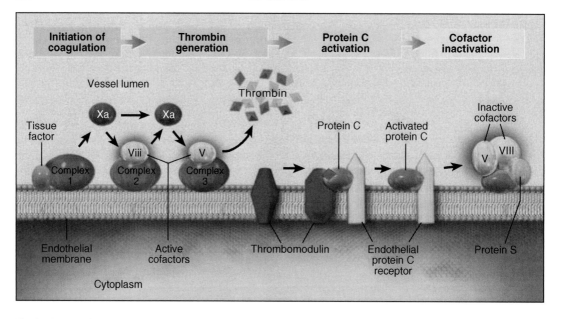

Fig. 2. The normal mechanism of activating protein C and the abnormalities induced by endothelial dysfunction in sepsis. During sepsis, there is endothelial damage, leading to thrombomodulin and endothelial protein C receptor detaching. The reduced endothelial thrombomodulin and endothelial protein C receptor prevent protein C from becoming activated. (*From* Faust SN, Levin M, Harrison OB, et al. Dysfunction of endothelial protein C activation in severe meningococcal sepsis. N Engl J Med 2001;345:408–16; with permission.)

of activated protein C in patients with an international normalized ratio greater than 3 or a platelet count of less than 30,000/mm^3. Currently, activated protein C is approved only for use in patients with sepsis who have severe organ compromise and the highest likelihood of death. Use of activated protein C is restricted in many hospitals to more seriously ill patients who meet the criteria for sepsis specified by the Acute Physiology and Chronic Health Evaluation (APACHE II) scoring system (APACHE Score >25).

Steroids

Administration of high doses of corticosteroids does not improve survival in patients with sepsis. It may worsen outcomes by increasing the frequency of secondary infections. In the late 1990s, several single-center studies of septic shock using stress (low) doses of steroids showed promising results [21]. In 2000, a prospective observational study used the response to a high-dose ACTH stimulation test to characterize the status of patients in septic shock [22]. The highest value of the two post-ACTH stimulation cortisols was compared with the baseline level and suggested that the inability to increase cortisol after the ACTH stimulation test was more predictive of a

poor outcome than the basal level itself. This group of patients was called "nonresponders" and was identified as having "relative adrenal insufficiency." Based on these findings, a multicenter, prospective, randomized, blinded study of stress-dose steroid therapy targeting this group of nonresponders was performed [23]. Patients with septic shock were randomized to receive either 50 mg of intravenous hydrocortisone every 6 hours plus 50 μg by mouth of the mineralocorticoid fludrocortisone every day or placebo. Treatment continued for 7 days. The primary analysis group was nonresponders to ATCH, defined as the failure to increase serum cortisol levels by 10 μg/dL or greater after ACTH stimulation. Use of stress-dose (low-dose) steroids in nonresponders was associated with decreased mortality and decreased vasopressor usage. There was no benefit of steroids in responders. There was *no* statistically significant difference in the 28-day mortality, but statistical significance was reached when logistic regression adjustment was done. Another worrisome aspect was the fact that patients who did not have adrenal insufficiency and who received corticosteroids had a slight, albeit not statistically significant, trend toward increased mortality.

A second issue that has been raised is the high mortality rate in the population of patients—63% in the placebo group. Although validation of this study is needed (and is being done in Europe), in the interim, it is reasonable to consider stress-dose steroids in patients who are requiring *high doses* of vasopressor therapy. In those patients, a reasonable approach would be to give dexamethasone, 4 mg intravenously every 6 hours (does not interfere with cortisol assay), until the high-dose ACTH stimulation test can be performed. Hydrocortisone and fludro-cortisone would be started and continued or discontinued based on the results of the ACTH stimulation test. If the ACTH stimulation test is not available, empirical stress-dose steroids should be considered. Some investigators question the choice of the 250-μg ACTH stimulation test for the evaluation of adrenal reserve in critically ill patients and judge it to be supraphysiologic and potentially overestimating of adrenal reserve. They recommend a 1- to 2-μg ACTH dose.

The proposed explanation for the physiologic response to corticosteroids (despite normal or elevated plasma cortisol levels) is desensitization of corticosteroid responsiveness with down-regulation of adrenergic receptors. Catecholamines increase arterial pressure through effects on adrenergic receptors of the vasculature; corticosteroids increase the expression of adrenergic receptors. Testing involving stimulation by adrenocorticotropic hormones may not be useful in identifying patients with relative adrenal insufficiency. Such patients may have markedly elevated baseline plasma cortisol levels and a blunted response to stimulation by ACTH.

Another more recent publication examining the role of free cortisol levels in critically ill patients further complicates the issue of stress-dose steroids in critically ill patients. Because more than 90% of circulating cortisol is protein bound, changes in the binding proteins can alter measured serum total cortisol concentrations without influencing free concentrations. The 10% free cortisol is the bioactive component. Of the 90% protein-bound cortisol, 20% is loosely bound to albumin, and 70% is tightly bound to cortisol-binding globulin. The binding to cortisol-binding globulin is nearly saturated at plasma cortisol levels in the range of 15 to 18 μg/dL. With stress and hypoalbuminemia, the maximal total cortisol measurement decreases to less than that measured in persons with a normal albumin concentration and, often below the traditional cutoff for the ACTH-stimulation test, even though the level of free, bioactive cortisol is appropriate for the clinical situation (Fig. 3) [24].

Hamrahian et al [25] investigated the effect of decreased amounts of cortisol-binding proteins on

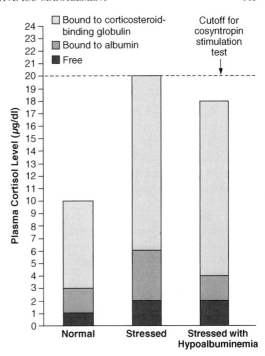

Fig. 3. Total and free-cortisol level in normal people, people with stress, and people with stress and hypoalbuminemia. (*From* Loriaux L. Glucocorticoid therapy in the intensive care unit. N Engl J Med 2004;350:1601–2; with permission.)

total and free cortisol concentrations during critical illness. They compared baseline serum total cortisol, ACTH-stimulated serum total cortisol, aldosterone, and free cortisol concentrations in critically ill patients and healthy volunteers. They found that the baseline and ACTH-stimulated total cortisol concentrations were lower in the patients with hypoproteinemia than in patients with near-normal serum albumin concentrations, but that baseline serum free cortisol concentrations were similar. They were several times higher, however, than the values in healthy volunteers. ACTH-stimulated total cortisol concentrations were subnormal in several patients, all of whom had hypoproteinemia. In all the critically ill patients, including patients who had hypoproteinemia, the baseline ACTH-stimulated serum free cortisol concentrations were high-normal or elevated. In this study, nearly 40% of critically ill patients with hypoproteinemia had subnormal total cortisol levels, even though their adrenal function was normal. They concluded that glucocorticoid secretion increases during critical illness, but that the increase is not discernible when only total cortisol concentration is measured. Free cortisol levels currently are not widely available, however. Until further studies of free cortisol in critically ill patients are done, the risks and benefits of cortisol therapy based on total cortisol levels has to be individualized, but critically evaluated in light of these important new findings.

New developments in ICU fluid therapy

Crystalloid versus colloid debate

Appropriate fluid management is important in critically ill patients and remains a controversial field. The Cochrane Injuries Group meta-analysis of randomized control trials examined the effect of albumin on mortality compared with crystalloid, no albumin, or low-dose albumin and found that the mortality was higher with albumin therapy [26]. In an effort to address the albumin controversy, a large Australian/ New Zealand randomized controlled trial (SAFE study) enrolled patients who required ICU admission to receive either albumin or normal saline [27]. The outcomes at 28 days were similar, including death, number of organ system failures, time in ICU/ hospital, time on mechanical ventilation, and days of dialysis. In the trauma subgroup, albumin was associated with increased morbidity, and in the severe sepsis subgroup, albumin was associated with a trend toward reduced mortality. Another interesting finding was that the commonly accepted rule of 3:1 crystalloid:colloid resuscitation did not hold up and that the actual ratio was 1.4:1.

Metabolic effects of fluid therapy

The choice of resuscitation fluid in the ICU has important metabolic consequences. Fluids that have high chloride concentrations cause hyperchloremic, non–anion gap metabolic acidosis. Although it historically has been thought to be benign, there is now increasing evidence that it impairs cellular mechanisms; decreases renal blood flow, gastric motility, and perfusion; and increases pulmonary artery pressure [28]. The greatest danger may be the reaction of clinicians, however, who may not recognize it or confuse it with other dangerous conditions (eg, anion gap acidosis and respiratory acidosis). In patients with compromised respiratory function and in patients receiving narcotics, both common situations after thoracic surgery, there is an impaired ability for compensatory hyperventilation, and severe acidemia may ensue.

Immunologic effects of fluid therapy

Fluid management also may have an effect on immune function [29]. Isotonic crystalloids cause immune activation, the effect being greatest with lactated Ringer's solution. Of the colloids studied, dextran and hetastarch cause the most pronounced neutrophil activation and cellular injury [30,31]. Efforts are being made to develop resuscitation fluids that eliminate lactate and substitute pyruvate as the base. Activation of the immune system has not been shown with fresh-frozen plasma and albumin.

Coagulation and fluid therapy

Fluid choice in the ICU also can affect the coagulation system. Nonprotein colloids are associated with impaired hemostasis, platelet dysfunction, and excessive bleeding [32–34]. Of the colloids, albumin has minimal effects on coagulation, although procoagulatory and anticoagulatory effects (eg, inhibiting platelet aggregation, enhancing the inhibition of factor Xa by antithrombin III) have been described. Dextrans affect hemostasis by decreasing VIIIR:Ag and VIIIR:RCo levels, leading to reduced binding to platelet membrane receptor proteins glycoprotein Ib and glycoprotein IIb/IIIa and decreased platelet adhesion. Gelatin-based plasma expanders (Gelofusine) have minimal negative effect on coagulation, although gelatin has been shown to impair thrombin generation significantly in healthy volunteers [35]. Changes in coagulation have been reported most often with hydroxyethyl starches (HES); the magnitude of the effect varies depending on the physiochemical properties of the HES preparation being used. These properties include concentration, degree of substitution, mean molecular weight, and ratio of hydroxyethylation [36]. Several HES preparations are available in Europe. In the United States, only the first-generation high-molecular-weight HES (Hetastarch 6%; 450/0.7) is approved. In Canada, only medium-molecular-weight HES (Pentastarch; HES 270/0.5) is available. HES has been associated with increased bleeding complications in cardiac surgery, but the effect depends on the type of HES [37]. The high-molecular-weight HES diminishes factors VIIIR:Ag and VIIIR:RCo more than a low-molecular-weight HES. Platelet aggregation abnormalities occur with high-molecular-weight HES, and fibrinolysis is accelerated.

All artificial colloids in large volumes potentially can cause increased bleeding, especially in patients with mild von Willebrand's disease. In contrast, crystalloids have been shown in some studies to induce a hypercoagulable state. It may increase the risk of deep venous thrombosis [38]; the postulated mechanism is hemodilution of antithrombin III [39].

Third space and edema

The volume of fluids used in ICU patients also has come under increasing scrutiny. In the 1960s, it was postulated that large volumes of fluid were required after some surgeries because of "third space" losses [40]. Giving large volumes of fluid is still common practice after esophageal surgery. Because of difficulties in measuring the fluid compartments, it is difficult to define accurately the amount of fluid needed. There is accumulating evidence, however, that the magnitude of extracellular fluid shifts may not be as large as previously thought. Studies on stress hormones show they generally cause fluid retention. Multiple abnormalities are induced in the normal Starling equation after major surgery, including changes in oncotic pressures and tissue capillary permeability. Large amounts of crystalloid cause deleterious tissue oxygenation and poor wound healing [41]. In one trial, patients undergoing colon surgery were randomized to receive standard therapy (which included replacing third space fluids) or restricted fluids (in which third space fluids were not replaced) [42]. Although there were some methodologic issues of concern, the restricted group had significantly fewer complications and had a trend toward fewer deaths. The development of postoperative intestinal edema and ileus has been associated with excessive crystalloid therapy and hypoalbuminemia, and the development of abdominal compartment syndrome may be more likely with massive crystalloid fluid resuscitation.

Pulmonary function, acute respiratory distress syndrome, and fluid therapy

Pulmonary function

Another significant problem of excess fluid therapy is pulmonary edema. A large fluid bolus has been shown to decrease pulmonary function acutely even in healthy patients, which can be corrected with furosemide [43,44]. Arieff [45] studied the incidence and morbidity of postoperative pulmonary edema in the United States and reported on 13 patients who died as a result of postoperative pulmonary edema. The autopsies showed no pathology other than pulmonary edema, and all patients had received high-volume fluid replacement. Of 8195 patients undergoing major operations, 7.6% developed pulmonary edema with a mortality of 11.9%.

Adult respiratory distress syndrome

There may be special consideration for choice of fluids in ARDS [46,47]. Hypoproteinemia is common in ARDS. Given Starling's law, it would seem logical to manipulate the forces to try to reverse fluid flux in the lungs. Mangialardi et al [48] found an independent association between hypoproteinemia and ARDS development and outcome, suggesting that colloid oncotic pressure may play a pathophysiologic role. In a randomized control trial comparing albumin and furosemide with standard therapy in patients with ARDS, diuresis and weight loss were better, as were the improvements in the PaO_2/FIO_2 ratio [49]. In the SAFE study, the subgroup with ARDS who received albumin did not do better, however [27].

Sepsis and the choice of fluids

The fluid choice in sepsis also is controversial, and prospective studies of choice of fluid resuscitation in septic shock are lacking. Meta-analysis of clinical studies comparing crystalloid and colloids in general and surgical patients indicates no clinical outcome difference; these studies would seem to be generalizable to septic patients [50,51]. The volume required is much larger for crystalloids; more fluid causes more edema, which may be deleterious for wound healing, gastrointestinal function, and tissue oxygen delivery. The SAFE study subgroup analysis suggested that albumin might be beneficial in septic patients. Albumin may have beneficial effects other than its volume effects, including its oncotic effects, transport functions, and free radical scavenging effects. In septic patients, resuscitation with HES and gelatin improves hemodynamics without increasing lung water or worsening oxygenation [52]. In a study of resuscitation in patients with septic shock, early goal-directed resuscitation resulted in a large mortality reduction; all patients in the study were resuscitated with crystalloids [6].

Blood transfusion strategies in the ICU

Minimal acceptable hemoglobin

Red blood cell transfusions are administered to increase oxygen carrying capacity, but what constitutes an acceptable trigger hemoglobin level is uncertain. Healthy animals can tolerate hemoglobin levels of 3 to 5 g/dL, but only levels of 7 to 10 g/dL in the presence of coronary stenosis before ischemia ensues. This situation is less well established in humans. Healthy volunteers undergoing isovolemic hemodilution develop ischemia at a hemoglobin level of 5 g/dL. There are reports, however, of humans tolerating hemoglobin levels of 4.5 g/dL. In Jehovah's Witness patients, healthy adults have been shown to survive without transfusion to hemoglobin of 5 g/dL [53]. Older patients with comorbidities are thought to tolerate anemia less well. Two retrospective studies, one in the perioperative period and one in critically ill patients, showed that severe anemia was associated with increased mortality in patients with cardiac disease [54,55]. In assessing transfusion in patients with cardiac disease, Hebert et al [55] showed that patients with cardiovascular and respiratory disease may have increased mortality when hemoglobin levels were less than 9.5 g/dL and that transfusion may result in significantly lower mortality. Similarly, in patients with acute myocardial infarction, transfusion is associated with a lower short-term mortality rate if the hematocrit on admission is 30% or less and may be effective in patients with hematocrit of 33%; mortality is increased, however, with hematocrit greater than 36% [56]. Elderly patients with hip fractures and comorbidities tolerated a hemoglobin of 8 g/dL [57]. In a European ICU study, the mean pretransfusion hemoglobin was 8.4 ± 1.3 g/dL, and transfusion was associated with a 33% increased risk of death [58].

Transfusion and outcomes

The CRIT study evaluated transfusion practice in 284 ICUs [59]. The investigators found that 44% of ICU patients still received blood and that transfusion practice had changed little during the last 10 years. The mean pretransfusion hemoglobin was 8.5 ± 1.5 g/dL. Only 30% of patients had a transfusion trigger of less than 8 g/dL, and in only 7.5% was the trigger less than 7g/dL. Several large cohort studies in England [60], Europe [58], and Australia [61] have shown similar transfusion triggers. These findings are surprising, considering the results of the TRICC trial [62] This randomized control trial assigned patients to either a liberal (hemoglobin 10–12 g/dL) or restrictive (hemoglobin 7–9 g/dL) transfusion strategy. The restrictive group received 54% less blood and had a lower in-hospital mortality. In the less severely ill patients and in patients younger than age 55, the restrictive group was half as likely to die within 30 days. In a follow-up study of patients in the TRICC trial with cardiorespiratory disease, overall mortality rates were shown to be similar in restrictive and liberal transfusion strategies, and the changes in multiple organ dysfunction scores were significantly less in the restrictive group [63]. In the subgroup of patients with severe ischemic heart disease, however, the restrictive group had a lower (but nonsignificant) absolute survival rate. The investigators concluded that a restrictive strategy is safe in most critically ill patients with cardiovascular disease except for patients with acute myocardial infarction or unstable angina. In patients requiring mechanical ventilation, hemoglobin levels did not affect duration of ventilation, although when adjusting for comorbidities, transfusion was associated with increased duration of mechanical ventilation and increased incidence of pulmonary edema and ARDS.

Why is liberal transfusion not associated with improved outcomes? Either anemia has beneficial effects, or transfusion has adverse effects. The adverse effects of transfusion include infections (including known and yet undiscovered agents), hemolytic reactions, contamination, allergic reactions, anaphylaxis, transfusion-related acute lung injury, fluid-overload pulmonary edema, and immune modulation. These complications all increase morbidity and mortality. The issue of transfusion-associated immune modulation has gained increasing attention. It is thought that transfused allogeneic leukocytes trigger an immune response, leading to an increased risk of infection, earlier recurrence of malignancy, and increased mortality. A significant association between the number of red blood cells transfused and the risk of nosocomial infections has been reported [64]. A study showed that the adoption of a universal leukocyte reduction pathway decreased hospital mortality [65]. Nosocomial infections did not decrease, but the frequency of posttransfusion fevers decreased significantly, as did antibiotic use. Other studies have not shown similar benefits, but many were limited by methodologic issues [66]. Universal leukocyte reduction is performed in Canada and many European countries, but remains voluntary in the United States. The only arguments against it are cost and the loss of 4% to 19% of red blood cells. Given that society has demanded policies that possibly increase blood safety, universal leukocyte reduction should become standard [67].

Blood storage

Another controversial area is the transfusion of old blood. Blood "storage lesion" refers to the depletion of 2,3-diphosphoglyceric acid and adenosine trisphosphate, with the subsequent changes to the cell membrane that reduce deformability. Oxygen delivery to tissues may be impaired by reduction of capillary flow and oxygen unloading from hemoglobin. One study supporting this view is an oxygen kinetics study that found a correlation between the transfusion of red blood cells stored for more than 15 days and a deterioration in gastric intramucosal pH [68]. In the CRIT study, the mean age of blood was 21 days, and in a European study, the mean age was 16 days. In the CRIT study, there was a trend toward worse clinical outcomes in patients who received relatively old blood. In another study, the transfusion of stored, leukocyte-depleted red blood cells to anemic, critically ill patients had no adverse effects, however, on gastric tonometry or global indices of tissue oxygen delivery [69].

Postoperative arrhythmias

Atrial arrhythmias are a common problem after thoracic surgery despite pharmacologic prophylaxis. The incidence of atrial tachyarrhythmias ranges from 10% to 30% after thoracic surgery [70], with atrial fibrillation (AF) being the most common arrhythmia. An analysis of more than 2500 patients undergoing noncardiac thoracic surgery over a 5-year period revealed a 12.3% incidence of AF [71], which is consistent with previous reports in this patient population [70]. Risk factors as described in this large study are listed in Table 1. Currently there are no consensus guidelines for the primary prevention of AF that are *specific* to thoracic or cardiac surgical patients. Digoxin, despite widespread use, has not been proved to reduce the incidence of postoperative AF and may be proarrhythmic [72]. Prophylactic *oral*

Table 1
Risk factors for atrial fibrillation after thoracic surgery

Significant variables	Relative risk (95% confidence interval)
Pneumonectomy	8.91 (4.59–17.28)
Bilobectomy	7.16 (3.02–16.96)
Age >70	5.30 (3.28–8.59)
Age 60–69	4.49 (2.79–7.22)
Lobectomy	3.89 (2.19–6.91)
Esophagectomy	2.95 (1.55–5.62)
History of CHF	2.51 (1.06–6.24)
Resection of mediastinal tumor or thymectomy	2.36 (0.95–5.88)
History of arrhythmias	1.92 (1.22–3.02)
Male sex	1.72 (1.29–2.28)
Age 50–59	1.70 (1.01–2.88)
History of peripheral vascular disease	1.65 (0.93–2.92)
Intraoperative transfusion	1.39 (0.98–1.98)

Data from Vaporciyan AA, Correa AM, Rice DC, et al. Risk factors associated with atrial fibrillation after noncardiac thoracic surgery: analysis of 2588 patients. J Thorac Cardiovasc Surg 2004;127:779–86.

amiodarone when given *before* cardiac surgery has been shown to be cost-effective and safe [73] and might be a reasonable preventive strategy in thoracic or other noncardiac surgical patients. The routine use of postoperative *intravenous* amiodarone may not be justified because of high cost and associated toxicities, including its proarrhythmic effects and potential for pulmonary toxicity. It may be cost-effective in selected patient groups only when there is a high predicted incidence of postoperative AF, such as in combined coronary artery surgery and valvular surgery with a predicted incidence of AF of greater than 30% [74].

Consensus practice guidelines for the management of new-onset or established AF, from the American College of Cardiology, American Heart Association, and European Society of Cardiology, recommend the use of β-blockers to treat AF, unless contraindicated [75]. Consideration for amiodarone and sotalol is given; however, the evidence for the recommendation is supported by only a few randomized trials with conflicting evidence or divergence of opinion about the usefulness or efficacy of the treatment among the task force members. More recent evidence supports the concept of *heart rate* control in AF, rather than *rhythm* control [75]. Immediate electrical cardioversion still is indicated whenever hemodynamic instability is present.

Left atrial appendage thrombus should be excluded with transesophageal echocardiography before *elective* cardioversion is used. Anticoagulation is recommended, however, for 3 to 4 weeks before and after cardioversion for patients with AF of unknown duration or with AF for more than 48 hours [75]. There is no solid clinical evidence that cardioversion followed by prolonged maintenance of sinus rhythm effectively reduces thromboembolism in AF patients. It is unclear at present whether efforts to restore and maintain sinus rhythm are justified for the specific purpose of preventing stroke. Recovery of mechanical function may be delayed for several weeks. This delay could explain why some patients with no demonstrable left atrial thrombus on transesophageal echocardiography before cardioversion subsequently experience thromboembolic events. Presumably, thrombus forms during the period of stunning and is expelled after the return of mechanical function [75].

Ventricular arrhythmias are much less common than atrial arrhythmias after thoracic surgery. Prophylactic suppression of nonsustained ventricular arrhythmias after cardiac surgery with lidocaine has not been shown to improve outcome. A detailed discussion of ventricular arrhythmias is beyond the scope of this section.

Strategies for management of respiratory failure after thoracic surgery

Lung-protective ventilation strategies: case for lower tidal volume ventilation

Acute lung injury and ARDS are common complications of sepsis and carry a mortality rate of almost 50% [76]. The use of lung-protective ventilatory strategies that use lower tidal volumes and reduced airway pressures has been shown to reduce morbidity and mortality.

Several large multicenter trials have been conducted to evaluate the effect of limiting ventilatory pressures by limiting tidal volumes [77–80]. There has not been consistent benefit shown in the studies, and this has been postulated to be due to the differences in airway pressures between the studies [80]. In the largest trial, the ARDS Network enrolled patients with acute lung injury in a multicenter, randomized trial. The trial compared traditional ventilation treatment, initial tidal volume of 12 mL/ kg predicted body weight and a plateau pressure (measured after a 0.5-sec pause at the end of inspiration) of 50 cm H_2O or less, with ventilation with a lower tidal volume, an initial tidal volume of 6 mL/kg, and a plateau pressure of 30 cm H_2O or less. The trial was stopped after the enrollment of 861 patients because mortality was lower in the group treated with lower tidal volumes than in the group treated with traditional tidal volumes (31% versus 39.8%; $P = .007$), and the number of days without ventilator use during the first 28 days after randomization was greater in this group [81]. Some controversy has surrounded this study, including a contention that 12 mL/kg could not be construed as "standard" therapy in view of what was known about volume and barotrauma at the time that the trial was conducted. Other elements were part of the protective ventilator strategy, such as permissive hypercapnia, variable levels of positive end-expiratory pressure, and low plateau airway pressures. Permissive hypercapnia as part of a lung-protective strategy has been shown to be safe in small, nonrandomized series [82,83].

A Cochrane collaborative systematic review of the literature concluded that the comparison between small and conventional tidal volume ventilation was not significantly different if a plateau pressure 31 cm H_2O or less was used in the control group. Mortality at day 28 was significantly reduced by lung-protective ventilation, whereas beneficial effect on long-term mortality was uncertain [84]. The impact from the possible adverse effects of smaller tidal volume

ventilation—acidosis and hypercapnia—on the development of organ failure and outcome is unclear. In a meta-analysis of low tidal volumes and outcome in ARDS, Eichacker et al [85] showed that the two trials showing benefit had an odds ratio of survival varying from 1.57 to 3.97 (confidence interval 1.28–7.7), whereas the odds ratio for surviving from the three nonbeneficial trials varied from 0.7 to 0.85 (confidence interval 0.48–1.28).

Prone ventilation

The role of the prone position in treating refractory hypoxemia is controversial. Patients improve their oxygenation in the prone position [86–88]; however, the prone position is labor intensive and can have serious complications, including loss of endotracheal tube and venous catheters, hemodynamic consequences from incorrect position, and pressure necrosis. In the study by Gattinoni et al [89] of prone positioning, there was no improvement in mortality rates, although there was a suggestion of improved mortality in a post-hoc analysis of the most critically ill patients. Until the effect of prone positioning on mortality is elucidated further, the benefit of improved oxygenation has to be weighed carefully against the risk, particularly in light of the potential role of selective pulmonary artery vasodilators in treating refractory hypoxemia (see later).

High-frequency oscillatory ventilation

The postoperative management of patients with high-output bronchopleural fistulas is a challenge in ventilatory and oxygenation management. Conventional positive-pressure ventilation (volume or pressure limited) often fails in these patients because of associated disease processes, such as decreased pulmonary compliance and bilateral diffuse airspace disease (ARDS), and persistent increased peak and plateau airway pressures. Applying positive end expiratory pressure in an effort to improve oxygenation invariably results in an increase in the bronchopleural fistula leak.

High-frequency ventilation first was introduced 30 years ago as a method for reducing intrathoracic pressure during thoracic and laryngeal surgery. High-frequency oscillation was developed in the 1970s for the treatment of lung disease of prematurity but now is used for acute hypoxemic respiratory failure in all ages—mostly as rescue therapy [90,91]. It has been described in the management of patients with ARDS and bronchopleural fistulas [92,93]. The simultaneous use of nitric oxide and high-frequency jet ventilation also has been safe and effective in this setting [94].

Extracorporeal membrane oxygenation

Extracorporeal membrane oxygenation (ECMO) first was introduced into clinical practice in the 1970s. Clinical trials to date have failed to show a mortality benefit in adult patients with ARDS. Several case reports describe successful outcomes, however, in patients in whom ECMO was used as rescue therapy [76,95]. Several advances have been made in ECMO technology, including heparin-coated membranes and circuits and the use of centrifugal as opposed to roller pumps and a better understanding of anticoagulation management. Some investigators report improved mortality rates in adult patients with refractory respiratory failure managed on ECMO compared with earlier experience with it [96]. There has been no published randomized clinical trial comparing current ventilatory treatment of ARDS with that of ECMO [76].

Role of selective pulmonary arterial vasodilators

Pulmonary hypertension, right ventricular dysfunction, and perioperative hypoxemia are common problems after thoracic surgical procedures requiring treatment in a cardiothoracic ICU. Inhaled nitric oxide (iNO) was the first agent shown to be a selective pulmonary artery vasodilator and has been shown to improve oxygenation in patients with acute lung injury and ARDS [97,98]. In a Cochrane review [99] and in a systematic review by Kaisers et al [100], the role of iNO in ARDS was addressed. Both reviews concluded that the use of iNO does not alter mortality or other clinically relevant end points (ventilator-free days, ICU stay), but that it does improve oxygenation and hemodynamics temporarily in the acute phase. These reviews proposed that iNO has a role only as "rescue therapy" in refractory hypoxemia associated with ARDS. iNO has become prohibitively expensive, however, and has several associated toxicities that require monitoring, which increases cost further [101].

As a result of these issues, there has been an ongoing search for other selective pulmonary artery vasodilators as an alternative and possibly complement to iNO. Several drugs administered via the *inhalational* route have been described in animal models and humans, including inhaled sodium nitroprusside, nitroglycerin, class 5 phosphodiesterase inhibitors (eg, zaprinast and sildenafil), milrinone,

prostaglandin E_1 (PGE$_1$) (alprostadil), prostaglandin I_2 (PGI$_2$) (prostacyclin), and iloprost (the stable analog of PGI$_2$) [102].

The use of intravenous PGI$_2$ was described first in 1978 [103]. As opposed to PGE$_1$, PGI$_2$ was shown not to have any pulmonary inactivation and was 10 times more potent as a systemic vasodilator even though its metabolite, 6-keto-prostaglandin $F_{1\alpha}$, had little systemic vasodilator properties. Intravenous PGI$_2$, as opposed to intravenous PGE$_1$, became an important pulmonary vasodilator in the treatment of pulmonary hypertension [104]. Systemic hypotension is a problem in patients with severe pulmonary hypertension in which large doses are required to lower pulmonary arterial pressures effectively. In 1993, Welte et al [105] reported that *inhaled* PGI$_2$ resulted in selective pulmonary artery vasodilation in dogs. It has been shown since to be as effective as iNO in reducing pulmonary vascular resistance in heart transplant candidates [106,107], in lowering pulmonary artery pressures in primary and secondary pulmonary hypertension [108], in improving right ventricular function in animals with hypoxic pulmonary vasoconstriction [109], and as a selective pulmonary artery vasodilator with improvement in oxygenation in patients with ARDS [110–112] and in patients with refractory hypoxemia after cardiothoracic surgery [113]. In patients with poor oxygenation, inhaled PGI$_2$ not only improves oxygenation, but also is effective as a pulmonary vasodilator while maintaining mean arterial pressure and cardiac output. It seems that there is no appreciable tolerance to any of the beneficial effects of inhaled PGI$_2$ after 4 to 6 hours of administration. Despite a theoretical concern about the potential antiplatelet effects of inhaled PGI$_2$, several studies have attested to its safety, with no increased risk of bleeding [113,114]. Compared with iNO, inhaled PGI$_2$ is less expensive, is easier to administer, is relatively free of side effects, and requires no special toxicity monitoring [113].

Special case of postpneumonectomy pulmonary edema

Zeldin et al [115] brought attention to the syndrome of PPPE in 1984. Using a dog study as corroboration, they concluded that the risk factors for this complication are right pneumonectomy, large perioperative fluid load, and high intraoperative and postoperative urine outputs. The exact definition and pathophysiology of PPPE still remains unclear, however. It probably is underdiagnosed. PPPE develops in approximately 5% of patients undergoing pneumonectomy or lobectomy and has a high associated mortality (>50%) [116]. Histologically, PPPE is indistinguishable from ARDS or acute lung injury. It is characterized by dyspnea, hypoxemia, diffuse infiltrates on chest radiograph, and rapid evolution often unresponsive to current conventional therapy. Acute lung injury occurs almost exclusively after pneumonectomy, usually within 3 days from surgery and without a preceding cause. Since the first description by Zeldin et al [115], many other factors have been implicated in its pathogenesis, including excessive fluid administration [117], perioperative administration of fresh-frozen plasma [118], alveolar injury during one-lung ventilation, pulmonary hypertension, impaired lymph drainage and trauma caused by surgical manipulation, right ventricular dysfunction, postoperative hyperinflation related to intercostal tube drainage modes, and possibly occult microaspiration. Bigatello et al [119] and Alvarez [120] have reviewed this subject.

Despite the initial emphasis on fluid overload, simple fluid overload is not entirely responsible for PPPE because diuresis is often unsuccessful in correcting the hypoxemia. Jordan et al [116] discussed the role of endothelial injury in the development of PPPE. They concluded that PPPE more likely represents the pulmonary manifestation of a panendothelial injury consequent to inflammatory processes induced by the surgical procedure, which involves collapse and re-expansion of the operative lung to permit hilar dissection and pulmonary resection. Animal studies have shown that pulmonary ischemia-reperfusion can result in edema formation, possibly secondary to the generation of pro-oxidant forces. Such evidence suggests that PPPE may be modulated by high inspired oxygen concentrations associated with one-lung ventilation or by ischemia-reperfusion injury. Tamura et al [121] showed that rats that underwent pneumonectomy had higher plasma and lung concentrations of atrial natriuretic peptide (ANP) and a higher expression of ANP receptor C. Similarly, Tayami et al [122] showed that ANP and B-type (brain) natriuretic peptide (BNP) are elevated after lobectomy and after pneumonectomy and that their concentrations correlated with the total pulmonary vasculature resistance after pneumonectomy. ANP and BNP correlate with the amount of lung tissue resected. Nesiritide is the recombinant form of endogenous human BNP. It is not dependent on endothelial function, cyclic adenosine monophosphate, or β-adrenergic receptors. It is currently used for decompensated heart failure and is a balanced arterial, coronary, and venous vasodilator with beneficial effects on the neurohormonal system, where it counteracts the effects of aldosterone, norepineph-

rine, and endothelin [123]. It remains to be seen if nesiritide has a role to play in patients with PPPE.

There is still no specific therapy for PPPE. Suggested measures in perioperative care include the meticulous maintenance of physiologic stability, judicious fluid restriction, and the limitation of ventilatory volumes and pressures [119]. Emphasis also is placed on a balanced underwater thoracostomy drainage system that prevents hyperinflation of the remaining lung. Cerfolio et al [124] showed in a prospective nonrandomized trial that compared with historical controls, 250 mg of methylprednisolone before pulmonary artery ligation prevented PPPE, decreased hospital length of stay, and yet did not increase the incidence of bronchopleural fistulas. Inhaled pulmonary vasodilators may ameliorate the hypoxemia by improving ventilation-perfusion matching [102,113].

Sedation and paralysis

Inappropriate use of sedation and paralysis significantly increases morbidity. There are no randomized control trials supporting the benefit of neuromuscular blockade over that of adequate sedation in patients with respiratory failure requiring mechanical ventilation. Neuromuscular blockade often is used in place of excellent sedation, analgesia, and "antidelirium" therapy. Routine use of neuromuscular blockade should be discouraged. Neuromuscular blocking agents should be used in the ICU to facilitate ventilation, manage increased ICP, treat muscle spasms, and decrease oxygen consumption only when all other means have been tried without success [118]. Practice guidelines now have been established for the use of sedation and neuromuscular blockade in the ICU (Fig. 4) [125–127]. "Rational-use guidelines" in the provision of continuous analgesia, sedation, and neuromuscular blockade to critically ill patients requiring ventilator management have been shown to be safe and cost-effective compared with baseline prescribing strategies. Direct drug costs, ventilator time, and lengths of stay are reduced as is the use of neuromuscular blockade [128].

In a study by Kress et al [129], the daily interruption of sedation in ICU reduced costs and decreased time on mechanical ventilation. In another study, the same group showed that this strategy also reduced the incidence of complications, such as ventilator-associated pneumonia, upper gastrointestinal hemorrhage, bacteremia, barotraumas, venous thromboembolic disease, cholestasis, and sinusitis requiring surgical intervention [130]. Propofol and midazolam

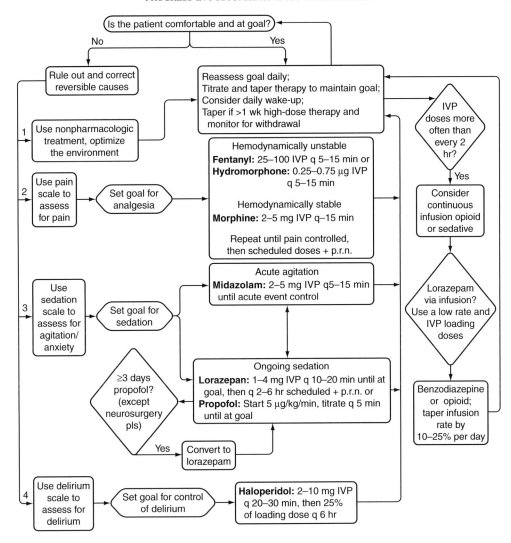

Fig. 4. Algorithm for the sedation and analgesia of mechanically ventilated patients. This algorithm is a general guideline for the use of analgesics and sedatives. Refer to the text for clinical and pharmacologic issues that dictate optimal drug selection, recommended assessment scales, and precautions for patient monitoring. Doses are approximate for a 70-kg adult. IVP, intravenous push. (*From* Jacobi J, Fraser GL, Coursin DB, et al. Clinical practice guidelines for the sustained use of sedatives and analgesics in the critically ill adult. Crit Care Med 2002;30:119–41; with permission.)

now are commonly used to achieve sedation in the ICU. Both drugs have been shown to achieve optimal sedation in a large fraction of patients when administered by specified dosing protocols. Propofol has a faster, more reliable wake-up time and provides for a more objective and reproducible assessment of time to awaken compared with midazolam [131]. Propofol infusion syndrome is a rare and often fatal syndrome occurring in critically ill patients undergoing high-dose propofol infusion. The syndrome consists of cardiac failure, rhabdomyolysis, severe metabolic acidosis, and renal failure. To date, 21 pedi-

atric cases and 14 adult cases have been described. The latter were mostly patients with acute neurologic illnesses or acute inflammatory diseases complicated by severe infections or even sepsis and receiving catecholamines or steroids in addition to propofol. Central nervous system activation with production of catecholamines and glucocorticoids and systemic inflammation with cytokine production are priming factors for cardiac and peripheral muscle dysfunction. High-dose propofol and supportive treatments with catecholamines and corticosteroids act as triggering factors. The syndrome can be lethal, and caution is suggested when using prolonged (>48 hours) propofol sedation at doses higher than 5 mg/kg/h [132].

Although still a common practice in the ICU, being intubated is not an indication for automatic "sedation." Many ICU sedation studies still rely on this premise, however. Each patient needs to be individualized, and with the appropriate nursing ratios, some patients require no psychoactive medications. Others may require only intermittent patient-requested analgesia, whereas the need of other patients may vary from a nocturnal sleep aide to anxiolysis, deep sedation, continuous analgesia, and treatment for delirium.

Glucose control

Van den Berghe et al [133,134] showed that intensive insulin therapy that maintained the blood glucose level at 80 to 110 mg/dL (4.4–6.1 mmol/L) resulted in lower morbidity and mortality among critically ill patients than did conventional therapy that maintained the blood glucose level at 180 to 200 mg/dL (10–11.1 mmol/L). Intensive insulin therapy reduced the frequency of episodes of sepsis by 46%. Patients with bacteremia who were treated with intensive insulin therapy had lower mortality than patients who received conventional therapy (12.5% versus 29.5%). Insulin therapy reduced the rate of death from multiple-organ failure among patients with sepsis, regardless of whether they had a history of diabetes. The protective mechanism of insulin in sepsis is unknown. The phagocytic function of neutrophils is impaired in patients with hyperglycemia, and correcting hyperglycemia may improve bacterial phagocytosis. Another potential mechanism involves the antiapoptotic effect of insulin. Insulin prevents apoptotic cell death from numerous stimuli by activating the phosphatidylinositol 3-kinase-Akt pathway [135]. Mesotten et al [136] showed, however, that the beneficial effects of insulin therapy on lipids, rather than on glucose control, independently accounted for the beneficial effects on morbidity and mortality. Insulin therapy increased low-density lipoprotein and high-density lipoprotein but suppressed elevated triglycerides. Regardless of mechanism, it seems reasonable to control blood glucose more tightly in critically ill patients. Clinicians must prevent hypoglycemic brain injury in attempting to maintain the blood glucose level at 80 to 110 mg/dL. Frequent monitoring of blood glucose is imperative, and studies are needed to determine whether less tight control of blood glucose (eg, a blood glucose level of 120–160 mg/dL [6.7–8.9 mmol/L]) provides similar benefits.

Evolving role of the pulmonary artery catheter in critical care

The use of a PAC in the care of critically ill patients is increasingly being questioned. In an important but controversial publication in 1996, the use of a PAC was associated with an increased risk of death (odds ratio 1.24) [137]. In an accompanying editorial, the question was raised whether or not there should be a moratorium on the use of the PAC [138]. In 2000, the National Heart, Lung and Blood Institute published a report on the role of the PAC and concluded that there was no compelling evidence that it improved outcomes and that its use was associated with significant risks and cost. The report concluded that a state of clinical equipoise existed regarding the use of the PAC in critically ill patients and that randomized studies on the its utility should be conducted. Richard et al [139] examined the use of the PAC in patients with shock and ARDS and found no effect on mortality, morbidity, and resource use. Sandham et al [140] examined the use of the PAC in patients after high-risk, noncardiac surgery. They found that there was no significant effect on mortality and that there was possibly increased morbidity with its use. Yu et al [2] examined the effect of the PAC in patients with severe sepsis and found no beneficial effect of mortality or resource use. There are many other less invasive techniques that can be used instead of the PAC to estimate or measure cardiac output and perfusion, including central venous oxygen saturation, transthoracic or transesophageal Doppler techniques, using the Fick principle for oxygen consumption (by estimating oxygen consumption or by measuring it using indirect calorimetry) and carbon dioxide production (using partial rebreathing of carbon dioxide and volumetric capnography), pulse contour analysis, dye dilution techniques, and bioimpedance techniques.

Intensivist-led multidisciplinary ICU team

The Leapfrog Initiative was established in January 2000 by the Business Roundtable (BRT) in response to the Institute of Medicine report on quality and safety of medical care. The BRT is composed of chief executive officers of US corporations representing more than 28 million employees, which aims to improve the safety and quality of health care to its member organizations in the United States. Leapfrog has proposed three hospital safety measures—computerized physician order entry, ICU physician staffing standards, and evidence-based hospital referral, which states that hospitals must meet certain volume/year criteria. Risk-adjusted mortality and process of care measures now augment or replace volume standards for some procedures [141].

Substantial data show that critically ill patients, when cared for in ICUs that have a multidisciplinary, intensivist-led team, have reduced morbidity and mortality [142]. High-intensity ICU physician staffing (ie, mandatory intensivist consultation or closed ICU—all care directed by intensivist) is associated with reduced hospital and ICU mortality and hospital and ICU length of stay compared with a model of low-intensity ICU physician staffing (ie, no intensivist or elective intensivist consultation only). This paradigm of care, which has been adopted widely around the world, has become an important focus for the Leapfrog group.

Summary

The clinical case presented in this article illustrates how many of the more recent advances in the management of critically ill patients apply to current clinical practice. Simple cost-effective general measures (eg, optimal sterile precautions during procedures; hand washing; early goal-directed resuscitation with appropriate fluids, inotropes, and antibiotics; and surgical source control of infected foci) still should form the basis of clinical practice, however. There has been renewed interest in blood transfusion therapy and its associated risks. Lower tidal volume ventilation now is practiced almost universally in patients with ARDS, and several new selective pulmonary vasodilators have extended the armamentarium when taking care of these patients. High-frequency oscillatory ventilation and ECMO remain challenging options in patients with refractory hypoxemia.

Appropriate patient selection is important when corticosteroid therapy is considered. Tight blood glucose control and monitoring improve outcome and should be part of ICU care of septic patients. The role of the PAC is controversial. Other techniques to measure cardiac output, hemodynamics, and perfusion are available and should be considered.

Sedation and analgesia form an integral part of critical care. Because of its immediate and long-term risks, neuromuscular blockade should be used sparingly and only when all other options have been exhausted. Ongoing education regarding sedation protocols and the effect of sedation on outcome is needed among physicians and nurses caring for these patients.

References

[1] Dellinger RP, Carlet JM, Masur H, et al. Surviving Sepsis Campaign guidelines for management of severe sepsis and septic shock. Crit Care Med 2004;32: 858–73.

[2] Yu DT, Black E, Sands KE, et al. Severe sepsis: variation in resource and therapeutic modality use among academic centers. Crit Care 2003;7:R24–34.

[3] Martin GS, Mannino DM, Eaton S, Moss M. The epidemiology of sepsis in the United States from 1979 through 2000. N Engl J Med 2003;348: 1546–54.

[4] Jimenez MF, Marshall JC. Source control in the management of sepsis. Intensive Care Med 2001; 27(Suppl 1):S49–62.

[5] Chastre J, Wolff M, Fagon JY, et al. Comparison of 8 vs 15 days of antibiotic therapy for ventilator-associated pneumonia in adults: a randomized trial. JAMA 2003;290:2588–98.

[6] Rivers E, Nguyen B, Havstad S, et al. Early goal-directed therapy in the treatment of severe sepsis and septic shock. N Engl J Med 2001;345:1368–77.

[7] Dellinger RP. Cardiovascular management of septic shock. Crit Care Med 2003;31:946–55.

[8] Rivers EP, Nguyen HB, Huang DT, Donnino M. Early goal-directed therapy. Crit Care Med 2004;32: 314–5.

[9] Natanson C, Danner RL. Early goal-directed therapy reduced mortality and multiorgan dysfunction in severe sepsis or septic shock. ACP J Club 2002;136:90.

[10] Dunser MW, Mayr AJ, Ulmer H, et al. The effects of vasopressin on systemic hemodynamics in catecholamine-resistant septic and postcardiotomy shock: a retrospective analysis. Anesth Analg 2001;93:7–13.

[11] Dunser MW, Mayr AJ, Ulmer H, et al. Arginine vasopressin in advanced vasodilatory shock: a prospective, randomized, controlled study. Circulation 2003;107:2313–9.

[12] Sharshar T, Blanchard A, Paillard M, Raphael JC, Gajdos P, Annane D. Circulating vasopressin levels in septic shock. Crit Care Med 2003;31:1752–8.

[13] Gattinoni L, Brazzi L, Pelosi P, et al. A trial of goal-oriented hemodynamic therapy in critically ill patients. SvO2 Collaborative Group. N Engl J Med 1995;333:1025–32.

[14] Hayes MA, Timmins AC, Yau EH, Palazzo M, Hinds CJ, Watson D. Elevation of systemic oxygen delivery in the treatment of critically ill patients. N Engl J Med 1994;330:1717–22.

[15] Hotchkiss RS, Karl IE. The pathophysiology and treatment of sepsis. N Engl J Med 2003;348:138–50.

[16] Faust SN, Levin M, Harrison OB, et al. Dysfunction

of endothelial protein C activation in severe meningococcal sepsis. N Engl J Med 2001;345:408–16.

[17] Bernard GR, Vincent JL, Laterre PF, et al. Efficacy
and safety of recombinant human activated protein C
for severe sepsis. N Engl J Med 2001;344:699–709.

[18] Bernard GR, Margolis BD, Shanies HM, et al.
Extended evaluation of recombinant human activated
protein C United States Trial (ENHANCE US):
a single-arm, phase 3B, multicenter study of drotrecogin alfa (activated) in severe sepsis. Chest 2004;
125:2206–16.

[19] Dhainaut JF, Laterre PF, Janes JM, et al. Drotrecogin
alfa (activated) in the treatment of severe sepsis
patients with multiple-organ dysfunction: data from
the PROWESS trial. Intensive Care Med 2003;29:
894–903.

[20] Dhainaut JF, Laterre PF, LaRosa SP, et al. The clinical
evaluation committee in a large multicenter phase
3 trial of drotrecogin alfa (activated) in patients with
severe sepsis (PROWESS): role, methodology, and
results. Crit Care Med 2003;31:2291–301.

[21] Bollaert PE, Charpentier C, Levy B, Debouverie M,
Audibert G, Larcan A. Reversal of late septic shock
with supraphysiologic doses of hydrocortisone. Crit
Care Med 1998;26:645–50.

[22] Annane D, Sebille V, Troche G, Raphael JC, Gajdos
P, Bellissant E. A 3-level prognostic classification in
septic shock based on cortisol levels and cortisol
response to corticotropin. JAMA 2000;283:1038–45.

[23] Annane D, Sebille V, Charpentier C, et al. Effect of
treatment with low doses of hydrocortisone and
fludrocortisone on mortality in patients with septic
shock. JAMA 2002;288:862–71.

[24] Loriaux L. Glucocorticoid therapy in the intensive
care unit. N Engl J Med 2004;350:1601–2.

[25] Hamrahian AH, Oseni TS, Arafah BM. Measurements of serum free cortisol in critically ill patients. N
Engl J Med 2004;350:1629–38.

[26] The Cochrane Injuries Group. Human albumin administration in critically ill patients: systematic review of randomised controlled trials. BMJ 1998;
317:235–40.

[27] Finfer S, Bellomo R, Boyce N, French J, Myburgh J,
Norton R. A comparison of albumin and saline for
fluid resuscitation in the intensive care unit. N Engl J
Med 2004;350:2247–56.

[28] Wilkes NJ, Woolf R, Mutch M, et al. The effects of
balanced versus saline-based hetastarch and crystalloid solutions on acid-base and electrolyte status and
gastric mucosal perfusion in elderly surgical patients.
Anesth Analg 2001;93:811–6.

[29] Rhee P, Koustova E, Alam HB. Searching for the
optimal resuscitation method: recommendations for
the initial fluid resuscitation of combat casualties.
J Trauma 2003;54(5 Suppl):S52–62.

[30] Deb S, Martin B, Sun L, et al. Resuscitation with
lactated Ringer's solution in rats with hemorrhagic
shock induces immediate apoptosis. J Trauma 1999;
46:582–9.

[31] Deb S, Sun L, Martin B, et al. Lactated Ringer's
solution and hetastarch but not plasma resuscitation
after rat hemorrhagic shock is associated with
immediate lung apoptosis by the up-regulation of
the Bax protein. J Trauma 2000;49:47–55.

[32] Knutson JE, Deering JA, Hall FW, et al. Does
intraoperative hetastarch administration increase
blood loss and transfusion requirements after cardiac
surgery? Anesth Analg 2000;90:801–7.

[33] Cope JT, Banks D, Mauney MC, et al. Intraoperative
hetastarch infusion impairs hemostasis after cardiac
operations. Ann Thorac Surg 1997;63:78–83.

[34] Boldt J. Fluid choice for resuscitation of the trauma
patient: a review of the physiological, pharmacological, and clinical evidence. Can J Anaesth 2004;51:
500–13.

[35] de Jonge E, Levi M, Berends F, van der Ende AE, ten
Cate JW, Stoutenbeek CP. Impaired haemostasis by
intravenous administration of a gelatin-based plasma
expander in human subjects. Thromb Haemost 1998;
79:286–90.

[36] de Jonge E, Levi M. Effects of different plasma substitutes on blood coagulation: a comparative review.
Crit Care Med 2001;29:1261–7.

[37] Wilkes MM, Navickis RJ, Sibbald WJ. Albumin
versus hydroxyethyl starch in cardiopulmonary
bypass surgery: a meta-analysis of postoperative
bleeding. Ann Thorac Surg 2001;72:527–34.

[38] Janvrin SB, Davies G, Greenhalgh RM. Postoperative
deep vein thrombosis caused by intravenous fluids
during surgery. Br J Surg 1980;67:690–3.

[39] Ruttmann TG, Jamest MF, Lombard EH. Haemodi-
lution-induced enhancement of coagulation is
attenuated in vitro by restoring antithrombin III to
pre-dilution concentrations. Anaesth Intensive Care
2001;29:489–93.

[40] Holte K, Sharrock NE, Kehlet H. Pathophysiology
and clinical implications of perioperative fluid excess.
Br J Anaesth 2002;89:622–32.

[41] Lang K, Boldt J, Suttner S, Haisch G. Colloids versus
crystalloids and tissue oxygen tension in patients
undergoing major abdominal surgery. Anesth Analg
2001;93:405–9.

[42] Brandstrup B, Tonnesen H, Beier-Holgersen R, et al.
Effects of intravenous fluid restriction on postoperative complications: comparison of two perioperative
fluid regimens: a randomized assessor-blinded multicenter trial. Ann Surg 2003;238:641–8.

[43] Polanczyk CA, Rohde LE, Goldman L, et al. Right
heart catheterization and cardiac complications in
patients undergoing noncardiac surgery: an observational study. JAMA 2001;286:309–14.

[44] Holte K, Jensen P, Kehlet H. Physiologic effects of
intravenous fluid administration in healthy volunteers. Anesth Analg 2003;96:1504–9.

[45] Arieff AI. Fatal postoperative pulmonary edema:
pathogenesis and literature review. Chest 1999;115:
1371–7.

[46] Martin GS, Mangialardi RJ, Wheeler AP, Dupont

WD, Morris JA, Bernard GR. Albumin and furosemide therapy in hypoproteinemic patients with acute lung injury. Crit Care Med 2002;30:2175–82.

[47] Gattinoni L, Caspani ML. Albumin and furosemide in acute lung injury: a little step forward? Crit Care Med 2002;30:2376–7.

[48] Mangialardi RJ, Martin GS, Bernard GR, et al. Hypoproteinemia predicts acute respiratory distress syndrome development, weight gain, and death in patients with sepsis. Ibuprofen in Sepsis Study Group. Crit Care Med 2000;28:3137–45.

[49] Quinlan GJ, Mumby S, Martin GS, Bernard GR, Gutteridge JM, Evans TW. Albumin influences total plasma antioxidant capacity favorably in patients with acute lung injury. Crit Care Med 2004;32:755–9.

[50] Schierhout G, Roberts I. Fluid resuscitation with colloid or crystalloid solutions in critically ill patients: a systematic review of randomised trials. BMJ 1998; 316:961–4.

[51] Cook D, Guyatt G. Colloid use for fluid resuscitation: evidence and spin. Ann Intern Med 2001;135:205–8.

[52] Molnar Z, Mikor A, Leiner T, Szakmany T. Fluid resuscitation with colloids of different molecular weight in septic shock. Intensive Care Med 2004; 30:1356–60.

[53] Hebert PC, Tinmouth A, Corwin H. Anemia and red cell transfusion in critically ill patients. Crit Care Med 2003;31(12 Suppl):S672–7.

[54] Carson JL, Duff A, Poses RM, et al. Effect of anaemia and cardiovascular disease on surgical mortality and morbidity. Lancet 1996;348:1055–60.

[55] Hebert PC, Wells G, Tweeddale M, et al. Does transfusion practice affect mortality in critically ill patients? Transfusion Requirements in Critical Care (TRICC) Investigators and the Canadian Critical Care Trials Group. Am J Respir Crit Care Med 1997;155: 1618–23.

[56] Wu WC, Rathore SS, Wang Y, Radford MJ, Krumholz HM. Blood transfusion in elderly patients with acute myocardial infarction. N Engl J Med 2001;345:1230–6.

[57] Carson JL, Duff A, Berlin JA, et al. Perioperative blood transfusion and postoperative mortality. JAMA 1998;279:199–205.

[58] Vincent JL, Baron JF, Reinhart K, et al. Anemia and blood transfusion in critically ill patients. JAMA 2002;288:1499–507.

[59] Corwin HL, Gettinger A, Pearl RG, et al. The CRIT Study: anemia and blood transfusion in the critically ill—current clinical practice in the United States. Crit Care Med 2004;32:39–52.

[60] Rao MP, Boralessa H, Morgan C, et al. Blood component use in critically ill patients. Anaesthesia 2002;57:530–4.

[61] French CJ, Bellomo R, Finfer SR, Lipman J, Chapman M, Boyce NW. Appropriateness of red blood cell transfusion in Australasian intensive care practice. Med J Aust 2002;177:548–51.

[62] Hebert PC, Wells G, Blajchman MA, et al. A mul

ticenter, randomized, controlled clinical trial of transfusion requirements in critical care. Transfusion Requirements in Critical Care Investigators, Canadian Critical Care Trials Group. N Engl J Med 1999;340: 409–17.

[63] Hebert PC, Yetisir E, Martin C, et al. Is a low transfusion threshold safe in critically ill patients with cardiovascular diseases? Crit Care Med 2001;29: 227–34.

[64] Fergusson D, Khanna MP, Tinmouth A, Hebert PC. Transfusion of leukoreduced red blood cells may decrease postoperative infections: two meta-analyses of randomized controlled trials. Can J Anaesth 2004; 51:417–24.

[65] Hebert PC, Fergusson D, Blajchman MA, et al. Clinical outcomes following institution of the Canadian universal leukoreduction program for red blood cell transfusions. JAMA 2003;289:1941–9.

[66] Carson JL, Berlin JA. Will we ever know if leukoreduction of red blood cells should be performed? Can J Anaesth 2004;51:407–10.

[67] Klein HG. Will blood transfusion ever be safe enough? JAMA 2000;284:238–40.

[68] Marik PE, Sibbald WJ. Effect of stored-blood transfusion on oxygen delivery in patients with sepsis. JAMA 1993;269:3024–9.

[69] Walsh TS, McArdle F, McLellan SA, et al. Does the storage time of transfused red blood cells influence regional or global indexes of tissue oxygenation in anemic critically ill patients? Crit Care Med 2004;32: 364–71.

[70] Amar D. Cardiac arrhythmias. Chest Surg Clin N Am 1998;8:479–93.

[71] Vaporciyan AA, Correa AM, Rice DC, et al. Risk factors associated with atrial fibrillation after noncardiac thoracic surgery: analysis of 2588 patients. J Thorac Cardiovasc Surg 2004;127:779–86.

[72] Amar D, Roistacher N, Burt ME, et al. Effects of diltiazem versus digoxin on dysrhythmias and cardiac function after pneumonectomy. Ann Thorac Surg 1997;63:1374–82.

[73] White CM, Giri S, Tsikouris JP, et al. A comparison of two individual amiodarone regimens to placebo in open heart surgery patients. Ann Thorac Surg 2002; 74:69–74.

[74] Mahoney EM, Thompson TD, Veledar E, Williams J, Weintraub WS. Cost-effectiveness of targeting patients undergoing cardiac surgery for therapy with intravenous amiodarone to prevent atrial fibrillation. J Am Coll Cardiol 2002;40:737–45.

[75] Fuster V, Ryden LE, Asinger RW, et al. ACC/AHA/ ESC guidelines for the management of patients with atrial fibrillation: executive summary. A Report of the American College of Cardiology/ American Heart Association Task Force on Practice Guidelines and the European Society of Cardiology Committee for Practice Guidelines and Policy Conferences (Committee to Develop Guidelines for the Management of Patients With Atrial Fibrillation): developed in

Collaboration With the North American Society of Pacing and Electrophysiology. J Am Coll Cardiol 2001;38:1231–66.

[76] Lewandowski K. Extracorporeal membrane oxygenation for severe acute respiratory failure. Crit Care 2000;4:156–68.

[77] Amato MB, Barbas CS, Medeiros DM, et al. Effect of a protective-ventilation strategy on mortality in the acute respiratory distress syndrome. N Engl J Med 1998;338:347–54.

[78] Stewart TE, Meade MO, Cook DJ, et al. Evaluation of a ventilation strategy to prevent barotrauma in patients at high risk for acute respiratory distress syndrome. Pressure- and Volume-Limited Ventilation Strategy Group. N Engl J Med 1998;338:355–61.

[79] Brochard L, Roudot-Thoraval F, Roupie E, et al. Tidal volume reduction for prevention of ventilator-induced lung injury in acute respiratory distress syndrome. The Multicenter Trial Group on Tidal Volume reduction in ARDS. Am J Respir Crit Care Med 1998;158:1831–8.

[80] Brower RG, Shanholtz CB, Fessler HE, et al. Prospective, randomized, controlled clinical trial comparing traditional versus reduced tidal volume ventilation in acute respiratory distress syndrome patients. Crit Care Med 1999;27:1492–8.

[81] The Acute Respiratory Distress Syndrome Network. Ventilation with lower tidal volumes as compared with traditional tidal volumes for acute lung injury and the acute respiratory distress syndrome. N Engl J Med 2000;342:1301–8.

[82] Hickling KG, Walsh J, Henderson S, Jackson R. Low mortality rate in adult respiratory distress syndrome using low-volume, pressure-limited ventilation with permissive hypercapnia: a prospective study. Crit Care Med 1994;22:1568–78.

[83] Bidani A, Tzouanakis AE, Cardenas Jr VJ, Zwischenberger JB. Permissive hypercapnia in acute respiratory failure. JAMA 1994;272:957–62.

[84] Petrucci N, Iacovelli W. Ventilation with lower tidal volumes versus traditional tidal volumes in adults for acute lung injury and acute respiratory distress syndrome. Cochrane Database Syst Rev 2004;2:CD003844.

[85] Eichacker PQ, Gerstenberger EP, Banks SM, Cui X, Natanson C. Meta-analysis of acute lung injury and acute respiratory distress syndrome trials testing low tidal volumes. Am J Respir Crit Care Med 2002;166:1510–4.

[86] Stocker R, Neff T, Stein S, Ecknauer E, Trentz O, Russi E. Prone positioning and low-volume pressure-limited ventilation improve survival in patients with severe ARDS. Chest 1997;111:1008–17.

[87] Lamm WJ, Graham MM, Albert RK. Mechanism by which the prone position improves oxygenation in acute lung injury. Am J Respir Crit Care Med 1994;150:184–93.

[88] Jolliet P, Bulpa P, Chevrolet JC. Effects of the prone position on gas exchange and hemodynamics in severe acute respiratory distress syndrome. Crit Care Med 1998;26:1977–85.

[89] Gattinoni L, Tognoni G, Pesenti A, et al. Effect of prone positioning on the survival of patients with acute respiratory failure. N Engl J Med 2001;345:568–73.

[90] Bohn D. The history of high-frequency ventilation. Respir Care Clin N Am 2001;7:535–48.

[91] Ferguson ND, Stewart TE. The use of high-frequency oscillatory ventilation in adults with acute lung injury. Respir Care Clin N Am 2001;7:647–61.

[92] Ha DV, Johnson D. High frequency oscillatory ventilation in the management of a high output bronchopleural fistula: a case report. Can J Anaesth 2004;51:78–83.

[93] Brambrink AM, Brachlow J, Weiler N, et al. Successful treatment of a patient with ARDS after pneumonectomy using high-frequency oscillatory ventilation. Intensive Care Med 1999;25:1173–6.

[94] Campbell D, Steinmann M, Porayko L. Nitric oxide and high frequency jet ventilation in a patient with bilateral bronchopleural fistulae and ARDS. Can J Anaesth 2000;47:53–7.

[95] Dunser M, Hasibeder W, Rieger M, Mayr AJ. Successful therapy of severe pneumonia-associated ARDS after pneumonectomy with ECMO and steroids. Ann Thorac Surg 2004;78:335–7.

[96] Frenckner B, Frisen G, Palmer P, Linden V. [Swedish experiences with ECMO-treatment with an artificial lung]. Lakartidningen 2004;101:1272–9.

[97] Rossaint R, Falke KJ, Lopez F, Slama K, Pison U, Zapol WM. Inhaled nitric oxide for the adult respiratory distress syndrome. N Engl J Med 1993;328:399–405.

[98] Fiser SM, Cope JT, Kron IL, et al. Aerosolized prostacyclin (epoprostenol) as an alternative to inhaled nitric oxide for patients with reperfusion injury after lung transplantation. J Thorac Cardiovasc Surg 2001;121:981–2.

[99] Sokol J, Jacobs SE, Bohn D. Inhaled nitric oxide for acute hypoxemic respiratory failure in children and adults. Cochrane Database Syst Rev 2003;1:CD002787.

[100] Kaisers U, Busch T, Deja M, Donaubauer B, Falke KJ. Selective pulmonary vasodilation in acute respiratory distress syndrome. Crit Care Med 2003;31(4 Suppl):S337–42.

[101] Weinberger B, Laskin DL, Heck DE, Laskin JD. The toxicology of inhaled nitric oxide. Toxicol Sci 2001;59:5–16.

[102] Lowson SM. Inhaled alternatives to nitric oxide. Anesthesiology 2002;96:1504–13.

[103] Kadowitz PJ, Chapnick BM, Feigen LP, Hyman AL, Nelson PK, Spannhake EW. Pulmonary and systemic vasodilator effects of the newly discovered prostaglandin, PGI2. J Appl Physiol 1978;45:408–13.

[104] Rubin LJ, Mendoza J, Hood M, et al. Treatment of primary pulmonary hypertension with continuous intravenous prostacyclin (epoprostenol): results

of a randomized trial. Ann Intern Med 1990;112: 485–91.

[105] Welte M, Zwissler B, Habazettl H, Messmer K. PGI2 aerosol versus nitric oxide for selective pulmonary vasodilation in hypoxic pulmonary vasoconstriction. Eur Surg Res 1993;25:329–40.

[106] Haraldsson A, Kieler-Jensen N, Ricksten SE. Inhaled prostacyclin for treatment of pulmonary hypertension after cardiac surgery or heart transplantation: a pharmacodynamic study. J Cardiothorac Vasc Anesth 1996;10:864–8.

[107] Haraldsson A, Kieler-Jensen N, Nathorst-Westfelt U, Bergh CH, Ricksten SE. Comparison of inhaled nitric oxide and inhaled aerosolized prostacyclin in the evaluation of heart transplant candidates with elevated pulmonary vascular resistance. Chest 1998; 114:780–6.

[108] Mikhail G, Gibbs J, Richardson M, et al. An evaluation of nebulized prostacyclin in patients with primary and secondary pulmonary hypertension. Eur Heart J 1997;18:1499–504.

[109] Max M, Kuhlen R, Dembinski R, Rossaint R. Effect of aerosolized prostacyclin and inhaled nitric oxide on experimental hypoxic pulmonary hypertension. Intensive Care Med 1999;25:1147–54.

[110] Walmrath D, Schneider T, Schermuly R, Olschewski H, Grimminger F, Seeger W. Direct comparison of inhaled nitric oxide and aerosolized prostacyclin in acute respiratory distress syndrome. Am J Respir Crit Care Med 1996;153:991–6.

[111] Zwissler B, Kemming G, Habler O, et al. Inhaled prostacyclin (PGI2) versus inhaled nitric oxide in adult respiratory distress syndrome. Am J Respir Crit Care Med 1996;154(6 Pt 1):1671–7.

[112] van Heerden PV, Barden A, Michalopoulos N, Bulsara MK, Roberts BL. Dose-response to inhaled aerosolized prostacyclin for hypoxemia due to ARDS. Chest 2000;117:819–27.

[113] De Wet CJ, Affleck DG, Jacobsohn E, et al. Inhaled prostacyclin is safe, effective, and affordable in patients with pulmonary hypertension, right heart dysfunction, and refractory hypoxemia after cardiothoracic surgery. J Thorac Cardiovasc Surg 2004;127: 1058–67.

[114] Haraldsson A, Kieler-Jensen N, Wadenvik H, Ricksten SE. Inhaled prostacyclin and platelet function after cardiac surgery and cardiopulmonary bypass. Intensive Care Med 2000;26:188–94.

[115] Zeldin RA, Normandin D, Landtwing D, Peters RM. Postpneumonectomy pulmonary edema. J Thorac Cardiovasc Surg 1984;87:359–65.

[116] Jordan S, Mitchell JA, Quinlan GJ, Goldstraw P, Evans TW. The pathogenesis of lung injury following pulmonary resection. Eur Respir J 2000;15:790–9.

[117] Parquin F, Marchal M, Mehiri S, Herve P, Lescot B. Post-pneumonectomy pulmonary edema: analysis and risk factors. Eur J Cardiothorac Surg 1996;10: 929–33.

[118] van der Werff YD, van der Houwen HK, Heijmans PJ, et al. Postpneumonectomy pulmonary edema: a retrospective analysis of incidence and possible risk factors. Chest 1997;111:1278–84.

[119] Bigatello LM, Allain R, Gaissert HA. Acute lung injury after pulmonary resection. Min Anestesiol 2004;70:159–66.

[120] Alvarez JM. Postpneumonectomy pulmonary edema. In: Slinger P, editor. Progress in Thoracic Anesthesia. A Society of Cardiovascular Anesthesioogists Monograph. Philadelphia: Lippincott Williams & Wilkins; 2004. p. 187–219.

[121] Tamura K, Takamori S, Mifune H, Hayashi A, Shirouzu K. Changes in atrial natriuretic peptide concentration and expression of its receptors after pneumonectomy in the rat. Clin Sci (Lond) 2000; 99:343–8.

[122] Tayama K, Takamori S, Mitsuoka M, et al. Natriuretic peptides after pulmonary resection. Ann Thorac Surg 2002;73:1582–6.

[123] de Denus S, Pharand C, Williamson DR. Brain natriuretic peptide in the management of heart failure: the versatile neurohormone. Chest 2004;125:652–68.

[124] Cerfolio RJ, Bryant AS, Thurber JS, Bass CS, Lell WA, Bartolucci AA. Intraoperative solumedrol helps prevent postpneumonectomy pulmonary edema. Ann Thorac Surg 2003;76:1029–35.

[125] Jacobi J, Fraser GL, Coursin DB, et al. Clinical practice guidelines for the sustained use of sedatives and analgesics in the critically ill adult. Crit Care Med 2002;30:119–41.

[126] Murray MJ, Cowen J, DeBlock H, et al. Clinical practice guidelines for sustained neuromuscular blockade in the adult critically ill patient. Crit Care Med 2002;30:142–56.

[127] Nasraway Jr SA, Jacobi J, Murray MJ, Lumb PD. Sedation, analgesia, and neuromuscular blockade of the critically ill adult: revised clinical practice guidelines for 2002. Crit Care Med 2002;30:117–8.

[128] Mascia MF, Koch M, Medicis JJ. Pharmacoeconomic impact of rational use guidelines on the provision of analgesia, sedation, and neuromuscular blockade in critical care. Crit Care Med 2000;28:2300–6.

[129] Kress JP, Pohlman AS, O'Connor MF, Hall JB. Daily interruption of sedative infusions in critically ill patients undergoing mechanical ventilation. N Engl J Med 2000;342:1471–7.

[130] Schweickert WD, Gehlbach BK, Pohlman AS, Hall JB, Kress JP. Daily interruption of sedative infusions and complications of critical illness in mechanically ventilated patients. Crit Care Med 2004;32:1272–6.

[131] Kress JP, O'Connor MF, Pohlman AS, et al. Sedation of critically ill patients during mechanical ventilation: a comparison of propofol and midazolam. Am J Respir Crit Care Med 1996;153:1012–8.

[132] Vasile B, Rasulo F, Candiani A, Latronico N. The pathophysiology of propofol infusion syndrome: a simple name for a complex syndrome. Intensive Care Med 2003;29:1417–25.

[133] Van den Berghe G. Beyond diabetes: saving lives

with insulin in the ICU. Int J Obes Relat Metab Disord 2002;26(Suppl 3):S3–8.

[134] van den Berghe G, Wouters P, Weekers F, et al. Intensive insulin therapy in the critically ill patients. N Engl J Med 2001;345:1359–67.

[135] Aikawa R, Nawano M, Gu Y, et al. Insulin prevents cardiomyocytes from oxidative stress-induced apoptosis through activation of PI3 kinase/Akt. Circulation 2000;102:2873–9.

[136] Mesotten D, Swinnen JV, Vanderhoydonc F, Wouters PJ, Van den Berghe G. Contribution of circulating lipids to the improved outcome of critical illness by glycemic control with intensive insulin therapy. J Clin Endocrinol Metab 2004;89:219–26.

[137] Connors Jr AF, Speroff T, Dawson NV, et al. The effectiveness of right heart catheterization in the initial care of critically ill patients. SUPPORT Investigators. JAMA 1996;276:889–97.

[138] Dalen JE, Bone RC. Is it time to pull the pulmonary artery catheter? JAMA 1996;276:916–8.

[139] Richard C, Warszawski J, Anguel N, et al. Early use of the pulmonary artery catheter and outcomes in patients with shock and acute respiratory distress syndrome: a randomized controlled trial. JAMA 2003; 290:2713–20.

[140] Sandham JD, Hull RD, Brant RF, et al. A randomized, controlled trial of the use of pulmonary-artery catheters in high-risk surgical patients. N Engl J Med 2003;348:5–14.

[141] Birkmeyer JD, Dimick JB. Potential benefits of the new Leapfrog standards: Effect of process and outcomes measures. Surgery 2004;135:569–75.

[142] Pronovost PJ, Angus DC, Dorman T, Robinson KA, Dremsizov TT, Young TL. Physician staffing patterns and clinical outcomes in critically ill patients: a systematic review. JAMA 2002;288:2151–62.

ELSEVIER
SAUNDERS

Thorac Surg Clin 15 (2005) 181–188

THORACIC
SURGERY
CLINICS

Index

Note: Page numbers of article titles are in **boldface** type.

Changing Your Address?

Make sure your subscription changes too! When you notify us of your new address, you can help make our job easier by including an exact copy of your Clinics label number with your old address (see illustration below.) This number identifies you to our computer system and will speed the processing of your address change. Please be sure this label number accompanies your old address and your corrected address—you can send an old Clinics label with your number on it or just copy it exactly and send it to the address listed below.

We appreciate your help in our attempt to give you continuous coverage. Thank you.

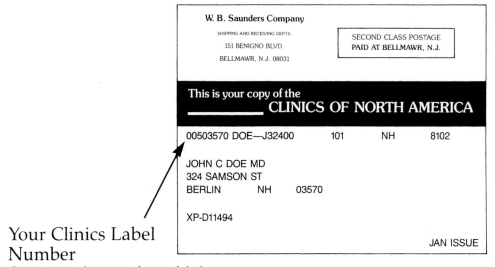

W. B. Saunders Company

SHIPPING AND RECEIVING DEPTS.
151 BENIGNO BLVD.
BELLMAWR, N.J. 08031

SECOND CLASS POSTAGE
PAID AT BELLMAWR, N.J.

This is your copy of the
CLINICS OF NORTH AMERICA

00503570 DOE—J32400   101   NH   8102

JOHN C DOE MD
324 SAMSON ST
BERLIN   NH   03570

XP-D11494

JAN ISSUE

Your Clinics Label Number
Copy it exactly or send your label
along with your address to:
W.B. Saunders Company, Customer Service
Orlando, FL 32887-4800
Call Toll Free 1-800-654-2452

Please allow four to six weeks for delivery of new subscriptions and for processing address changes.